Sick Societies

Sick Societies
Responding to the global challenge of chronic disease

Edited by

Dr David Stuckler
Department of Sociology,
University of Cambridge, UK
Department of Public Health and Policy,
London School of Hygiene & Tropical Medicine, UK

Ms Karen Siegel
Laney Graduate School & Rollins School of Public Health,
Emory University, Atlanta, GA, USA

OXFORD
UNIVERSITY PRESS

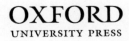
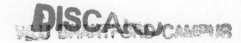

OXFORD
UNIVERSITY PRESS

Great Clarendon Street, Oxford ox2 6DP

Oxford University Press is a department of the University of Oxford.
It furthers the University's objective of excellence in research, scholarship,
and education by publishing worldwide in

Oxford New York

Athens Auckland Bangkok Bogotá Buenos Aires Cape-Town
Chennai Dar-es-Salaam Delhi Florence Hong-Kong Istanbul Karachi
Kolkata Kuala-Lumpur Madrid Melbourne Mexico-City Mumbai Nairobi
Paris São-Paulo Shanghai Singapore Taipei Tokyo Toronto Warsaw
with associated companies in Berlin Ibadan

Oxford is a registered trade mark of Oxford University Press
in the UK and in certain other countries

Published in the United States
by Oxford University Press Inc., New York

British Library Cataloguing in Publication Data
Data available

Library of Congress Cataloging in Publication Data
Data available

Typeset in Minion by Cenveo, Bangalore, India
Printed in Great Britain
on acid-free paper by
Ashford Colour Press Ltd, Gosport, Hampshire

ISBN 978–0–19–957440–7

10 9 8 7 6 5 4 3 2 1

Oxford University Press makes no representation, express or implied, that the drug dosages in
this book are correct. Readers must therefore always check the product information and clinical
procedures with the most up-to-date published product information and data sheets provided by
the manufacturers and the most recent codes of conduct and safety regulations. The authors and the
publishers do not accept responsibility or legal liability for any errors in the text or for the misuse
or misapplication of material in this work. Except where otherwise stated, drug dosages and
recommendations are for the non-pregnant adult who is not breastfeeding.

Preface: Epidemiology of modern society

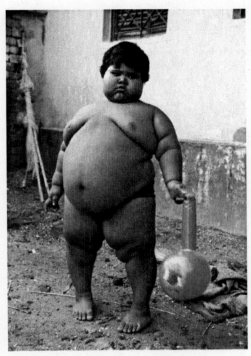

Reproduced with kind permission of Amba
Horton, Barcroft Media, the copyright holder.

When you come face-to-face with an image of an obese child like Suman, you may not know
whether to laugh or to cry. You are instantly confronted by Suman's near-nakedness, but you may
not immediately be drawn to think that it could be that no one makes clothes to fit children her
size. We are all aware of poverty, but may fail to consider that her problem is deeper and is linked
not only to development but to broader issues of public health and human rights. While it is likely
that Suman has a genetic predisposition, where she is from one out of every five children is overweight or obese: there are millions of children like her in India alone. She is but one face of a
modern epidemic.

Over the past decade, concerned people have invested more than $50 billion dollars in nutri-
tion supplements, vaccines, and immunizations, aiming to conquer the world's deadliest and
most avoidable diseases. Malnutrition, starvation, and HIV/AIDS are on the decline (although
they still remain highly concentrated among the poor), but these hard-fought gains are now being
threatened by an unforeseen and equally dangerous trend. An epidemic of chronic diseases—
heart disease, common cancers, respiratory disease, and diabetes—place in peril many of the
health gains made across the past century.

Your first reaction may be that these obese children urgently need medical attention. But all the drugs, money, and technology in the world cannot solve a problem that is engineered by the societal conditions in which we are born, live, work, and play (1). Such unhealthy circumstances are beyond the control of individuals.

No matter how hard such a child tries to exercise or be healthy, he or she cannot overcome the powerful forces that make them more likely to die too young from diabetes or heart disease. Before they were born, their bodies were at much greater risk of becoming ill, 'pre-polluted' by toxic exposures in the womb. By the time they become adolescents, their blood pressure will be too high, their arteries calcified with plaque and fatty streaks, and their chance of developing 'adult-onset diabetes' will be significantly elevated.[1] These conditions will cause their bodies and organs to age at a pace five times faster than the previous generation, reducing their life expectancy by over 10 years. These children need more than just a magic bullet, quick fix solution to help them live a full and happy life.

Sick Societies argues that we are building environments that are poorly designed for our bodies: we create societies where tobacco, alcohol, and foods containing high levels of salt, sugar, and fats are the easiest, cheapest, and most desirable choices, while fruits, vegetables, and exercise are the most expensive, inaccessible, and inconvenient options. The rise in chronic diseases is the result of a model of societal development that is out of control: a model that puts wealth before health. While the faces of chronic disease are numerous and diverse, the threat these diseases pose is truly global: they are a challenge for all of us.

A threat to human development

Chronic diseases are not only attacking the affluent and old—they are not simply a consequence of an ageing society or a sign of progress—but increasingly afflicting the young, poor, and most marginalized groups in society. Worldwide, more than 30 million people die each year because of chronic diseases, a number projected to rise to more than 50 million deaths each year by 2030. Four out of five of these deaths will be in low- and middle-income countries. Of course everyone must die of something, but people are dying too young: more than half of the rise in chronic disease deaths will occur among people in their early- and middle-stages of life when they still have their greatest contributions to make to societies.

The consequences of chronic diseases for human development, however, will be even greater in the very poorest countries where these rises will add to the unfinished challenge of fighting hunger, HIV/AIDS, and tuberculosis. When parents smoke, children go hungry and tuberculosis spreads; when men drink dangerously, women are at risk of abuse and can end up in hospitals. The main risks of heart disease, such as tobacco, indoor smoke, and diabetes, are also leading threats in tuberculosis epidemics; similarly, antiretroviral therapy, which has allowed many people with AIDS to stay alive, also has the undesirable side effect of increasing risks of diabetes and heart disease. Increasingly we have come to realize that the causes of poor health, be they chronic or infectious, have common roots and interconnected consequences. Until we begin to address comprehensively the risks that confront people living in resource-poor communities, which are increasingly becoming chronic, we will fail to achieve our basic goals to improve the health of the poorest and most vulnerable groups.

We stand at the cusp of a perilous moment for human development and health, similar to the crossroads we stood at during the 1980s when faced with the HIV epidemic. Now, as then, we can see a grim future: massive losses of human life; heavy tolls on economies of the world's poorest populations; and the indignity of suffering that can be avoided at a low cost. Will the world once again be delinquent in its duty to care for the world's most ill and vulnerable populations?

Neglecting chronic diseases to our peril

How have we responded to the global challenge of unhealthy societies so far? Mostly, we have pointed the finger at sick individuals and focused on developing expensive medical procedures and genetic technology. One example of this biomedical approach is bariatric surgery, a complicated and costly procedure which restricts the stomach and intestines to help people resist food temptations.[2] As society breeds more disease, our response has been to redesign our bodies to fit our increasingly unhealthy environments.

While it is easy to blame victims of chronic disease, *Sick Societies* suggests that their choices are not as free as we would first believe. As John Donne put it, 'No man is an island'; people make choices but not in the circumstances of their own choosing. The choices to eat poorly, drink dangerously, smoke to cope with stress, and the lack of time or money for exercise are all strongly shaped by the world around us. As a few examples, in India, cell phones are now more abundant than toilets; ice cold Coca-Cola is more widespread than insulin to treat diabetes; and Western supermarkets and food companies are taking over traditional farmers' jobs and markets, forcing workers to migrate to the cities or other countries in search of work, often ending up in slums. In these rapidly changing circumstances, the capacity for individuals and parents to make real, free choices is limited.

The net result is a deeply unfair and unequal situation. The World Health Organization (WHO) has labelled such avoidable inequalities in health as a 'social injustice' (1). To quote Martin Luther King, of all the forms of inequality, injustice in health care is the most shocking and inhumane. But not all social injustices are given equal treatment, even by the world's institutions committed to saving lives, such as WHO. The world's main social agenda to help developing countries become like developed countries by fighting poverty and eradicating illness is set out in the Millennium Development Goals. These global goals do not include a target for reducing chronic diseases. As we will show in Chapter 5, according to the world's richest countries a death that follows years of suffering from a chronic disease in a resource-poor country is worth less than one-seventh of a death caused by an infection, which is the exact opposite of how the rich countries invest their health resources to serve their population's health needs.

This 'us' and 'them' mentality prevents global diseases, including chronic diseases, from becoming a priority. Importantly, though, the way that people in 'developed' countries have chosen to build their society is the model for 'developing' countries. Can poor societies then be said to have chosen to be unhealthy? From the growing dependency of Indian women's diets on bankers' decisions about where to invest on Wall Street; from a devastating in epidemic in Russia to a fisherman's plague in a small Pacific island of Nauru, people decisions about diets and lifestyles are coming to depend on the incentives created by the investment patterns of Western corporations and financial institutions. Rich countries, through the global system of aid and healthcare, are shaping resource-poor countries in their own image, but then leave them to their own devices when it comes to chronic disease. This 'help' with strings attached essentially traps resource-poor societies in cycles of poverty and illness.

Ironically, the rising burden of chronic diseases is now being recognized as a key reason why the United Nations' Millennium Development Goals are not being met (2). Chronic poverty, poor child health, tuberculosis, and HIV/AIDS, share common risk factors with chronic diseases. But the risk factors that cause these chronic diseases appear very rarely on the agenda.

The origins of this situation are traceable back to the colonial period. When Europeans colonized the rest of the world, they brought a raft of modern diseases with them, in some cases wiping out entire civilizations. In an effort to protect their troops from indigenous sicknesses in the tropics, they set up large colonial hospitals to care for the emergency needs of military personnel who would soon go back to Europe. Today, rich countries follow a similar model, and while this is only rarely through direct force, it is now through a radical model of free-market development and medicine. Vast sums of aid money have set up health systems that focus mainly on a narrow set of infectious diseases posing a threat to the global North. When it comes to protecting poor people from the conditions that cause their greatest avoidable suffering—that is, human-produced, chronic disease—there is no budget, there is no will.[3]

Resource-poor societies cannot afford to continue along the path they are going. Expensive medicines, like those used in Global North, are typically unavailable and when they can be found, the price will often break the bank. Diabetes treatment, where available, can cost over US$10,000 per year. How can the governments of Brazil and India care for their diseased populations with less than US$100 of health funding available per person? With no health insurance, sick people in these unhealthy societies face a dilemma: chronic poverty or a slow, painful death.

The good news is that chronic diseases are among the easiest killers to prevent. More than half of all premature death and suffering due to chronic disease can be averted by reengineering the most toxic aspects of society that we have created. For example, a few basic interventions to reduce salt, sugar, fat, and tobacco, as well as providing cheap essential medicines, could save up to 36 million lives and more than $500 billion within a decade—a sum that could lift half of Africa's population out of poverty (3). It seems like an obvious win–win situation.

Social injustice driven by powerful vested interests

Why, then, have we not made greater progress? Part of the problem is that powerful corporations, and vested interests which influence them, benefit from the status quo. They emphasize the importance of expensive pharmaceutical and genetic solutions, and the central role of responsible consumer behaviour and physical activity to limit ever-growing consumption of nutritionally-defective products and design of toxic environments. Meanwhile, tobacco companies see the next big market in selling 'nicotine—an addictive product effective in the release of stress mechanisms' to young women in resource-poor countries; food companies have begun hiring the world's leading neuroscientists and psychologists to 'create demand through marketing' for products that their food chemists have engineered to be more addictive by preying on people's biological predispositions to high salt, fat, and sugar content; and pharmaceutical companies have placed heavy bets on the potential to design a pill to cure obesity, while seeking to influence trade agreements to keep cheap generics out of resource-poor, high-diabetes environments.

This scenario sounds like a perfect corporate conspiracy—tobacco companies get people to start smoking, pharmaceutical companies manufacture medical devices to help people quit—except this corporate arrangement is the exact opposite of a conspiracy. Food, tobacco, and pharmaceutical companies collude in the light of day. Food and pharmaceutical companies make headlines when they team up to create 'nutra-ceuticals': foods that deliver medicines. Fortified soft drinks are being used as vehicles to address micronutrient deficiencies, and cholesterol-lowering drugs are proposed as condiments at fast-food restaurants. These companies have begun hiring the world's top experts working previously at the US Centers for Disease Control and WHO as part of their strategies to pursue 'innovative models of business development'.

The influence of these companies extends beyond the products they create. Key partners and funders of the Gates Foundation, Global Alliance for Improved Nutrition, Global Alliance for Vaccines and Immunizations, and UNAIDS are food companies. Part of the good these organizations do to save lives, such as providing free electricity as part of so-called 'horizontal' global health programmes to enable doctors to deliver refrigerated vaccines to deprived communities, have a flip side: the logistic routes they create are instantly used to deliver ice-cold fizzy drinks to the most nutritionally-deprived environments of the world. Belatedly, these multinational companies have started to improve the nutrition content of their foods in rich societies (under pressure of government taxation or regulation), but so far they have done little to change their portfolios in resource-denied communities where pressure from government leaders is absent.

In other words, the battle against chronic diseases is no longer a technical issue. Cost-effective strategies are available; governments can even save money by taxing tobacco, alcohol, and unhealthy foods. Instead, the problem is a political one. The threat these diseases pose is truly global—they are a challenge for all of us—and therefore they demand a global political response. There is a better way if we, as members of a global community, choose to take it.

Why did we write this book?

Why would two public health scholars who work in universities and are principally concerned about monitoring statistics write this book about global chronic disease? Because we have spent more than a combined two decades working on the greatest and most unfair challenges in global health, seeking to find ways that we can improve the world in which we live with the resources we have. Increasingly these statistics about what is killing and disabling the poor are revealing a devastating rise in chronic disease and a gross failure to respond.

For many of us, the causes of chronic diseases are personal. Exercise would feel great, but most of the day is spent sitting in front of a computer. Eating healthy foods would be ideal, but at every turn the least healthy foods are the cheapest and easiest to find. Quitting smoking would no doubt make life better, but life is so stressful today that perhaps it is better to wait until tomorrow. To most of us, tomorrow never comes.

The consequences of chronic disease will also be real to those who have cared for a parent or family member with cancer. Fear, anxiety, and hopelessness: chronic diseases cause suffering that extends beyond a person's body, into their mind, soul, and spirit, and ultimately spills over to leave a permanent impact on their families, communities, and entire societies.

As university professors and researchers, we have also been approached by students passionate about global health who seek to understand the underlying issues driving the epidemic of global chronic diseases. Many are already aware of the rising toll of chronic diseases, but are looking for practical suggestions about how to have an exciting career in global health that can begin to address some of our society's most deeply embedded and intractable health challenges. As we scanned the available texts and course materials, we found numerous and detailed treatments about epidemiology, medicine, and clinical methodologies. A handful of books covered chronic diseases as one chapter in a global health book that sequentially treated diseases in isolation. Rapidly we came to realize that no text exists that comprehensively addresses the range of perspectives needed to understand and address an issue as complex and grounded in our models of societal development as global chronic diseases. Our book aims to fill this gap.

To our knowledge, this book is the first to integrate the required perspectives from epidemiology, economics, management, medicine, political economy, sociology, and governance about global chronic diseases into one text. In this regard, the book is a continuing work in progress. By the time it is published, it will already be out of date; the statistics it contains are likely to have become worse. Inevitably, some areas have been given a less detailed or technical treatment than some readers may have preferred. To the extent possible we have included references and endnotes so that the interested reader can find sources which address key material and methodologies in greater depth. Much detailed information and recommended further readings can be found in the book's endnotes and Appendix, which we would encourage interested readers to pursue.[4]

As the intended audience ranges from graduate students in public health and medicine to interested professionals in other fields, the language has been kept as accessible as possible, and less technical. The introduction and conclusion have especially been written for a more general audience. The epidemiology and economics chapters include more complex material, and so in these sections we have resorted in several cases to a more technical discussion.

What this book includes

Sick Societies is written in five main parts. Each part contains one or several chapters. They all contain a series of clues about the causes and consequences of chronic diseases. Towards the later chapters, we identify potential and practical ways that readers can address these harms and include a series of strategies and tactics. Each chapter includes policy and practice points. Inevitably there is a degree of overlap between them. Overall, the policy points are aimed at a wider, non-specialist audience, while the practice points are mainly intended to provide practical suggestions to those working in public health on addressing chronic diseases.

In this book we use the term chronic diseases, although often the phrase chronic noncommunicable diseases or the abbreviation NCDs is applied. Indeed, in the first version of the text NCDs was used throughout until, at the request of our editor, this was revised to chronic diseases. These multiple terms cause confusion for policymakers and students alike (for more details see our discussion in the first chapter of how diseases are classified). Unless otherwise specified, in this book the terms chronic diseases can be used interchangeably with NCDs.

In the first part of the book, we aim to understand what are the causes and consequences of chronic diseases on a global level. Chapter 1 sets out the four leading killers—heart disease, common cancers, respiratory disease, and diabetes—and their main behavioural risk factors—tobacco use, unhealthy diet, physical inactivity, and alcohol. This chapter reveals a clear picture of a world where all people in all nations, rich and poor, and young and old, will be at risk, although the consequences will be the greatest among the youngest, poorest, and most vulnerable groups. This chapter is essential reading for setting out what chronic diseases are and the main behavioural risks that give rise to them. The rest of the book aims to understand and modify these unhealthy factors and outcomes.

Chapter 2 explains why so many people all over the world are becoming at greater risk of chronic diseases. The chapter traces back the links from a slum-dweller in India eating an unhealthy diet to the ultimate powerful forces in places like Washington DC who determine what is 'good' for development. The chapter shows how people's decisions about whether to use tobacco, drink dangerously, or eat unhealthy diets are strongly influenced by their price, availability, and marketing. As the chapter demonstrates these market forces are making unhealthy choices increasingly the economically smarter choices.

Stepping back one link further in the causal chain, the chapter reveals how behind these changing market circumstances lie the vested interests of multinational corporations. They lobby governments to subsidize oils, fats, and sugars, while at the same time putting rural farmers in poor countries out of business. Product marketing teams employ sophisticated tactics developed by scientists and engineers to 'slip below the radar' of people's conscious thought, influencing their preferences, desires, and, eventually, their choices. As an ultimate link in the causal chain, the chapter investigates who controls these societal determinants of chronic disease. It reveals how the dominant 'neoliberal' model of economic development which places priority on economic growth, and a radical set of free-market conditions of deregulation, privatization, and liberalization in pursuit of it, has made it easy for multinational food and tobacco companies to achieve these profitable market changes in low-income countries (where their efforts are currently concentrated), while at the same time weakening the ability of concerned people and government leaders to respond.

To illustrate the power of these societal forces, the chapter concludes with three country case studies. During the 1990s, Russian policymakers chose to pursue radical free-market policies (so-called 'Shock Therapy'), ultimately causing more than 3 million excess deaths due to heart disease and alcohol-related deaths—the world's worst mortality crisis in the past half-century. On the other hand, when the economies of Japan, Finland, and Cuba crashed, their people returned to eating traditional, healthier foods, and some of the most unexpected and remarkable reductions in chronic disease ever recorded took place. In the final and the most extreme case of Nauru, an entire society's traditional way of life is disappearing, partly due to chronic diseases and a development model that built an unsustainable society in the hasty pursuit of wealth.

Chapter 3 uses economic perspectives to look beyond the impact of chronic diseases on health to understand how they affect people's families, communities, and broader societies. What are the consequences of chronic diseases—not just in terms of money but in people's suffering and overall well-being? How do we measure these costs? Who is being affected most? Healthcare is often regarded as a cost to be contained, but this chapter makes a case that providing these services and investing in health could save money. The chapter first shows that chronic diseases are extremely costly, not just in terms of healthcare expenses but also in the labour market. In the United States (US), where at the time of this writing there were over 45 million uninsured people, they are a leading cause of bankruptcy, insurance costs literally put companies out of business. Then, the chapter shows how people who have or are at risk for chronic diseases tend to earn less money and are more likely to be unemployed. These harms combine to significantly impact the economy, reducing workers' productivity as well as people's incentives to seek education and save money.

The chapter further illustrates social consequences of chronic diseases. The ways in which families respond to chronic diseases when there are no social supports and healthcare insurance create a much greater set of social and economic costs many years later. When people with few resources and little health support get a chronic disease, their child may end up leaving to school to early to work to help the family survive while women are often forced into traditional, care-giving roles. When parents spend money on tobacco, alcohol, or chronic care, they use money that could have otherwise been used to provide food and clothing to their children. In the world's poorest countries, chronic diseases can trap families in poverty for generations, creating a vicious cycle of deprivation and illness.

In concluding, Chapter 3 uses economic perspectives to evaluate the role of markets as a potential risk factor of chronic diseases. It documents a series of cases of market failure, identifying situations when it may be appropriate for governments to intervene, but also points out how these interventions can have unexpected, and sometimes risky, consequences for chronic diseases.

In the second part of the book, we identify approaches for preventing and managing chronic diseases. The question is simple: What are the best ways to reduce the burden of chronic diseases? The answers are far from straightforward. Chapter 4 is split into two halves, focusing on how to care for persons who have chronic diseases before identifying ways to prevent people from getting sick in the first place.

The first half of Chapter 4 shows how healthcare systems, set up in a period when infectious diseases were dominant, have locked in a focus on treating acute-care episodes. It further shows how global health has come to focus a narrow set of low-cost, magic-bullet solutions, based on historical successes in eradicating smallpox. The chapter argues that these healthcare systems and this smallpox paradigm are inappropriate for caring for people who have chronic, long-term illnesses, and reveals an alternative model of 'liberatory medicine' based on chronic care models that could improve patients' outcomes at lower cost. The chapter then identifies a series of historical barriers to achieving this transformation of the way medical practice is done and care is delivered. It concludes on a sceptical note about the potential benefit of healthcare and pharmaceutical development to improving human development.

The second half of Chapter 4 reveals that public health initiatives have been skewed towards medical interventions rather than preventative approaches. This has manifested itself in major gaps in the research base for understanding how chronic diseases can be prevented at low cost. Nevertheless, the chapter argues that, despite gaps in the evidence base, there are a clear set of proven strategies to reduce the suffering and occurrence of chronic diseases in an entire population. These most effective strategies involve fiscal and regulatory changes to reverse engineer society towards healthier development. However, these 'best practice' strategies are often the most difficult politically, confronted by vested interests—both powerful corporations and the medical community. The chapter concludes by recommending a community-driven model of engagement, to experiment while expanding the evidence base, as a viable alternative to the dominant Western model whereby scientists define the costs, benefits, and appropriate solutions (often perpetuating the smallpox paradigm).

In the third part of the book, we consider the power and politics in global health that have stymied an effective response to chronic disease. The first part of Chapter 5 evaluates what is currently being done to address chronic diseases by a range of key groups, including governments, public health and development agencies, the United Nations (UN), the World Bank, and WHO. This is difficult to do because, as the chapter shows, more than one-third of all global health money comes from private foundations or development agencies which drive the global health agenda. Many of these private donors have potential conflicts of interests, as they are in close contact with, sit on the boards of, or own substantial shares in food and pharmaceutical companies. As the chapter shows, a worrisome irony is that many of these global health philanthropists have close links with powerful businesses whose products and ethically questionable business practices spread chronic disease. Much of the money they donate is channelled through global budgeting systems that are inconsistent and difficult to track, and close to one-third of all global health money is spent on unidentifiable purposes.

The chapter documents how, within all of these institutions, powerful vested interests appear to be driving the agenda. This process has been dramatic over the past few years, in what is referred to as the privatization of global health. The net effect of additional aid resources, the chapter shows, has been to lock in the acute-care, smallpox paradigm, while transferring capacity to control chronic diseases away from governments and to private donors (along with the vested interest they serve). The first part of the chapter concludes that the capacity to decide what is relevant in global health and how it will be addressed is held in the hands of a very few powerful institutions and decision-makers. In other words, global health is ruled by a few private donors who make decisions behind closed doors. The chapter makes the case that failure to prioritize and act on chronic diseases is a political, rather than a technical issue. It proposes that a challenge for global health is to identify these interests and bring them to the light of day, holding them to standards of transparency and public accountability.

The second half of Chapter 5 then describes how a social movement to influence the political priority and action on chronic diseases might be created. Using a sociological model of the political process, this chapter draws insights from the success and failure of a range of social movements, from climate change to HIV/AIDS, to civil rights campaigns. The chapter identifies three main strategies for strengthening a social movement on chronic diseases: reframing the debate, creating and identifying political opportunities, and mobilizing resources. Within each strategy, the chapter proposes a series of tactics that can be taken by concerned people to address the currently inequitable situation of chronic diseases.

In the fourth part of the book, the themes from the first three parts come into focus through a series of invited contributions from leading public health experts. In the first section, authorities with differing viewpoints share their vision for the appropriate roles of the private sector, with a focus on food companies. The first set of contributors include leading public health experts who have worked at the Centers for Disease Control and Prevention and led the chronic disease cluster at WHO, but who are currently leading PepsiCo's global health and wellness strategy. They argue that food companies have been and will continue to invest in health as part of their efforts to be socially responsible. Not only is it the right thing to do, they argue, but it can be highly profitable, creating co-benefits for business and health. In response, the author of *The Bottom Line or Public Health: Tactics Corporations Use to Influence Health and Health Policy, and What We Can Do To Counter Them*, critiques the food industry's strategies, drawing analogies to tactics used by tobacco companies to distort public health research, undermine effective interventions, and influence legislation. The analysis concludes with a series of tactics and recommendations for public health practitioners to avoid potential conflicts of interest while placing pressure on the private sector to improve its public health performance.

In the second section, public health experts contribute a series of country case studies about social change and chronic diseases in five rapidly-emerging economies: Brazil, China, India, Mexico, and South Africa. These countries were chosen because they have undergone very rapid transformations to their ways of life in the past decade. Each is set to become a world power. Their economies have been growing at record pace. Yet, each shares a common threat of rising chronic diseases that risks the stability and sustainability of their development.

These case studies are structured in a comparative way, addressing each of the themes from the first five chapters of the book so as to enable readers to draw insights from their successes and failures. While each country faces significant differences in their key risks and drivers of chronic disease, their stories are remarkably similar: substantial and inequitable rises in chronic diseases threaten to slow economic growth, in the context of resource-deprived public health systems that are already operating at capacity to address infectious disease, with little capacity or resources for addressing the societal drivers of chronic diseases.

These chapters offer an additional key insight. The way they talk about chronic disease and strategies for change offer a clue into how public health experts identify the causes, consequences, and opportunities for preventing chronic diseases. At times, concerned scientists and advocates have unintentionally spread myths that chronic diseases are diseases of the rich; individual choices that should not be changed; or inevitable consequences of ageing and social progress. In placing blame for little global action being taken to reduce chronic diseases, we (current authors included) must also point the finger at ourselves.

In the fifth part, we take a reflective view, looking at our societies' current and future health as a mirror that reveals who we are and who we are becoming. Looking into the mirror, the chapter argues, we see unhealthy societies, and a model of development that threatens human welfare. Looking beyond the mirror—if we dare—the chapter argues we can imagine a more egalitarian world where reducing human suffering—be it chronic or infectious—is the principal objective of social policy. While this approach may seem novel and untried, in medicine it traces back to an historical era of the 19th century, where drugs were ineffective but the public health community was nevertheless able to greatly reduce suffering due to infectious diseases. Today we stand at the opposite end of the spectrum: we have gained medical know-how and technology, but lost the public health imagination that could achieve remarkable health gains. Drawing on these insights, the conclusion provides a series of practical suggestions for how readers can help contribute to a healthier, fairer world, where suffering due to chronic diseases is managed, prevented, and controlled.

This book is intended to be a useful tool. The final part of the book sets out a model of pragmatic and imaginative solidarity, building on the work of the famous non-governmental HIV advocacy organization Partners in Health, wherein the struggles of the rich and poor to survive are united by a common cause and shared goals. Whether this book and its recommendations have an effect will ultimately depend on what you do with it.

Many thanks

We could not possibly have hoped to cover an entire field without the support of many brilliant colleagues. As Isaac Newton famously said, 'If I have seen far it is because I have stood on the shoulders of giants' (never mind that he was responding to his main competitor who happened to be a dwarf). We have benefited tremendously from the comments and criticisms of experts from many walks of public health life. Our sincerest appreciation goes to Denise Stevens, Sanjay Basu, Martin McKee, Sandeep Kishore, Lawrence King, Derek Yach, Shah Ebrahim, Venkat Narayan, Roberto De Vogli, Chris Lockamy, Robert Geneau, Stig Pramming, Richard Smith, Sarah Steele, Diane Martinez, Devi Sridhar, Gauden Galea, Katy Cooper, Mike Pratt, Prachi Bhatnagar, Pete Scarborough, Pam Dyson, Kathleen O'Connor Duffany, Adam Coutts, Richard Garfield, Rajaie Batniji, Janet Voute, Fiona Wong, Greg Martin, David Korn, Pedro Hallal, Juan Rivera, Yue Gao, Jun Lv, Mohammed Ali, Robert Beaglehole, Christine Hancock, and Rajeev Gupta. We are both grateful to our friends and families for constant support and encouragement. Special thanks go to Georgia Pinteau, who decided the book would be a good idea, and to Nicola Wilson and Jenny Wright who ended up with the task of seeing it through. Their guidance has been invaluable. When you reach the book's conclusion, know that these experts are your colleagues.

Endnotes

1 See Chapter 1 for more details. Children show signs of fatty streaks in their arteries, previously thought to occur in people's adult stages of life. More than one in five children living in South African or Chinese cities is overweight or obese.

2 See Chapter 7, Part 4 about the dangers of Western medical solutions. See also reference 4, Yach et al. (2005).

3 See Chapter 4, Part 2 reflecting the perspectives of health ministers and Chapter 5 about the critical lack of financing from Western donors.

4 Readers will note that the book draws heavily on research conducted in the US and UK. This is because these two countries are the largest funders of research about chronic diseases. To the extent possible, we have tried to focus on developing countries where the greatest rise in chronic disease is predicted to occur.

Contents

Contributors

Tara Acharya
PepsiCo, USA

V.S. Ajay
Centre for Chronic Disease Control
New Delhi, India
and CARRS Center of Excellence
Public Health Foundation of India
New Delhi, India

Simon Barquera
Instituto Nacional de Salud Pública (INSP)
Mexico

Sanjay Basu
University of California
San Francisco, CA, USA

Debbie Bradshaw
Medical Research Council, UK

Tania Cavalcante
National Tobacco Control Program
National Cancer Institute (INCA)
Ministry of Health, Brazil

Amy C. Fuller
Global Health Policy
PepsiCo, USA

Yubei Huang
Peking University Health Science Center
China

Rebecca Kanter
Johns Hopkins Bloomberg School of
Public Health
Baltimore, MA, USA

Lawrence King
University of Cambridge
Cambridge, UK

Sandeep Kishore
Weill Cornell/The Rockefeller University/
Sloan-Kettering Institute, Tri-Institutional
MD-PhD Program
New York, NY, USA

Estelle V. Lambert
University of Cape Town
Rondebosch, South Africa

Naomi Levitt
University of Cape Town
Rondebosch, South Africa

Sandra M.M. Matsudo
Center of Studies of the Physical Fitness
Research Laboratory from São Caetano
do Sul (CELAFISCS)
São Paulo, Brazil

Victor K.R. Matsudo
Center of Studies of the Physical Fitness
Research Laboratory from São Caetano
do Sul (CELAFISCS)
São Paulo, Brazil

Martin McKee
Department of Health Services Research
and Policy
Faculty of Public Health and Policy
London School of Hygiene and Tropical
Medicine, London, UK

George A. Mensah
Heart Health and Global Health Policy
PepsiCo, USA

V. Mohan
Madras Diabetes Research Foundation
Chennai, India

Kathleen O'Connor Duffany
Yale University School of Public Health
New Haven, CT, USA

Barry Popkin
Carolina Population Center
University of North Carolina at Chapel Hill
Chapel Hill, NC, USA

Dorairaj Prabhakaran
Centre for Chronic Disease Control
New Delhi, India
and CARRS Center of Excellence
Public Health Foundation of India
New Delhi, India

K.S. Reddy
CARRS Center of Excellence
Public Health Foundation of India
New Delhi, India

Karen Siegel
Emory University
Atlanta, USA

Sarah Steele
University of Cambridge, Christ's College
Cambridge, UK

Denise Stevens
Yale University and Matrix Public Health
Solutions, Inc
New Haven, CT, USA

Krisela Steyn
Medical Research Council, UK
and University of Cape Town
Rondebosch, South Africa

David Stuckler
University of Cambridge
Cambridge, UK

Marc Suhrcke
University of East Anglia
Norwich, UK

K.R. Thankappan
Sree Chitra Tirunal Institute for Medical
Sciences and Technology
Thiruvananthapuram, India

K.M. Venkat Narayan
CARRS Center of Excellence
Public Health Foundation of India,
New Delhi, India
and Rollins School of Public Health/School
of Medicine, Emory University
Atlanta, GA, USA

Roberto De Vogli
University of Michigan
Ann Arbor, MI, USA

William H. Wiist
Northern Arizona University
Flagstaff, AZ, USA

Yangfeng Wu
The George Institute and Peking University
Health Science Center
Beijing, China

Derek Yach
Global Health Policy
PepsiCo, USA

Lijing L. Yan
The George Institute
Beijing, China

Chen Ying
The George Institute and Peking University
Health Science Center
Beijing, China

Chapter 1

Evaluating the health burden of chronic diseases

- What is the current and future impact of chronic diseases on health?

David Stuckler and Sanjay Basu

Key policy points

1 Chronic diseases are long-term conditions often brought on by our living environments and the choices we make about the design of our communities.

2 In 2010, four chronic diseases—heart disease, respiratory disease, common cancers, and type 2 diabetes—claimed more than 35 million lives; that is, about three out of every five deaths in the world. Close to half of these deaths are premature (before age 70). Nearly 80% of these deaths occur in low- and middle-income countries, where these chronic diseases claim around 80% more lives than do the total of all infectious causes.

3 If societies continue on their current path, the number of premature deaths and years of live lived with disability caused by chronic disease will triple by 2030.

4 Globally, youth tobacco use and obesity rates are greater than 20%. An increasing number of children have been identified with high blood pressure and damage to their arteries, especially in lower-income settings. Left unaddressed, these risks in youth will carry into adulthood, causing a potential threat of a generation that for the first time will live fewer years than their parents.

5 Chronic diseases are diseases of poverty: the most impoverished people living in resource-deprived societies have the greatest risk of dying and suffering due to chronic diseases.

6 More than half of all deaths due to chronic diseases can be avoided by increasing access to essential medicines, reducing tobacco use, and improving people's diets (such as by reducing sugar, fat, and salt intake).

Key practice points

1 Substantial and rising inequalities in chronic disease rates within geographic regions indicate that they are socially determined and therefore, at least theoretically, avoidable.

2 Myths that chronic diseases are 'diseases of the rich' or 'diseases of ageing' in part stem from common misunderstandings about chronic disease epidemiology.

Key practice points *(continued)*

3 Rising co-incidence of infectious and chronic diseases reflects a set of common and interrelated causes of poor health. For example, high prevalence of undernutrition and overnutrition within the same household results from an underlying issue of poor nutrition. Major chronic disease risks such as tobacco and indoor air pollution increase risks of tuberculosis (TB); conversely, infections such as Chagas disease can cause heart disease and HIV/AIDS medications can elevate risk of heart disease and diabetes.

Epidemiology of chronic disease

A group of foreign doctors working in a rural farming community in South Asia decided to set up a small community clinic. Their objective was to provide basic primary care services: splinting broken bones; providing antenatal vitamins and delivering newborns; treating common conditions like diarrhoea, tuberculosis, and malnutrition; and administering vaccines. Once the clinic opened, the physicians kept track of the diagnoses they made and how their patients were doing, as part of their routine to determine how many medications and supplies to buy each month, and what ailments to be aware of in their community.

After only a few weeks, it became clear that one of the top diagnoses was one commonly found in the US and Europe—chronic obstructive pulmonary disease (COPD)—the manifestation of emphysema and chronic bronchitis that develops typically after years of smoking tobacco. In the first year of practice, 173 cases of COPD had been diagnosed, particularly among working-aged adults who were coming to the clinic with severe shortness of breath, requiring immediate treatment with oxygen masks and aerosol medications.

'Surely, the farmers had taken up smoking', the doctors realized.

Determined to nip this new addiction in the bud, the doctors set out to find the sources of tobacco in the community. They wandered to the central market, and found a few food stands selling unpackaged cigarettes for a couple cents apiece. Most of their customers were truck and bus drivers passing through the transit station, buying bread or a few chips and a handful of cigarettes for their shirt pockets. But these men weren't the farmers in the community; they were migrant workers who hadn't come to the clinic and were usually just passing through. The few food stalls selling individual cigarettes also could not account for the large volume of patients who showed up out of breath at the clinic's doorstep, or the curious finding that men weren't the principal patients being diagnosed with COPD. Instead, middle-aged women were being carried by their friends and neighbours, sometimes for hours on the hilly back pathways around farming fields, to get oxygen treatment and ease their wheezing.

The doctors were puzzled. When they asked the women coming to the clinic if they smoked, they said 'never'. Was this a cultural stigma, a refusal to acknowledge secret tobacco use? No—even the gossipy neighbours of these women agreed that the patients had never smoked. Was this second-hand exposure? It didn't appear so; the women denied that their husbands smoked, or that anyone else in their houses ever did.

Flabbergasted, the doctors sent respected women in the community to the homes of some of these women. These respected women were previously trained as mobile nurses for the clinic, who served as community health workers, roaming from house to house in the villages farthest from the clinic. Often they would travel these long distances, sometimes over dangerous terrain, in order to provide follow-up care for patients in need of basic care such as contraceptives, prenatal vitamins, or check-ups to ensure recovery from a recent illness treated at the clinic. This time, when they visited these women, they had a simple question in mind: what could be causing their cases of COPD?

The community health workers followed these women through their workdays to figure out their possible environmental exposures. At 4 a.m., the women woke and went outside to tend to wheat and rice fields, spending the early hours of the morning to plant and pick before the sun's heat made the work unbearable. They ventured out with axes to the nearby forests around noon, cut timber, and carried large sacks of wood on top of their heads back home to cook for their families, using the firewood in large stoves.

Here, the community health workers spotted the most important clue: the women would lean above these wood-burning stoves for 6 to 8 hours a day while preparing the major evening meal, boiling slow-cooked foods like dal (legumes) and hard root vegetables. The stoves were simple clay stands with holes into which to place pots, beneath which a wood-burning fire emitted smoke that filled the single-room homes of these women, often wafting straight into their faces and those of the children tied to their backs. The smoke lingered for hours to stain the walls and ceilings of their homes.

Could these smoky stoves be shortening the breath of these women?

Turning to the medical literature, the physicians found dozens of studies demonstrating that indoor cooking with 'dirty' wood-burning stoves increased the risk of COPD by as much as 80%, particularly in poor communities that could not afford cleaner petroleum-based fuels. The doctors also found that the chronic smoke exposure among women produced a 30% greater risk of cataracts (5), a 2.5-fold greater risk of experiencing active TB (6), and more than twice the risk of upper respiratory tract infections (7) as compared to unexposed individuals.

The doctors also learned that there was a low-cost solution. During the early 1990s, numerous clinical trials in Latin America and sub-Saharan African countries demonstrated that simply connecting tin chimneys from the stove to an outside window, or using alternative cleaner and healthier stoves that could be produced at low cost, could dramatically reduce the risk of dying and suffering from respiratory disease (not to mention help the environment). Overall, the World Health Organization (WHO) estimates that about 700,000 out of 2.7 million global deaths due to COPD in 2004 were caused not by smoking, but by indoor air pollution (8).

The mysterious case of respiratory disease among women in this region was essentially no mystery at all.

In these first two chapters we will draw on the principles that the doctors in the small farming community used to detect the hazardous cooking stoves, but apply them to entire populations to study the global burden of poor health caused by chronic diseases. In medicine, doctors are taught to ask, 'why is this patient seeking my help with this problem at this time?' (9). Like a well-trained physician, we too can start by taking our patient's medical history—except in this case our focus is not just on the patient but entire populations. In public health, we act as doctors of the masses, so we must ask, 'why is this entire population experiencing this burden of disease at this time?'.

Epidemiology will be our guide. It is the study of the distribution and determinants of diseases and their risks in society. In other words, epidemiology is like detective work. It involves searching for clues about disease that can help researchers and policymakers figure out what the culprits are and how to respond.

To address these key questions, we start by setting out what we mean by chronic diseases. Then, we summarize the scope of the problem: how many people are getting sick, who is dying, and what diseases are they dying from? As we fill out these populations' medical charts, we will be on the lookout for several unusual features. These puzzles offer clues about why people are at risk as well as insights about what we can do to reduce these risks, points to which we will return throughout the book. In the concluding section, we discuss a few limitations of what we know and highlight areas where we need more information.

Table 1.1 General characteristics of acute and chronic diseases

Characteristic	Acute diseases	Chronic diseases
Onset	Rapid	Gradual
Duration	Short term	Long term
Causation	Isolable agent causation	Multivariate causation
Diagnostic and prognostic accuracy	High	Low
Treatement modality	Curative	Palliative
Therapeutic options	Specific; self-limited	Multiple; undulating course
Medical technology	Less invasive; highly effective	More invasive; high toxicity
Level of uncertainty	Low	High
Professional-patient relationship	Asymmetric: physician highly knowledgeable, patient inexperienced	More symmetric: physician and patient equally knowledgeable

What is the scope of the problem? Rising chronic diseases . . .

Before we begin evaluating the health burden of chronic diseases we must first set out what exactly is included in this disease category.

Chronic diseases are long-term conditions. They are typically not caused by a virus or infection, but by exposure to multiple, often human-produced hazards (hence they are often labelled 'non-communicable'). Long lag periods occur between when a person is exposed to a hazard and when he or she actually shows signs of clinical illness. The four main chronic non-communicable diseases (NCDs) are cardiovascular disease, malignant neoplasms (cancers), respiratory disease, and diabetes mellitus (mainly type-2). Other important chronic NCDs include digestive diseases, neuropsychiatric conditions, genitourinary disease, endocrine disorders, musculoskeletal disease, skin disease, congenital anomalies, sense organ diseases, and oral conditions (see Tables 1.1 and 1.2).

Placing diseases into broad categories is a complex task. The terms *infectious* and *chronic* are often juxtaposed, even though they describe different dimensions of disease (e.g. some diseases can be both chronic and infectious, such as HIV/AIDS). This simple taxonomic division between infectious and chronic diseases has become increasingly problematic for epidemiologists and policymakers alike (see Annexure for a further discussion). Whichever classification system is used has limitations and it is possible to argue that there are exceptions. Thus, in this book, for historical reasons, we continue the WHO classification as our starting point, focusing on the four main chronic diseases which account for four-fifths of all deaths due to all chronic NCDs (hereafter referred to as chronic disease).[1]

Evaluating the mortality burden of chronic diseases

Modern societies have undergone profound societal and demographic changes that have shifted the fundamental risks to human health. In the past half-century, child mortality decreased and life expectancy increased by 20 years. Improvements in child survival led to declining fertility rates, the slowing of population growth, and created the potential for greater investments in health and education. Rapid increases in economic productivity, achieved through technological advances and industrialization, resulted in mass migration of people from the countryside to the cities. Meanwhile, countries invested their newfound wealth to build public health infrastructure (including, amongst other things, modern sewage and sanitation systems) along with providing basic primary healthcare services.

Table 1.2 Morbidity and mortality rates for chronic non-communicable diseases

Chronic non-communicable diseases	Percentage mortality	Percentage DALYs
Cardiovascular disease		
Rheumatic heart disease, hypertensive heart disease, ischaemic heart disease, cerebrovascular disease, inflammatory heart disease	49.90	21.23
Malignant neoplasms		
Mouth and oropharynx cancers; oesophagus cancer; stomach cancer; colon and rectum cancers; liver cancer; pancreas cancer; trachea, bronchus, lung cancers; melanoma and other skin cancers; breast cancer, cervix uteri cancer; corpus uteri cancer; ovary cancer; prostate cancer; bladder cancer; lymphomas; multiple myeloma; leukemia	21.23	10.83
Respiratory diseases		
Chronic obstuctive pulmonary disease, asthma	11.04	7.90
Digestive diseases		
Peptic ulcer disease, cirrhosis of the liver, appendicitis	5.87	6.66
Neuropsychiatric conditions		
Unipolar depressive disorders, bipolar disorder, schizophrenia, epilepsy, alcohol use disorders, Alzheimer's and other dementias, Parkinson disease, multiple sclerosis, drug use disorders, posttraumatic stress disorder, obsessive-compulsive disorder, panic disorder, insomnia, migraine, lead-caused mental retardation	3.32	27.70
Diabetes mellitus	2.95	2.32
Genitourinary diseases		
Nephritis and nephrosis, benign prostatic hypertrophy	2.53	2.18
Endocrine disorders	0.72	1.14
Other neoplasms	0.44	0.25
Musculoskeletal diseases		
Rheumatoid arthritis, osteoathritis, gout, low back pain	0.32	4.32
Skin diseases	0.21	0.54
Congenital anomalies		
Abdominal wall defect, anencephaly, anorectal atresia, cleft lip, cleft palate, oesophageal atresia, renal agenesis, Down syndrome, congenital heart anomalies, spina bifida	0.15	3.92
Sense organ diseases		
Glaucoma, cataracts, age-related vision disorders, adult-onset hearing loss	0.01	9.94
Oral conditions		
Dental caries, periodontal disease, edentulism	0.01	1.06
Total CVD, DM, COPD, cancer	85.12	42.29

Source: Author's calculations, based on World Health Report 2004 and Global Burden of Disease Statistics, World Health Organization.

Notes: CVD is cardiovascular disease; DM is diabetes mellitus; COPD is chronic obstructive pulmonary disease; and cancer is malignant neoplasms.

As infectious diseases fell substantially in most regions of the world,[2] chronic diseases increased and continued to rise. This phenomenon is commonly referred to as 'epidemiologic transition' (16), as depicted in Figure 1.1. While the precise reasons for these changing disease patterns are not fully understood, in general the declines in mortality are thought to relate to advances in medical care, public health interventions such as sanitation and hygiene, and improved social and economic conditions interventions (8); the debates over these factors are returned to throughout the book (especially in Chapters 2 and 4).

Reflecting these major health changes, in 2004 three out of five deaths in the world were due to the four main chronic diseases, totalling more than 35 million deaths. Eighty per cent of these deaths occurred in low- and middle-income countries, where they accounted for four out of every five deaths. Over the past decade, rises in chronic diseases have been most greatly concentrated in developing countries and, in the case of diabetes, have outpaced epidemiologists' 'pessimistic scenario' forecasts (11, 17, 18).

If nothing is done, chronic diseases will increase by a further 18% before 2015, most markedly in low- and middle-income countries. At regional levels, the highest increases in deaths from chronic disease are projected to occur by 2015 in the WHO regions of Africa (24%), Eastern Mediterranean and South East Asia (23%), Western Pacific (21%), the Americas (16%), and Europe (6%). By 2030, the pattern of deaths in low-income countries will resemble high-income countries, as chronic diseases will account for about 59% of all deaths by 2030, or more than 37 million lives a year (a 64% increase) (18, 19). As shown in Figure 1.1, above $3500 income per capita, chronic diseases overtake infectious disease to become the leading killers (20).

Although clearly something must be the leading cause of death, the increased risk of chronic disease mortality is not simply a result of a reduction in infectious disease mortality. In East Asia and the Pacific countries, for example, the expected rise in chronic disease mortality rates will be more than five times the expected drop in infectious disease mortality rates. In sub-Saharan Africa, where the HIV/AIDS epidemic is the worst and remains highly prevalent, infectious disease mortality rates are expected to drop by 40% over the next 20 years while chronic disease mortality rates are expected to rise by 12% (see Figures 1.2 and 1.3). As a result, in low- and middle-income countries these rapid rises in chronic diseases are combining with high rates of infectious diseases to create a 'double burden' of disease, exacerbating the consequences of both (see country Chapters 7.1–7.5 for more examples) (21).

People are also dying too young from these chronic diseases, especially in the poorest countries where the burden is the greatest but the resources to respond are the least. As shown in Figure 1.3, in 2004, about 9 million deaths due to chronic diseases occurred in people below the age of 60; close to four million of these were in low-income countries. About 15 million premature deaths occurred in people below the age of 70. On average, the age of death due to a chronic disease in low-income countries was about a decade younger than in high-income countries.

This analysis leads us to our first set of clues:

Clue 1: In all regions of the world, even in low-income countries, the chronic diseases will be the major killers.

Clue 2: Chronic diseases are increasing at a faster rate in poor countries than in rich countries.

Clue 3: Rises in chronic diseases have tended to outpace the falls in infectious diseases, creating a double-burden of disease in resource-poor countries.

Clue 4: People living in poor countries tend to die at younger ages from chronic diseases than do persons in rich countries.

When people seek good health, they want more than just to avoid death, but to be free from sickness (a topic returned to in Chapter 3 which discusses the economics of chronic diseases).

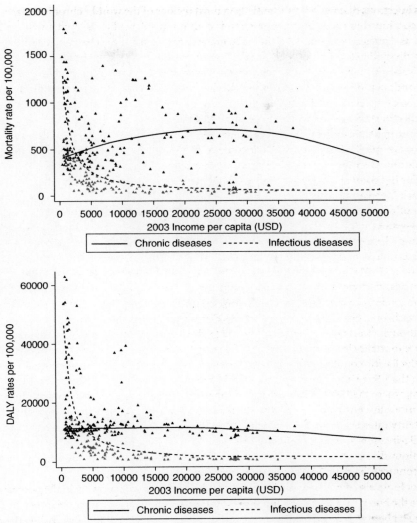

Fig. 1.1 Trends in mortality and disability-adjusted life year rates for chronic and infectious diseases, by income level, 2003/2004 data.
Notes: Chronic diseases are based on the WHO type II category; Infectious diseases are based on the WHO type I category. For more details and data sources see World Health Organization. *Mortality and burden of disease estimates for WHO Member States in 2004.* Geneva: World Health Organization, 2009. Each dot represents one country.

In continuing our search for clues, we now turn to ways to identify the full extent of human suffering caused by chronic diseases.

Evaluating the morbidity burden of chronic disease

Because of their long-term, cumulative nature, death from a chronic disease often occurs after extended periods of suffering and illness. This suffering, commonly referred to as 'morbidity' (22), is difficult to measure, because suffering or disability are socially defined and thereby not

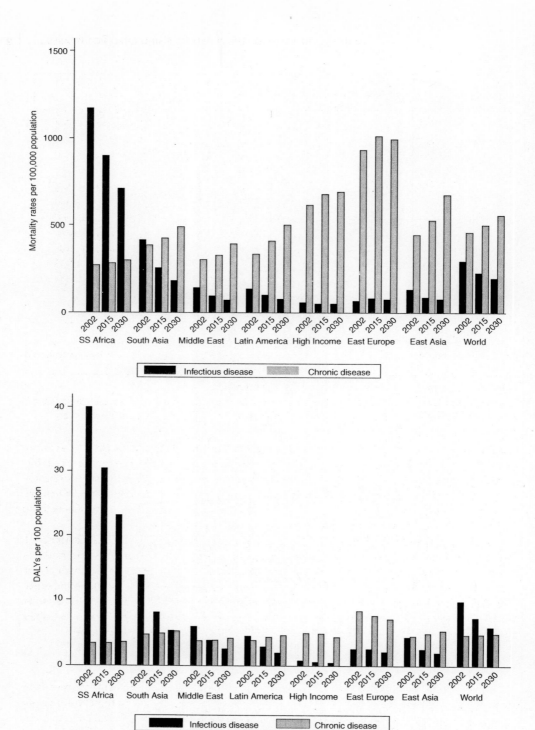

Fig. 1.2 Evolution of the global burden of mortality and disability-adjusted life years, 2002 to 2030. *Notes:* Infectious disease classification is based on WHO's type 1 burden of disease cluster. Chronic disease classification is based on cardiovascular disease, cancers, respiratory disease, and diabetes mellitus subcategories of WHO's type 2 burden of disease cluster. Appendix 1 further describes the data sources, disease classifications, and calculations.

Source: Author's calculations based on Mathers and Loncar 2006 and WHO's Global Burden of Disease projections.

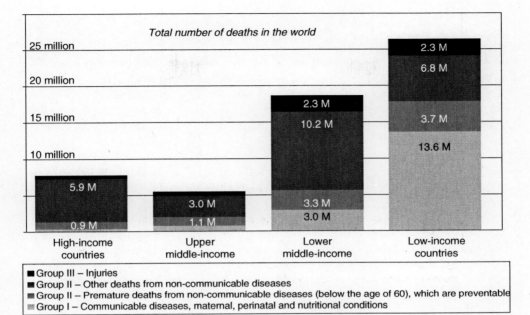

Fig. 1.3 Global mortality burden of mortality, WHO estimates, 2004.
Source: Reproduced from World Health Organization. *Mortality and burden of disease estimates for WHO Member States in 2004.* Geneva: World Health Organization, 2009, with permission.

directly comparable or objective qualities. Often researchers try to estimate the extent and duration of life's quality foregone because of the disease based on people's perceptions of the suffering associated with disease. This perceived suffering is used to calculate broader measures of health than death counts, such as the years of life lived with disability and premature deaths, which are combined to estimate disability-adjusted life year. Box 1.1 provides a short summary of how these adjustments are made to estimate disability-adjusted life years.

According to these broader measures of human suffering, chronic diseases accounted for about half of the global burden of disease in 2004, again concentrated heavily in low- and middle-income countries. Each death due to a chronic disease was, on average, associated with about 1.2 years of disability in a rich country (based on years of life lived with disability); on the other hand, in a poor country, this figure was about 12.5 years: the experience of chronic disease (such as breast cancer or heart disease) causes about 10-times more human suffering for those affected people living in the poorest regions of the world. This also provides an additional clue:

Clue 5: People living in poor countries have greater rates of suffering due to chronic disease than people in rich countries.

In spite of our best attempts to quantify the disease burden, these measurements of years lived with disability are unable to capture the entirety of the disease experience (a topic to which we return in Chapter 3 where we assess the social and economic consequences of NCDs). In the case of prostate cancer, the disease can literally metastasize into people's social lives, leading to divorce (when men's wives divorce them because of sexual complications), poverty (because of costly treatments), or depression (when people lose hope). As anyone who has had a sick relative will know, the experience of illness not only harms affected individuals, but also causes suffering to families, communities, and entire societies.

Box 1.1 Techniques for assessing human suffering caused by illness: disability- and quality-adjusted life years

The most commonly used assessments of morbidity are surveys that ask people to grade their abilities to perform usual life tasks (e.g. ability to walk up stairs without pain or shortness of breath, ability to obtain groceries, etc.). Summing up answers to these questions is used to generate a health score, used as a measure to provide a 'quality-adjusted' or 'disability-adjusted' assessment of how good or bad it is to live a year of life with a particular disease. These scores provide a series of weights to age-specific mortality rates, which are then integrated using life-table methods to calculate a 'quality-adjusted' or 'disability-adjusted' life year (QALY or DALY, respectively). For example, a year of life with terminal lung cancer may only be 0.4 DALYs, as compared to 1 DALY for a year of life as a healthy 21-year-old. The QALY measure is the basis of many cost-effectiveness analyses, which seek to determine how many QALYs can be gained by a particular amount of spending (a 'cost-effectiveness ratio' is expressed as dollars per QALY gained).

The DALY measure, applied in the Global Burden of Disease study, simultaneously accounts for both premature mortality and the prevalence (which do not specifically address morbidity), duration, and severity of the non-fatal consequences of disease and injury, enabling comparative analysis of diseases, injuries, and major risk factors.

Although these measures mark a significant advance in understanding 'morbidity' (22), its estimation is one of the most controversial elements of the Global Burden of Disease initiative, primarily because these measures can make some diseases appear less policy-relevant than others. The main problem is the lack of robust reproducibility. One person's experience of terminal lung cancer can widely differ from another's. Yet the calculations made with QALYs and DALYs can be very sensitive to slight changes in these scores (as the calculations usually have a difference between two scores as the denominator of a cost-effectiveness ratio, so that $100/0.2 QALYs is very different than $100/0.3 QALYs).

Who makes these perceptions and how much they actually know about the condition can skew their judgement. For example, who can assess the quality of life experienced by a person suffering from schizophrenia? It is not straightforward to ask this person himself, nor can a doctor or the general public reliably assess this person's quality of life. Nonetheless, the approach is used for most diseases, relying on populations to assess how much suffering they perceive a disease to carry.

Many other disease metrics exist, such as years of life lived with disability, years of productive life lost, or healthy life expectancy; interested readers can find such measures from WHO's Statistical Information System (20). Sometimes advocacy groups selectively report the disease metric that gives rise to the most striking figures. For example, life expectancy gives prominence to burdens of cardiovascular disease and cancer, working age mortality emphasizes injuries, and disability levels gives higher weight to musculoskeletal disorders and mental illness.

Four main chronic diseases: heart disease, cancer, chronic respiratory disease, and diabetes

So far we have provided a helicopter view of the health burden of chronic diseases. However, these headline statistics can hide important patterns. It is necessary to zoom in to evaluate specific chronic diseases in specific populations, as otherwise, for example, we run the risk of mistakenly thinking the main cause of COPD among women in poor communities to be smoking, because that is what we tend to see on average in rich communities where there are more data.

In this section, we describe the health burden attributable to four main chronic diseases and their key known risk factors (see Table 1.3).

Cardiovascular disease

In 2010, heart disease killed more than 17 million people (18), which is about 30% of all deaths. These deaths are projected to rise to 23 million each year by 2030. Deaths due to cardiovascular disease tend to occur about a decade earlier in low- than high-income countries in poorer settings (23). Significant fractions of cardiovascular disease deaths are reported among people below the age of 65 (41% in South Africa, 35% in India, and 28% in Brazil, compared to only 12% in the US and 9% in Portugal) (23, 24).

Cancer

Cancer deaths are projected to rise from 7.4 million in 2004 to 11.8 million in 2030 (18). Lung cancer is the most common form of cancer worldwide, highly fatal, and mostly due to tobacco and indoor air pollution (8). As with diabetes and heart disease, cancer-related deaths also tend to occur at younger ages in resource-deprived countries. For example, in India, 40% of patients who present to clinics with lung cancer are less than 50 years of age and 11% are less than 40 years (25).

Chronic respiratory disease

Chronic respiratory diseases cause between 8% and 10% of global deaths (8). Their two primary risk factors—tobacco and indoor air pollution—are disproportionately concentrated among the poor. Over half of COPD deaths in women in high-mortality regions such as Sub-Saharan Africa are due to indoor smoke from solid fuels (8).

Diabetes mellitus

Diabetes is expected to double from 285 million to 439 million cases over the period 2000–2030 (26). Diabetes affects 2–3% of sub-Saharan African adults, a figure that is underestimated because

Table 1.3 Top 10 causes of death, WHO estimates, 2004

Low-income countries	Middle-income countries
1 Lower respiratory infections	1 Stroke and cerebrovascular disease
2 Coronary heart disease	2 Coronary heart disease
3 Diarrhoeal disease	3 Chronic pulmonary disease
4 HIV/AIDS	4 Lower respiratory infection
5 Stroke and cerebrovascular disease	5 Trachea, bronchus, and lung cancers
6 Chronic pulmonary disease	6 Road traffic accidents
7 Tuberculosis	7 Hypertensive heart disease
8 Neonatal infections	8 Stomach cancer
9 Malaria	9 Tuberculosis
10 Premature and low birth weight	10 Diabetes mellitus

people often die quickly without access to essential diabetes medicines, such as insulin. Because antiretrovirals to treat HIV/AIDS increase the risk of diabetes (as well as heart disease), public health doctors expect to see a marked rise in the cases of diabetes over next few decades in the region. Currently, China and India have the greatest number of people living with diabetes: they are the 'diabetes capitals' of the world (see Chapters 7.1 and 7.2). More than 113 million people were living with diabetes in Asia in 2007, a large proportion of whom were young and middle aged (19).

Four main behavioural risk factors: tobacco use, unhealthy diet, physical inactivity, and alcohol use

What is causing these deaths among individuals?

Here we will need to draw on a working model of chronic disease epidemiology to begin tracing back the risks from the causes of death to the risks borne in people's conditions of daily living. But choosing a model to describe a specific disease and its determinants is not easy. There are many dimensions to consider.

This complexity recalls a classic Buddhist tale. In the story, a king tells three blind men to feel a different part of an elephant, then asks, 'Well, blind man, have you seen the elephant? Tell me, what sort of thing is an elephant.' The man who felt the ear said the elephant was like a wicker basket. The man who felt the tusk said it was like a solid pipe. The man who felt the tail said it was like a brush. All the blind men were right, and yet all were wrong. So it is in chronic disease epidemiology.

Reality includes complex, tangled webs of interrelated causal factors that contribute to individual chronic disease outcomes (27, 28). The burden of disease in a population reflects the influence of a series of interacting factors lying along a causal pathway. In the case of chronic diseases, they additionally have specific determinants of development and decline that can have different effects at various stages of life. Attempts to capture the richness of this complexity in two dimensions quickly turn into bowls of noodles, as shown in the Web appendix depicting a diagram of the risks of obesity, popularly known as the 'Spaghetti Monster'. One simple way to conceptualize the determinants of health is in terms of immediate, proximal, and underlying factors (a distance metric), acting at different levels of influence (e.g. individual, family, community, and population), and carrying varying degrees of power (a strength metric).[3]

A large body of (mostly Western) evidence has identified a relatively small set of proximal risk factors of chronic diseases. These include individual-level, behavioural risks of chronic diseases— unhealthy diet, physical inactivity, tobacco use, and hazardous drinking—which in turn increase the likelihood of a person becoming obese or overweight,[4] or developing high blood pressure, high cholesterol, or other biological risks. In other words, the way people live can literally 'get under their skin' to cause serious health problems due to chronic diseases.

There are close interrelationships among people's behavioural and clinical risks and their resulting experience of chronic diseases. Extensive documentation of these linkages can be found elsewhere (8); here, we briefly describe the four main behavioural risks: tobacco use, unhealthy diet, physical inactivity, and alcohol use.

1 Tobacco use and exposure (about 17% of all NCD deaths)

Tobacco kills about half of the people who use it, roughly half of whom will die before retirement (on average about 15 years early) (29). In 2004, tobacco caused 1 in 10 deaths worldwide (about 4 million people each year), making it the greatest avoidable killer. Tobacco use has been implicated in the risks of numerous diseases, ranging from infectious diseases (such as TB and HIV/AIDS), to heart disease and lung cancer. In 2010, researchers estimate that 6.3 trillion cigarettes—or more than 900 cigarettes for every person on the earth—will be consumed (23). Tobacco-attributable deaths are projected to decline by about 10% in high-income countries over the next two decades, but to double from 3.4 million to 6.8 million in low- and middle-income countries (19). In 2010 there were estimated to be more than 1.3 billion smokers. The world's top tobacco epidemiologists have projected that, if currents trends continue, tobacco will kill as many as 1 billion people in the 21st century, many in their middle-stages of life (29).

2 Unhealthy diet (>40% of all NCD deaths)

Unhealthy diet is linked to heart disease, certain cancers, diabetes, and many other chronic diseases. Biological risks arise from eating diets high in total calories, in saturated fats, salt, and sugar, as well as low intake of fruits and vegetables, folic acid, and omega-3 fatty acids (found in fish oils). Salt, for example, is a leading cause of high blood pressure. Saturated fats result in high cholesterol and elevated lipids. Low fruit and vegetable intake has been implicated in the rise of several kinds of cancer and heart disease.

3 Physical inactivity (about 10% of all NCD deaths)

There is strong evidence that physical inactivity is linked to heart disease, independent of the effects of diet (23), dating back to research in the 1950s comparing sedentary bus drivers with active bus conductors (30). Many studies have since found that increasing physical activity can decrease the risk of coronary heart disease, stroke, and some cancers (mainly colorectal and breast cancer), type 2 diabetes, osteoporosis, high blood pressure and high cholesterol (23).

4 Alcohol use (about 7% of all deaths)

Alcohol has been identified as a cause of more than 60 types of disease and injury (28, 31, 32). Overall it causes about 1.8 million deaths (3.2% of all deaths) and accounts for 58.3 million lost DALYs (about 4% of all DALYs). Alcohol is estimated to cause between 20% and 30% of cases of oesophageal cancer, liver cancer, liver cirrhosis, homicide, epileptic seizures, and motor vehicle accidents worldwide. It is the leading risk factor among men in eastern Europe (31, 33).

As mentioned above, these risk factors, acting both in isolation and combination, result in a few main clinical risk factors, such as high blood pressure, high blood glucose, insulin resistance, and high blood cholesterol. One example is obesity, a result of an energy imbalance (too much energy in and too little energy out). Therefore, an unhealthy, high calorie diet and decreased physical activity are the most important drivers of obesity (with most studies emphasizing the rise in calories as the overwhelming cause of rising rates of obesity, discussed further in Chapter 2). Currently, more than 1.1 billion adults are overweight worldwide, and 312 million of them are obese.

Of the top-10 global risk factors of poor health, eight relate to chronic diseases (including high blood pressure, tobacco, high blood glucose, physical inactivity, overweight and obesity, high cholesterol, alcohol use, and indoor smoke from solid fuels, see Figure 1.4). Epidemiologists working at WHO estimate that if these risks could be completely eliminated, as many as four out of every five premature deaths due to heart disease, stroke, and type 2 diabetes, and up to 40% of all cancers could be prevented (34). In Chapters 7.1–7.5, these leading NCDs and their key risk factors are described in greater detail in Brazil, China, India, Mexico, and South Africa.

Who is dying and suffering from chronic diseases?

Rising prevalence of risks and disease in children

An important feature of chronic diseases is that their risks accumulate over all stages of life, starting as early as the prenatal period. These risks result from a mother's tobacco use, dietary and physical activity behaviours, overweight and obesity, and other adverse childhood experiences.

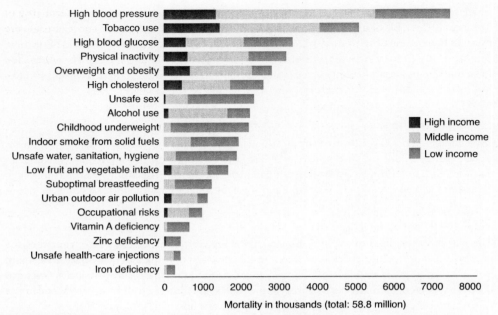

Fig. 1.4 Deaths attributable to 19 leading risk factors, by country income level, 2004 WHO estimates. *Notes:* Data are from World Health Organization. *Mortality and burden of disease estimates for WHO Member States in 2004.* Geneva: World Health Organization, 2009. Key chronic disease risk factors include high blood pressure, tobacco use, high blood glucose, physical inactivity, overweight and obesity, high cholesterol, alcohol use, indoor smoke from solid fuels, low fruit and vegetable intake, and urban outdoor air pollution. Each dot represents one country.

At each stage of life—infancy, childhood, education, work and retirement periods—exposures to risk may have adverse effects that do not occur when exposed at other stages (35). The now extensive body of research known as 'life-course' epidemiology can identify how exposures to a hazard that occur at any stage of life could increase risks of disease much later. This is important because some NCDs require decades of exposure to hazards such as tobacco before manifesting as clinical illness (latency period).[5]

Using life-course techniques, studies have documented how many of the major risk factors for cardiovascular disease are established in childhood and adolescence (23). Life-course investigations conducted in the US and Europe have shown how poverty and social instability in childhood are linked to greater risks of cardiovascular disease later in life.

Many of the risks of chronic disease are manifesting in children at early ages. About 10% of boys and girls in the Seychelles, a middle-income African country, were found to have elevated blood pressure, putting them at risk of organ damage and early heart disease (36). Close inspection of the data from the Seychelles revealed that prevalence was greater among younger than older children, indicative of growing risks (36). Similar patterns of elevated blood pressure were observed among children in diverse settings ranging from the Ashanti region of Ghana (37) to Pakistan (38). Fatty streaks and inflammation in arteries, which in the past were the signature of old age, are also being identified in children, especially obese ones (39, 40). These risks track from adolescence into adulthood (41).

Obesity is driving these risks to children. Worldwide, overweight and obesity affect 10% of children age 5–17 years. In the US, the world leader in child obesity rates, about 35% of youth are overweight or at risk of being overweight (42); 17% of children between 2 and 19 years of age were clinically obese (body mass index (BMI) >30). Rates are rapidly rising in resource-poor countries. In China, obesity rates in children under the age of 15 rose from 15% in 1982 to 27% in 2004 (43). In Mexico, about 17% of children between ages 5 and 11 were overweight and about 9% were obese. In South Africa, about 22% of schoolchildren were found to be overweight or obese (4).

Rising prevalence of childhood obesity is, in turn, fuelling an epidemic of diabetes. Once considered primarily a disease of adulthood ('adult-onset diabetes'), type 2 diabetes was diagnosed in only 1–2% of diabetes cases in children two decades ago (44). Type 2 diabetes has recently begun surfacing in children at alarming rates, in some countries representing up to 80% of all diabetes cases reported in the paediatric population (44, 45). One in three children born in the US in 2000 are projected to develop type 2 diabetes during their lifetime as a result of obesity (46).

Rates of tobacco use are unacceptably high among children in all regions of the world. As shown in Figure 1.5, the risks are the greatest among lower- and middle-income countries where tobacco companies are investing to take advantage of rising incomes and relatively unregulated markets. Data from 2008 surveys of youths aged 13–15 in South Africa and Mexico reveal that more than one-quarter currently smoke cigarettes. This situation continues in spite of a global legislative agreement, the Framework Convention on Tobacco Control, to curb tobacco use among children.

As a result of these growing risks of chronic disease in society, one recent study finds that, if current trends continue, for the first time the gains in life expectancy in rich countries such as the US will be reversed (47).

Clue 6: Rates of chronic diseases and risk factors have risen significantly among youth.

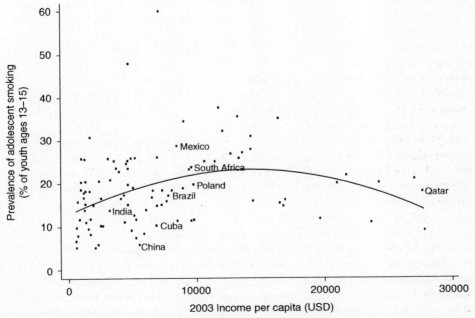

Fig. 1.5 Global youth tobacco rates, latest available data, by income. Each dot represents one country.

Inequalities in chronic diseases and diseases of poverty

Although the precise combination of risks of NCDs differs across regions and communities, they share an important common feature in all settings: the risks of dying and suffering from a chronic disease are by far the greatest among the poor.

Comparing high- and low-income countries reveals that in every age group, persons in low-income countries have about twice of the risk of dying and tend to die at earlier ages from NCDs than persons in high-income countries. As shown in Figure 1.6, this is a quite general pattern: the lower a country's income, the greater its age-standardized mortality and DALY rates from chronic diseases.[6] This observation reflects a key public health theorem:

Public Health Theorem 1: The greatest risks of poor health occur among the poorest and most vulnerable segments of the population.

Chronic diseases cause marked inequalities both within and across entire populations. For example, a person living in Russia has about a 50% higher risk of dying from a chronic disease than a person living in Poland, despite relatively similar levels of income per capita (see Figure 1.6). Similarly, residents of Nauru, a small Pacific island, have nearly double the risk of NCDs as citizens of China, despite both having similar income levels of about $5000 per capita. At the high-income end of the spectrum, people living in Qatar have more than double the risk of NCDs as people living in Japan. Qatar's society is at risk of becoming the next case of Nauru, where chronic diseases contributed to the undoing of an entire society's way of life (see Chapter 2).

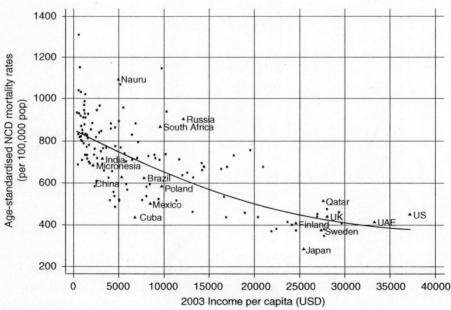

Fig. 1.6 Age-standardized rates of mortality due to chronic diseases, 2004, by income.
Notes: Age-standardized mortality rates presented for selected country cases referenced throughout the book. Best-fit line represents average of all countries. Chapter 2 includes Cuba, Finland, Japan, Micronesia, Nauru, Poland, Russia, and Sweden. Chapter 7 includes Brazil, China, India, Mexico, and South Africa. Each dot represents one country.

What can explain these substantial differences in the risks borne by entire societies? We know that individual behavioural risks play a significant role. But why are they rising in some societies faster than in others?

Returning these important questions to Chapter 2, here we note that these population-based inequalities reveal that the risks of chronic diseases are largely created by societies in which we live. Importantly, this means that a high burden of chronic disease is not inevitable, but instead is highly avoidable. These data imply that the greatest opportunity for acting to reduce avoidable chronic diseases is occurring now in the poorest countries (23), where the highest levels of risk in the world can be prevented from manifesting as a very high burden of disease.

These observations echo a key point, emphasized by Geoffrey Rose's famous public-health theorem:

Public Health Theorem 2: A large number of people exposed to a small risk may give rise to more cases of disease than a small number of people who are exposed to a large risk.

Although chronic diseases are clearly diseases of poverty, in the very poorest countries the health gap between the rich and the poor continues to be largely driven by infectious diseases and maternal health challenges. After adjusting for differing age-structures, we see that once an economy passes about US $1000 income per capita,[7] chronic diseases become leading causes of death and disability. In an analysis of what accounts for the gap in deaths between rich and poor countries, chronic diseases accounted for about one-third of this gap in the world's two poorest quintiles of countries (48). The poor are about twice as likely to die from a chronic disease as the rich (based on age-standardized mortality rates), but they are about 20 times more likely to die from infectious causes.[8]

How do we know that chronic diseases can be prevented?

In 2005, the prestigious medical journal *The Lancet* and WHO jointly issued a call to reduce chronic disease deaths by 2% each year over the next several decades, which was predicted to avert about 36 millions deaths and save about 500 million years of life between 2006 and 2015 (3). How did researchers arrive at these numbers?

It is difficult to estimate the extent to which any disease is preventable, because the burden of disease reflects a complex combination of risks, ranging from fixed biological factors, such as genetics, to macroeconomic factors, such as taxation. Four main concepts are commonly used to describe the extent to which a disease can be prevented: avoidable, premature, excess, and modifiable.

The first concept is based on a strict categorization of deaths that should not occur in the presence of effective medical care, referred to as 'avoidable mortality' (or at times amenable mortality). This category incorporates one-half of all ischaemic heart disease deaths as well as several other NCDs such as cerebrovascular disease, chronic rheumatic heart disease, hypertensive disease, diabetes (ages 0–49), and several cancers (49).

Premature deaths are those that occur before the average life expectancy of a given population. The assumption is that if someone dies before the average population member, then something went wrong that could have been avoided. One limitation in using this approach is the difficulty in comparing countries because each has a different average lifespan; for example, a suicide at age 60 would be considered premature in the US where life expectancy is above 75 years but not in Russia, where life expectancy is below 70 years. To overcome this problem, age 70 is a frequently used global cut-off for assessing whether a death is premature. About 16 million chronic disease deaths were estimated to occur before age 70 in 2005; hence about one-half of chronic disease deaths are premature (50).

The third approach is to analyse 'excess mortality', or deaths that are over and above historical trends. For example, the rapid rise of chronic diseases in eastern Europe during the 1990s indicates that, in some populations, a considerable portion of chronic disease risk is 'excess'. The date used as the reference point for assessing excess risk is inevitably a subject of debate. A related approach, confusingly, referred to at times as avoidable mortality, uses a reference population's age-specific rates of disease as a comparison. For example, one could ask how many deaths could be avoided if men aged 30–44 had the same risk as women of that age group to acquire diabetes. Another option would be to compare a country like Russia to its neighbour Belarus, or to compare chronic disease risk in African American populations in the US to white US populations. Clearly, here the greatest difficulty is selecting an appropriate reference population. One strategy to overcome this issue is to choose the lowest set of age-specific risks from within a block of countries that are similar geographically and economically. In part the 2% prevention of chronic disease goal was based on the insight that chronic disease rates had dropped in several high-income countries by as much as 6% per year, indicating that such reductions were possible to achieve.

A fourth approach is based on assessing the modifiability of risk factors. Often epidemiologists presume that the common risk factors associated with people's lifestyles are partially modifiable, making the disease they cause preventable. This is clear in the case of the tobacco—the world's leading cause of preventable death; an individual can decide not to smoke and reduce risk to zero (barring second-hand tobacco smoke). Obesity is also highly preventable, apart from cases arising from genetic susceptibility such as thyroid dysfunction. Salt, cholesterol, and alcohol intake can also be averted through dietary interventions (51). One recent estimate is that at least 80% of heart disease, stroke, and type 2 diabetes and 40% of cancer could be avoided through healthy diet, regular physical activity, and avoidance of tobacco use (52). In 2007 *The Lancet* specified that three simple actions could achieve the goal to reduce chronic disease mortality rates by 2% each year: 1) scaling-up a multidrug regimen for the prevention of cardiovascular disease; 2) reducing salt intake in the population by 15%; and 3) implementing four key elements of the WHO Framework Convention on Tobacco Control.

Thus, whichever approach is taken to assess preventability, it is clear that a substantial fraction of death and disability due to chronic disease can be averted. Preventing disease may be biologically feasible, but not economically or politically, a point taken up again in Chapter 3 about cost-effectiveness and in Chapter 5 about political economy of chronic disease interventions.

Where do the data come from? A scandal of ignorance . . .

The epidemiologic trends depicted in the above section sound worrisome: deaths and disability will rise significantly, largely due to avoidable causes, with the greatest impacts on the poorest members of populations in low- and middle-income countries. But we must ask, how do we know whether any of this is true? Where do these numbers come from?

A key problem is that a substantial portion of the data used in these models is often fabricated. The truth is, we do not know how many people worldwide died from chronic disease or any other disease for that matter. Most data come from a series of statistical models, based on a combination of data sources about what people died from, including estimates from sentinel sites and population registers of death certificates. As one of the authors of the Global Burden of Disease study notes, 'while most countries have some information about prevalence, incidence and mortality from some diseases and injuries, it is generally fragmented, partial, incomparable and diagnostically uncertain' (53).

This lack of data has been called a 'scandal of invisibility' (54). Worldwide, about one-third of all children are unregistered, totalling about 48 million missing children. In sub-Saharan African countries, less than half of all births are recorded. Only two small African island states of Mauritius and the Seychelles have complete registration of births, deaths, and cause of death data. South Africa is the only other African country in which registration of births and deaths is high, but large proportions of deaths are still attributed to undetermined causes. The situation is only slightly better in South East Asia and Latin America.

In the context of these missing vital statistics, most of the Global Burden of Disease information is created using demographic models or projections from local surveys. Box 1.2 describes how adult mortality is estimated where there are no data. The predictive value of the forecasts depends on the validity of the underlying models of chronic disease mortality rates. In the past, because these models excluded key individual explanations of chronic disease risk, such as obesity, they were poor predictors of rises in diabetes mortality. Subsequent Global Burden of Disease analyses have been done, taking advantage of greater availability of data from the year 2004; however, the basic population statistical model used to estimate chronic diseases remains inaccurate (17, 18).[9]

How do epidemiologists estimate chronic disease data where there are none? About 56 countries monitored by WHO's surveillance teams resort to estimating chronic disease mortality either from data from similar countries where there are data or, in cases where there are sufficient child mortality data, using them to estimate adult deaths. Excellent vital registration data exist for only five low- and middle-income countries—Chile, Costa Rica, Cuba, Singapore, and Sri Lanka—making it possible to analyse trends in adult mortality since 1950.

Even where there are data, there can be serious classification errors, especially when persons suffer from multiple chronic diseases, referred to as co-morbidities. Most people will have more than one chronic disease in their lifetime (see Chapter 4 for implications for managing NCDs). When a person dies due to cardiovascular disease and has type 2 diabetes, it is difficult to identify which factor initiated the causal chain resulting in death, resulting in either under- or over-reporting of cardiovascular disease or diabetes. An eleventh update to the International

Box 1.2 Examples of estimates of adult mortality where there are no data

No sources of nationwide mortality data in Nigeria existed until the World Bank conducted a Demographic & Health Survey in 1990. Prior to that time, the United Nations (UN) estimated Nigeria infant mortality rates based on small-scale surveys in one or two states in the 1970s and mortality levels of neighbouring countries. The UN demographers describe their estimation as a 'qualitative review of the data', not a quantitative analysis. Using these estimates of infant mortality, the UN generated a hypothetical age pattern of mortality at all other ages using the model life table 'North'. These estimates in the mid-1970s were used to generate the current estimates by assuming that life expectancy improved by 2 years every 5 chronological years. In turn, the World Bank combined the UN results for the infant mortality rate and life expectancy with the model life table North to calculate yet again the age pattern of adult mortality based on the Bank's projection model. Put simply, for most of the world's poorer countries the empirical basis for estimates of adult mortality is tenuous.

Source: Murray CJL, Yang G, Qiao X. Adult mortality: levels, patterns, and causes. In Feachem RGA, Kjellstrom T, Murray CL, Over M, Phillips MA (eds) *The health of adults in the developing world*, pp.23–111. Oxford: Oxford University Press, 1992.

Classification of Disease (ICD-11) aims to improve the harmonization of these death coding procedures across countries.

In summary, despite the air of scientific authority these estimates can sometimes project, it is important to bear in mind these very significant caveats to them. Nonetheless, it is generally better to make judgements and set priorities in the presence of data, however weak, than without them. Further, the process of using these data can also reveal key weaknesses in surveillance systems and encourage better data collection, as well as help stimulate attention to the issue of rising chronic diseases (see Chapter 5 about how surveillance is an important advocacy tool).

Insights from community-based studies and national investigations

Small-scale investigations of the burden of disease, such as those conducted by the doctors and community health workers about respiratory disease among women in the South Asian farming community, provide important insights into the chronic disease epidemic. One example comes from an ongoing demographic surveillance programme in a rural region of Bangladesh called Matlab. Researchers examined causes of death obtained from 'verbal autopsies' covering 19,000 deaths that occurred between 1986 and 2006 (55). Despite inherent difficulties involved in translating a history of symptoms into reliable cause of death information (53), the study revealed a clear progressive shift in the burden of disease from infectious to chronic causes of death, as depicted in Figure 1.7 (55).

In the mid-nineties, the WHO Adult Morbidity and Mortality Project team reported that Tanzanian men (56), aged 15–64, were dying from stroke at three to six times the rate of their counterparts in the UK. A more a recent study of 45 villages in the Andhra Pradesh Rural Health Initiative found that chronic diseases accounted for 55% of all deaths (57).

Surveys have also found household evidence of an emerging double-burden of disease. In Brazil 44% of families with an undernourished member also had an overweight member, with high prevalence also observed in China (23%) and Russia (58%) (58). A survey of very-low-income populations in Maceio, Brazil found that 30% of all families had both an underweight and overweight-obese member living under the same roof (59) (see country Chapters 7.1–7.5 for more details).

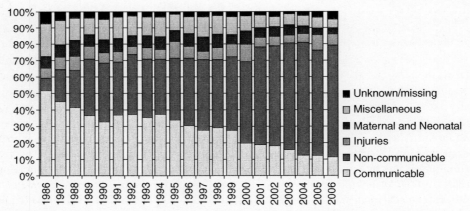

Fig. 1.7 Change in broad causes of death for both sexes in Matlab Government service area, 1986–2006.

Source: Reproduced from Karar et al. 2009. *Global Health Action* v2, with permission. Available at http://www.globalhealthaction.net/index.php/gha/article/view/1904/2301.

New insights on the importance of chronic diseases are also being obtained from studies that track health expenditure in families (as opposed to most studies which track hospitals or clinics). Household surveys of families in South Africa found that 74% of reported health problems were 'chronic', 48% of which had received no treatment in the previous month. In a linked follow-up of households, among subjects with chronic illness, only 62% had an allopathic diagnosis and only 35% were receiving regular treatment (60). A study in India found that chronic diseases represented 17.7% of illnesses but 32% of costs. Although hospitalizations were the single most costly component on average, they accounted for only 11% of total costs, compared to drugs, which accounted for 49% of total costs (61).

Risk factor data are even more limited than the mortality data. One recent review of the available surveillance of blood pressure found there were a total of 703 country-year data points (mostly from the US, Japan, and western Europe). About 1% of Africa's population were covered by cancer registries. Despite these gaps, there is clear evidence that populations in resource-poor countries are being increasingly exposed to risk factors of chronic disease. Another recent report from WHO's surveillance team found that 9 out of 10 people in 21 countries in Africa had one major NCD risk factor; about one-third of populations had between three and five risk factors at once (62).

In sum, these detailed studies of population subgroups provide evidence that paint a consistent picture of marked rises in chronic diseases, concentrated in resource-deprived settings.

Summary

We can return to where we started: what are chronic diseases? Who is being affected? Why are rates of chronic disease rising?

Chronic diseases are long-term conditions. They are typically not caused by a single infection, but by exposure to multiple, often human-produced hazards. Decades can pass between the original exposure to a hazard and the eventual onset of clinical illness.

In 2010, four main chronic diseases—heart disease, common cancers, respiratory disease, and diabetes—claimed more than 35 million lives, accounting for about three out of every five deaths in the world. Four out of five of these deaths and years of life lived with disability occurred in low- and middle-income countries, where chronic diseases caused an 80% greater burden of death and disability than infectious diseases.

The outlook is no better: if nothing changes, chronic disease deaths will more than triple over the next two decades. The bulk of this increase in death and disability will occur in low- and middle-income countries, most greatly in Sub-Saharan Africa and Latin America, where there continues to be a high burden of infectious disease. In many of these regions, the rises in chronic diseases have outpaced the falls in infectious diseases, creating a 'double-burden of disease' and worsening the ability of resource-deprived countries to address both.

The rising co-incidence of infectious and chronic diseases reflects the common and interrelated causes of poor health. For example, there has been a rising prevalence of undernutrition and over-nutrition in the same household, a problem that relates to an underlying problem of poor nutri-tion. Several chronic diseases and their risk factors are known causes of infectious diseases; tobacco, alcohol abuse, indoor air pollution, and diabetes increase risks of TB. Conversely, infections and their medications can cause heart disease or diabetes (such as HIV/AIDS or Chagas disease).

There is clear evidence that chronic diseases are diseases of poverty. Like all forms of poor health, the poorest and most vulnerable members of the population are at the greatest risk. In the case of chronic diseases, there is delay between a hazardous exposure and the development of disease, so that only after a period of time does the actual health burden come to be visibly concentrated among the poor. The fact that the poor often die prematurely from an acute cause can hide the reality that the risks of chronic disease are always the greatest among the poor (giving rise to a myth that chronic diseases are 'disease of affluence'). As we have demonstrated, at all points in time and within every age group, the poorer a person is and the poorer their society, the greater their risk of death due to a chronic disease.

Chronic disease can cause extended periods of suffering and disability, not to mention financial expense (see Chapter 3), before a victim ultimately succumbs. In higher-income countries, an afflicted person suffers for about 1 year of life lived with disability before dying from a chronic disease. This contrasts with the situation in low- and middle-income countries, where people live almost 12 years of life with disability for each chronic disease death.

There are strong links between chronic diseases and the ways in which society is organized. One reflection of our society's development is the health of our youth. In recent years, rising rates of high blood pressure and type 2 diabetes have begun to manifest in children. Examination of their arteries reveals signs of atherosclerosis and inflammation, which were once considered to be considered hallmarks of old age. These risks in turn derive from unacceptably high rates of youth tobacco use and obesity, which are globally above 20%. In other words, the lag period between exposure to a behavioural risk of chronic diseases, such as physical inactivity or unhealthy diets, and the development of heart disease appears to have shortened—the pace of ageing of these children has unnaturally increased.

Left unaddressed, these risks in youth forebode even greater rises in chronic diseases than the forecasts presented above, which could not account for them. This insight is corroborated by recent studies of children which have provided evidence of how, if current trends continue, there could be a potential reversal of life expectancy in the most affected countries. These high-risk societies include many countries, but at present those at greatest risk include the US and Mexico, where more than one out of every four youth are overweight or obese.

Many of these deaths among the poor will continue to be invisible, what has been called a scandal of ignorance (54). Often the poor's only voice to Western audiences, their statistics and body counts, remain hidden by current systems. An overarching global health challenge is to 'make everyone count by counting everyone'; that is, by increasing the populations covered by surveillance systems. Not only does inadequate or inaccurate information impede effective disease control and planning, but they also prevent a political priority being placed on chronic diseases (see Chapter 5). Despite gaps in the evidence base in local settings, recent data from sentinel sites do confirm the global picture of a rapidly rising burden of chronic diseases in resource-poor settings.

How can we reduce these risks? Returning to our key clues reveals, crucially, that the ultimate causes of rising chronic diseases are beyond the control of individuals, relating instead to the choices we are making about how to design our communities and living environments. Estimates that take account of this issue suggest that, in theory, more than half of the overall suffering and death caused by chronic diseases can be prevented through population-wide measures to improve diets, reduce tobacco, and enhance access to quality healthcare (a topic to which we return in Chapter 4). This creates a window of opportunity to act to prevent and control chronic disease risks, especially in the low-income countries where the risks are at present the greatest but, because of the delay between exposure and disease, can still be prevented from becoming costly and disabling. Without significant change, their patterns of societal development will lock-in trajectories of rising rates of death and disability due to chronic diseases.

In the next chapter, we continue investigating the changing societal circumstances that are influencing people's choices in greater detail, in search of further clues about what can be done to reduce the risks of chronic diseases.

Endnotes

1 Among chronic disease community, including government departments, academics, and non-governmental organizations, there are ongoing debates about what chronic NCDs should be called and what specific syndromes the classification should include. Some argue for focusing on just a few key diseases (heart disease, diabetes, respiratory disease, common cancers), while others seek a broader classification including mental health. Others dispute the appropriate terminology for chronic diseases, calling for NCD, chronic non-communicable disease (CNCD), or chronic disease (CD) as labels. Indeed, in inviting contributors to this book, we received all three interpretations of what was understood by chronic diseases. The focus on the main four diseases can be justified because they have strong links to a common set of risk factors (unhealthy diet, physical inactivity, tobacco, and alcohol) and account for the greatest number of deaths. Although musculoskeletal disorders and mental health burdens are leading causes of chronic disease-related disability, it is likely that, if other NCD risks were addressed, these high morbidity CNCDs would also improve. It has also has been argued that more lives could be saved by focusing on common risk factors of chronic disease.

2 With the important exception of sub-Saharan Africa and eastern Europe, resulting from major rises in HIV/AIDS in the former and tuberculosis in the latter.

3 Another system focuses on the level of an exposure: risks can be undertaken by individuals (choosing to drink and smoke) and by societies (determining how much to charge individuals to drink and smoke), with multiple levels falling between, such as households, schools, firms, communities, countries, regions, or continents (a level metric). Within each level, there are layers of people's identities, such as age, gender, ethnicity, education, social class, and status (a sphere metric). Complex chains of these preceding systems can form a unique pathway, such as taxation of tobacco (societal level, underlying) leading to greater tobacco use (individual level, proximal) and, decades later, ultimately greater lung cancer deaths (individual level, immediate). Each of these chains can be characterized as having a certain strength (a power metric), acting over periods of time spanning moments to centuries (a time metric). Together, these six metrics—distance, level, pathways, power, sphere, and time—can fully characterize the determinants of the burden of disease. Such metrics relate fundamentally to the criteria used for assessing the causality of potential relationships between risk exposures and disease outcomes. Classically these criteria have been set out by Bradford-Hill; they include biological plausibility, experimental evidence, coherence, strength of association, analogy, temporality, and specificity (62a).

4 Obesity is frequently cited as a risk factor for chronic diseases, but can also be regarded as a 'chronic disease' in its own right. For the purposes of this book we will consider obesity as a risk factor. Persons with a BMI over 30 kg/m^2 are considered obese, while those with a BMI over 25 kg/m^2 but less than 30 kg/m^2 are considered overweight.

5 This dynamic approach could be fruitfully extended to other spheres to provide insight into the social contexts of chronic diseases risk. For example, the life-course of communities could study how communities structure chronic disease risks from their inception, when people move to the community, to their ageing, when the communities' population composition and size changes, perhaps resulting in ultimate growth (as in mega-Indian cities), stagnation (as in British 1960s peripheral urban communities), or decline (as in low-fertility Italian villages).

6 Policymakers are mostly concerned about disease burdens; epidemiologists are principally concerned about disease risk. None of the crude mortality or morbidity measures presented thus far has accurately accounted for who is at greatest risk of chronic diseases. The problem is that, because there is a long latency period between exposure to risk and disease outcome, often lasting decades, chronic diseases begin showing up clinically during in middle- and later-stages of life. If, like some acute diseases, risk produces disease incidence or mortality very rapidly, possibly immediately, the 'crude' measures used above to describe the burden of disease would accurately characterize risk. In most cases, to capture disease risk epidemiologists cannot simply trust what meets the immediate eye; an adjustment for age needs to be made to the disease burden to identify the actual risk of chronic diseases occurring in a population.

7 There is a delay for this to manifest in the crude burden. In terms of crude mortality rates, as shown in Figure 1.1, the crossover point is at about $3500 per capita.

8 Another measure of the disease burden is the morbidity:mortality ratio, often regarded as a measure of economic costs. It indicates how much suffering from a chronic disease is associated with a death due to chronic disease. This ratio is greater in low-income countries, compresses slightly in middle- and high-income countries (reaching the narrowest point at about 33,000 USD per capita), and then expands in the very highest-income countries.

9 In the first Global Burden of Disease (GBD) study, conducted in 1996 out of Harvard, the analysts estimated regression models of chronic disease mortality rates as a function of a country's income, population size, age distribution, and the percentage of the population using tobacco (equation 1).

WHO Global Burden of Disease regression model structure:

$$\ln M_{a,k,i} = C_{a,k,i} + \beta 1 \ln\gamma + \beta 2 (\ln\gamma)^2 + \beta 3 \ln HC + \beta 4 \ln SI + \beta 5t$$

Here a is age group, k is sex, and i is cause of death. γ is GDP per capita, M is the mortality level, HC is human capital, SI is an index of smoking impact, and t is a linear time trend. Model parameters were estimated using ordinary least squares regression separately for each age-sex-cause group for 106 countries for death data from 1950–2002.

Annexure

Challenges in attempting to categorize diseases

Diseases can be classified in many ways, but the two main taxonomic divisions are by their duration (acute/chronic) and mode of transmission (communicable/non-communicable) (see Table 1.1). Historically, the WHO has collapsed this 2×2 framework into three categories: a 'type I' cluster comprising acute/communicable diseases and maternal and child health conditions; a 'type II' cluster comprising chronic/NCDs; and a 'type III' cluster comprising acute/non-communicable injuries and violence (10, 11). Advances in medical knowledge have called this classification into question.

Consider type 1 diabetes, a disease that can originate when a virus infects a genetically predisposed individual. In this case, the diabetes disease process is clearly non-communicable (the virus has done the damage and cleared the body), but some of the long-term complications, such as skin ulcers, are clearly infectious. Another example is HIV/AIDS. The virus is clearly infectious but gives rise to disease processes, such as Kaposi's sarcoma, that are non-infectious. Furthermore, antiretrovirals for treating HIV/AIDS greatly increase the risk of cardiovascular disease: HIV/AIDS is both infectious and chronic (12).

Many NCDs have infectious origins: cervical cancer is caused by human papillomavirus; stomach cancers are predominantly caused by *Helicobacter pylori* (13); heart disease in Latin America is caused by Chagas disease, a neglected tropical disease; in Africa and the Middle East, kidney failure is largely caused by schistosomiasis (14).

Conversely, NCDs and their risk factors can increase the risk of infectious disease spread. For example, in the case of TB, WHO notes that 'risk factors that seem to be of importance at the population level include poor living and working conditions associated with high risk of tuberculosis transmission, and factors that impair the host's defence against tuberculosis infection and disease, such as HIV infection, malnutrition, *smoking, diabetes, alcohol abuse, and indoor air pollution*' (emphases added) (15).

This interconnected nature of disease risks and outcomes defies simplistic attempts to classify the disease burden (and to intervene, as we return to in Chapter 4). As shown in Web Appendix, chronic diseases correlate with nearly all causes of death at a population level, and have many associations which have a causal biological or socioeconomic basis. For example, tobacco–TB, diabetes–TB, HIV–cardiovascular disease, neglected tropical diseases–chronic diseases, and stunting–obesity, are just a few of the range of interactions between chronic diseases and other conditions that occur at both biological and socioeconomic levels.

Ultimately, separating diseases into categories is a social process. It creates a symbolic understanding of disease burdens which, in turn, influences how programmes are developed, targets are set, and progress is monitored.

Chapter 2

Sick individuals, sick populations: The societal determinants of chronic diseases

- What are the social causes of rising chronic diseases?

David Stuckler, Karen Siegel, Roberto De Vogli, and Sanjay Basu

Key policy points

1 Societies in which people are born, live, work, and age create risks of chronic disease. Health is largely determined by factors outside of the healthcare system.

2 About half of all deaths due to chronic diseases relates to tobacco use, unhealthy diet, alcohol use, or physical inactivity.

3 People's choices about these unhealthy behaviours depend strongly on circumstances beyond their immediate control. By influencing the price, availability, and marketing of unhealthy products, social and economic circumstances affect people's perceived costs and benefits—two powerful determinants of choice.

4 Reductions in the price of unhealthy foods, alongside increases in their availability and marketing, are making nutritionally-poor choices become the easier, more desirable, and economically smarter choices. Similarly, declining opportunities for movement make it more difficult for people to be physically active.

5 Opening markets to trade can increase the price of traditional, healthy foods in resource-poor countries and potentially price them out of the market. When rich countries subsidize oils, fat, and sugar, they put farmers and small businesses in poor countries at a competitive disadvantage as well as provide incentives for people to make unhealthy dietary choices.

6 Remarkable gains in health could be achieved if broader social forces were harnessed to ameliorate the societal risks of chronic diseases.

Key practice points

1 Much of a person's risk of chronic disease can be attributed to a few common risk factors. This narrow set of risk factors can account for a large fraction of the population-wide burden of disease mainly because they reflect the broader societal conditions in which people live.

2 Knowing about the main chronic disease risk factors can help us identify who is at risk, but tells us little about why people have them or how to intervene. In the future, greater insights will come from identifying the specific biological hazards associated with these risks ('zooming in') or developing a better understanding of the underlying societal determinants of chronic diseases and their risks ('zooming out').

3 Overemphasizing the most common risks of chronic disease in rich countries—such as tobacco, high blood pressure, and obesity—could divert attention from the main risk factors operating in low-income settings—such as indoor air pollution—where the greatest risks of death and disability due to chronic disease have been observed.

4 Public health experts should seek to identify and address what is driving unhealthy ageing, urbanization, and growth processes: they must concentrate on the 'causes of the causes' and 'risk factors of the risk factors'.

5 Dietary dependency is a process by which food choices comes to depend on choices of governments, producers, and multinational companies. This dependency is fostered by models of economic development emphasizing trade liberalization, export-oriented agriculture, and foreign direct investment in foods and beverage sectors, especially in the context of unregulated marketing and government subsidies.

What can explain rising chronic diseases? Leading population explanations . . .

Why are some populations becoming sicker while others are remaining healthy?

In the 1970s Geoffrey Rose threw down the gauntlet to public health to identify not just the causes of poor individual health, but the 'causes of the causes' influencing the health of entire populations. As he put it, there are 'Sick individuals and sick populations', and it is necessary to address the causes of both (9).

At the time Rose was writing, tremendous strides were being made in identifying the key individual risks of heart disease: alcohol, tobacco, physical inactivity, and obesity and their medical correlates, diabetes, high blood pressure, and high cholesterol. But to Rose, it was clear that this approach was not gaining ground toward the key goal for public health—to understand and improve the health of entire populations.

This remains an unmet challenge. As one example, consider the trends in mortality rates due to ischaemic heart disease (IHD) in four European countries—Spain, France, Sweden, and the UK—over the past three decades, depicted in Figure 2.1. Remarkable inequalities exist, both across countries and over time. These variations raise a number of questions: How did France, despite starting out with higher rates of IHD than Spain, reach a figure half of Spain's present rate? How did Sweden reduce rates of IHD by two-thirds within three decades? What happened in the UK so that liver cirrhosis rates tripled while in France and Spain they fell by over 60%?

Or, as another example, take a look at the trends in mortality in Western and Eastern Europe since the 1980s, shown in Figure 2.2. As Central and Eastern European countries began 'returning to Europe' following the collapse of the Soviet Union in 1989 (63), the health of its people began to converge with their neighbours in Western European countries. However, the former Soviet countries experienced an explosive rise in chronic disease, resulting in more than three million excess deaths. What can explain such remarkable differences between these populations?

Such marked rises, falls and fluctuations in the mortality of entire societies cannot simply result from a series of disconnected changes by individuals. Did people suddenly become personally

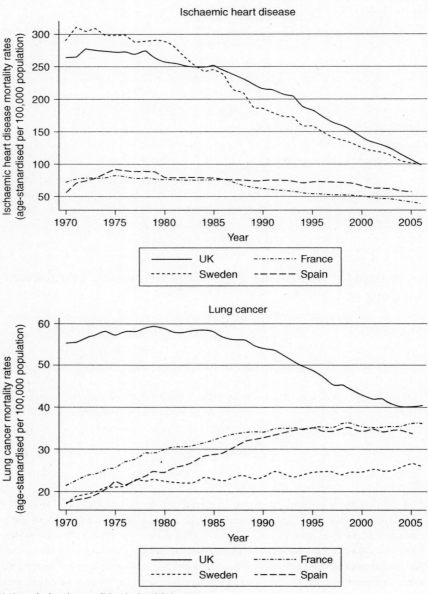

Fig. 2.1 Population inequalities in health in Europe.

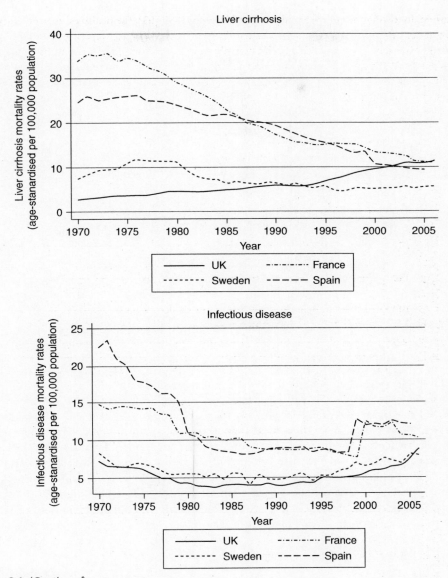

Fig. 2.1 (*Continued*)

irresponsible in Eastern Europe? Or more responsible in Sweden than France? If so, why? Would it be helpful to tell people in the UK that they should really take better care of themselves like people in France and Spain decided to do? Whenever substantial changes in an entire population's risk take place, they are not ultimately a result of preferences, willpower, or even genetics but of factors beyond the control of individuals. To understand why some populations are becoming more or less healthy, we need to examine the societal conditions that create population risks of chronic diseases.

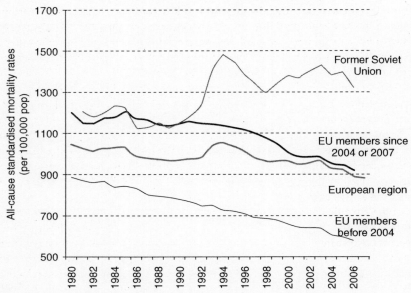

Fig. 2.2 Trends in age standardised all-cause mortality rates, Europe 1980–2007.
Source: WHO European Health for All Database HFA-MDB 2008 edition.

In this chapter we continue our previous search from Chapter 1 for the reasons why chronic diseases have risen so markedly over the past several decades. We begin by assessing the contribution of individual risk factors to the disease burden. Then we evaluate the social and environmental context of these risks using a theoretical framework that spans individual and population levels. We provide a series of case studies to illustrate the importance of major societal changes to population risks of chronic diseases, including political choices in Eastern Europe's transition from communism, the sudden wealth of the Western Pacific islands, and the periods of prolonged economic hardship experienced in Finland, Japan's 'double-dip' recession, and Cuba's 'Special Period.' In concluding, we revisit the leading population theories of health, health transition, risk factors, and population ageing, in the context of the societal determinants of health.

In search of a few common risks: individual risk factors of chronic disease

The vast majority of chronic disease research, both epidemiological and biological, has focused on a few common risk factors in the aetiology of many chronic diseases. These risk factors include genetic and environmentally determined physiological factors, such as lipid and blood pressure levels. These are in turn influenced by proximal factors, sometimes referred to as behavioural risk factors. Examples of the latter include unhealthy diet, alcohol and tobacco use, and physical inactivity, as well as biological factors that can, to varying degrees, be attributed to the proximal factors (often interacting with genetic susceptibility), such as high blood pressure and cholesterol. Proximal and immediate risks frequently interact with certain personal behaviours, thereby increasing the risk of a variety of diseases acting through different biological mechanisms.

One example is tobacco use, whereby those who smoke (or inhale tobacco smoke from others) are exposed to substances such as nitrosamines, which act as carcinogens creating genetic mutations. Concurrently, carbon monoxide displaces oxygen from haemoglobin while other components of smoke impair endothelial function (a thin layer of cells that enable the heart to pump blood further), increasing the risk of coronary artery disease.

In the 1950s Doll and Hill showed the critical importance of tobacco for lung cancer (64). Since that time, tobacco has been implicated in cardiovascular disease (CVD) and chronic obstructive pulmonary disease (generally tobacco-induced emphysema and chronic bronchitis), two diseases which account for about 60% of all chronic diseases. (This has created an apparent puzzle, for example, that Japan has very low rates of CVD in spite of having one of the highest rates of tobacco use—see Figure 1.6 in Chapter 1—although this is likely to be, in part, due to partial protection conferred by the very healthy Japanese diet.) Tobacco also is known to contribute to risks of diabetes as well as of mouth, oesophageal, stomach, and liver cancers.

Much of the chronic disease burden is thought to result from a few common clinical and behavioural risks: the smoking epidemic in the 20th century, the contemporary imbalance between excess calorie intake and reduced physical activity, and, especially among men, growing rates of alcohol consumption (see Chapter 1). How much could these individual risks matter to the population's overall risk of chronic disease? As described in Chapter 1, WHO scientists calculated that the total global chronic disease experience attributable to eight main individual risk factors totalled about 76%. Life expectancy could substantially be increased, by as much as a decade, if these risks were reduced.

Almost every scholarly paper about chronic diseases begins with a citation of these numbers (or some variation of the enormity of the health burden). However, before we, too, point to the gross unfairness of how easily we could modify these risks and heroically save millions of lives, we pause to ask a couple of questions. How could estimates of the population-level causes be performed if we do not know how many people died from chronic diseases in low- and middle-income countries? How did these models attributing risks to specific factors differentiate the contributions of obesity and physical inactivity? How did estimates account for delays between exposure and disease? Can we assume these risk factors have similar health consequences in all populations of the world?

Let's take a moment to look at the assumptions that lie behind these numbers. To calculate the population attributable risk of an individual risk factor, it is necessary to know how many people were exposed and the magnitude of the risk caused by the exposure. Both can be difficult to assess. In the case of tobacco, there are consumption-based measures of tobacco use and surveys implemented in many countries. With regard to fruits and vegetables, however, much less is known, so researchers resort to extrapolating information to countries where there are no data. For example, in the 2000 edition of the Global Burden of Disease, data for the Asia region were extrapolated from Singapore.

In the next step of estimating population-attributable risk it is necessary to assess the relative risk of disease, calculated as the ratio of disease rates in exposed and unexposed persons. The WHO estimates draw heavily from the WHO-MONICA (Multinational monitoring of trends in determinants of CVD) study of risk factors in 21 countries among persons aged 25–64, tracking 10 million men and women across the 1980s and 1990s. A second case–control study, INTERHEART, assessed nine major risk factors among 15,000 matched cases (deaths due to CVD) and controls (CVD-free persons) covering 52 countries. They asked those who had survived heart attacks (thus excluding sudden deaths) questions about their health and lifestyles, such as whether they smoked and were physically active, and took physical measurements of people's BMI and performed blood tests. By comparing they could assess the reasons why persons had greater risk than others. The researchers estimated that, combined, nine risk factors—smoking, raised ApoB/ApoA1 ratios (a measure of abnormal lipids that is unaffected by fasting), history of hypertension, diabetes, abdominal obesity, psychosocial factors, fruit and vegetable intake, alcohol use, and physical inactivity—accounted for 90% of the population attributable risk of myocardial infarction (65).

Getting the right relative-risk estimate for each risk factor is a difficult task. It requires assessing causality. This is often done using multivariate models that adjust for potential observed confounders in order to isolate the contribution of each factor while also accounting for interactions among them. This involves estimating the 'extra attributable risk', the portion that can be attributed exclusively to the specific risk factor. In case–control studies, the matching process assumes all else is the same between the case and controls except for the variables being studied, eliminating key confounders (66). Rarely is the technique perfect. In observational studies assessing causality is even more challenging because it is difficult to construct statistical 'matches' to hold constant such confounding variables.

Nonetheless, many studies do not adjust estimates of relative risks for potential confounders. In many cases, a meta-analysis is performed so as to generate a better measure of the relative risk. Even when studies do adjust for potential confounders, they sometimes overadjust in biologically implausible ways. For example, how do we differentiate the effect of physical inactivity from that of obesity? Clearly physical inactivity leads to obesity, but it could have additional biological risks independent of obesity. If models try to estimate physical inactivity and obesity at the same time, they underestimate the population risk of the more distal factor (in this case physical inactivity). In other words, the WHO risk factor study should clarify that its estimate of the population attributable risk (PAR) for physical inactivity is adjusted for high cholesterol; its estimate of PAR for tobacco is adjusted for hypertension. If PARs are estimated separately for each unadjusted risk factor, however, risks will be double-counted, overestimating the effects of each.

Some have argued that estimates of relative risk calculations can be viewed as 'biological constants' (67), varying little by region or population group. Arguably, the more proximal a factor to the individual biological process, the more constant the relative risk estimates will be across populations. It is also important to note that the more proximal a factor is to the biological process being studied, the greater the estimate of attributable risk will be, ultimately reaching 100%.

Nonetheless, there are significant variations in the effects of risk factors across populations. The INTERHEART study found that the nine risks being considered accounted for a high proportion of the PAR in every ethnic group studied (Europeans, 86%; Chinese, 90%; South Asians, 92%; black Africans, 92%; Arabs, 93%; and Latin Americans, 90%) (65). However, the effect sizes of the risk factors did vary significantly across regions. It also found, in contrast to Western studies, that in South Asia alcohol had no protective effect on CVD (that is, alcohol was adverse to health at all levels of consumption).

Further, the combination of major risk factors of chronic diseases that drive higher rates among the poor differs across countries. Evidence that non-traditional risk factors likely play a key role in chronic disease burdens of low- and middle-income countries is revealed in the comparison of the trends in age-standardized versus crude death rates due to chronic diseases. If the prevalence of conventional risk factors, like tobacco and obesity, appear to increase or follow an inverse U-shaped pattern with rising incomes pattern with rising incomes, as shown in Figure 2.3, why are the highest rates of death due to chronic diseases among the poorest populations (see Figure 1.5 in Chapter 1)? Clearly, other factors must be driving these risks.

In cases where interactions among risk factors play a key biological role in the disease process, it is necessary to account for them. Taking one example, eating fruits and vegetables may confer protection against a smoker's risk of cancer. But the extent of this protection could differ in countries where the soil provides rich nutrient content, and the nutritional content of fruits varies greatly depending on where they are grown and how they are stored. Further, the differential use of

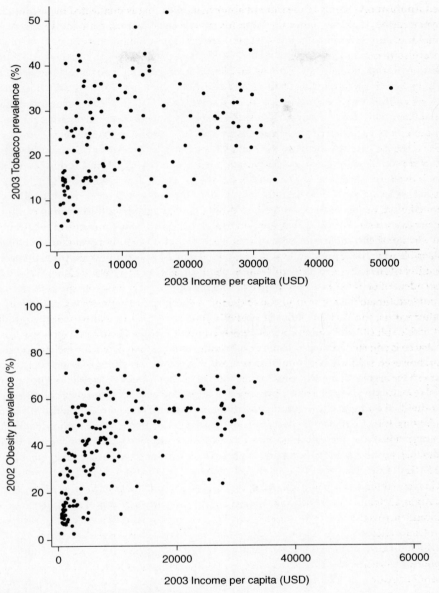

Fig. 2.3 Income-NCD risk factor patterns, 2003.

pesticides could create additional risks of cancers as a result of fruit and vegetable intake. Yet, these interactions, albeit well known to exist and exert effects, are rarely addressed. For example, the INTERHEART study reports 'by summation of model coefficients [estimates of each of the nine relative risks] . . . the combined effect of combinations of exposures can be estimated'. This is only correct when there are no interactions among exposures. Estimating interactions raises another challenge: which estimate of attributable risk is assigned the interactive effect? Is smoking's attributable risk higher because of low fruits and vegetable intake, or the other way around?

Studies also can end up with inconsistent estimates, depending on how the relative is calculated and the measures used to assess the prevalence of the exposure. For example, one study estimated the burden of disease attributable to low fruit and vegetable consumption, reporting 2.6 million deaths due to IHD, stroke, and four types of cancer (68). This estimate was about 1 million greater than the number of deaths estimated by the WHO to have occurred due to low fruit and vegetable intake. Other studies of risk factors have even greater deviation. Studies by Peto and colleagues identified that tobacco accounted for about half of all TB deaths in India (69). Yet, WHO estimates that, worldwide, tobacco accounted for about 6% of all TB deaths. This suggests revisiting their hazard ratios of tobacco–TB or their methods to estimate the contribution of tobacco to the disease burden.

Estimates of PAR are widely used to suggest how many lives could be saved. Beyond the issue of whether such targets indeed are feasible (such as *The Lancet*'s 2% target described in Chapter 1), they can be misleading for a few reasons.

First, they lack a 'what if' analysis to suggest what could happen if the goals were achieved.

For example, in the study assessing the PAR of increasing fruit and vegetable consumption to 600g per day could reduce the global burden of disease by 1.8%. Besides the interactions of fruit and vegetables with other disease risks that were not considered, it is important to ask about the potential risk of eating more fruit and vegetables (high in sugar) to obesity. Will people prepare these vegetables using recipes that call for the use of palm oil, ghee, or excessive salt? Or what will people eat less of as a result of consuming up to half a kilo of additional fruits and vegetables each day?

Second, it is often unclear over what time period the benefits could accrue, because the risk factor estimates often are measured based on a lifetime of risk accumulation. For example, the INTERHEART study measured current exercise reports, such as whether a person was 'regularly involved in moderate (walking, cycling, or gardening) or strenuous (jogging, football, and vigorous swimming) exercise for 4 hours or more a week'. But, as we know from lifecourse epidemiology, described in Chapter 1, the sequence, timing, and cumulative amount of risks and protective factors over many years could be crucial modifiers of the estimates of additional relative risk of disease. Importantly, reducing the consumption of fruits and vegetables today will be unlikely to save these lives anytime soon (although its effects on endothelial function might result in immediate benefits), a fact accounted for in biological models of infectious disease but often not for chronic disease.

Thus, our review has identified a first key insight about how to respond to the global challenge of chronic diseases.

Strategy 1: Epidemiologists cannot assume that reducing a behavioural risk factor will achieve significant population health benefits without considering the societal context in which people engage in these risks.

In search of further strategies, we explore a few more limitations to focusing narrowly on individual risks.

Limitations of risk factors for public health practice

Countless studies have been undertaken on common proximal risk factors and diagnoses, both individually and in combination: obesity and breast cancer; obesity and diabetes; tobacco and diabetes; diabetes and heart disease (see Appendix). How much has this body of knowledge contributed to the improvement of public health?

Irrespective of the precise magnitude of the PAR, if the WHO estimates are correct that about nine in every ten deaths due to chronic diseases relate to a few individual risk factors, the implications are profound. It is clear that there is very little explanatory payoff to studying these individual risks further. They no longer respond to the longstanding challenge put forward by Rose—to understand why entire populations are sick.

Focusing attention on these individual risk factors could be counterproductive from a public-health policy standpoint. They could, for example, divert attention from non-traditional risk factors, such as urban pollution, especially important in low-income countries. Most risks arise from distinctive cultural, societal, and environment aspects of daily living in resource-poor settings. For example, policymakers have been slow to recognize the importance of smoke from indoor cooking stoves in poor households, creating high risks of respiratory disease among women and their children, overall accounting for about half of chronic obstructive pulmonary disease deaths in low-income countries (see also Chapter 1, the mysterious case of the women with respiratory disease).

Clue 1: The highest risks of death due to chronic disease observed in the lowest income countries reveal a need to identify a series of non-traditional risk factors (such as indoor air pollution).

Finally, while knowing these individual risks helps us to identify who is at risk, this tells us nothing about why people have them (or how to intervene). People make choices but rarely do so entirely in the circumstances of their own choosing. For example, studies of Japanese migrants to the US reveal how important societal factors can be to risks of diseases. Over generations, these migrants adopted American values, diets, lifestyles, and, ultimately, disease rates (70). Another example comes from the Pima Indians living in the US and Mexico; while the two groups are similar genetically, those living in Mexico have much lower rates of diabetes than the group living in the US, largely attributable to differences in their diets (Box 2.1). Choice depends on circumstance.

Box 2.1 The case of the Pima Indians: environmental risks of chronic disease

At the time of the Spanish conquest, the Pima Indians inhabited northern Mexico and what is now southern Arizona. Their descendents were split into separate populations: the Mexican Pima, residing in a remote region in the Sierra Madre Mountains only accessible by road, and the US Pima Indians, who live mainly in the desert regions of Arizona.

Both groups have a similar genetic make-up but very different lifestyles and, as a result, varying risks of chronic diseases (a type of natural experiment).

The Mexican Pima live in a subsistence economy, mainly farming and growing their own food and getting around on horseback. Their environment builds in chronic disease prevention: their work involves considerable physical activity; their meals are typically prepared at home and consist largely of beans, wheat flour tortillas, corn tortillas, and potatoes, creating diets that are naturally high in fibre and low in fat. The US Pima Indians, albeit once traditional farmers, now follow a more typical of rural US lifestyle, relying on motorized transit, jobs which do not involve physical activity, and eating food purchased at local supermarkets and restaurants.

The chronic disease rates of the Mexican Pima are much closer in magnitude to their neighbouring Mexicans (who have a different genetic background) than the American Pima Indians who live in Arizona. Among Pima Indians living in the US, diabetes prevalence is 34.2% for men and 40.8% for women, about five times higher than in Mexican Pima (5.6% for men and 8.5% for women) and non-Pima (<1% for men and 5% for women). Obesity, in part, explains such differences; Mexican Pima have relatively low levels of obesity (6.5% for men and 19.8% for women), like the Mexican non-Pima (8.7% for men and 26.7% for women), while the Pima Indians living in the US have rates of obesity—63.8% for men and 74.8% for women, similar to the rest of the country.

Source: Schulz, L. O., P. H. Bennett, et al. (2006). *Effects of traditional and western environments on prevalence of type 2 diabetes in Pima Indians in Mexico and the U.S. Diabetes Care,* **29**(8): 1866–1871.

Another example of how choice depends on the environment is seen with the case of smoking. Smoking rates are strongly socially patterned, at present concentrated among the poor and the least well educated in rich countries and among young urban dwellers in poor countries. These social patterns reflect the interplay of a wide range of distal factors acting at both individual and societal levels, including social norms, health beliefs, economic and employment circumstances, and marketing by tobacco companies.

Clue 2: Individual risk factors of chronic disease account for a large fraction of the burden of disease mainly because they reflect the embodiment of the common social conditions in which people live.

Strategy 2: There is little additional return to continuing to study conventional individual risk factors of chronic disease. Potential insights will come from either focusing on the more immediate biological hazards associated with these risks ('zooming in') or by focusing on the underlying societal determinants of these risks ('zooming out').

In this next section, we begin to zoom out from the experience of an at-risk individual to understand how the broader societal environments in which he/she lives can literally 'get under their skin' to cause chronic diseases.

Putting individual risks in their social context: the built environment

Case of a US factory worker

Imagine the following scenario, based on a true story, set in the Midwestern USA involving a middle-aged, lower-middle class, male factory worker—Eli Peterson (name changed to conceal identity).

For 20 years Eli worked on an automotive factory line. His job involved performing repetitive motions. Working days were long; the few breaks Eli had to do things 'for himself' were on smoke breaks, catching a few laughs with workers off the factory floor. His unhealthy diet, combined with a lack of physical activity, over the years contributed to Eli becoming overweight at around 30 years of age. His doctor began warning him about the risks of developing type 2 diabetes unless he began exercising and lost weight. But Eli had a hard time changing his lifestyle: the musculoskeletal problems provoked by his job made exercise difficult; his long working day and family responsibilities led him to eat out frequently instead of cooking at home; and his low salary made it difficult to afford healthy food options.

While Eli may have been genetically predisposed to diabetes, this explanation cannot account for why so many people like Eli around the world are becoming physically inactive, eating unhealthy diets, and being diagnosed with diabetes. Have people like Eli suddenly become less personally responsible? In fact, socioeconomic factors, like his class background and relatively low education, constrained the scope of job opportunities available to Eli. Ultimately, within the choices available to him, Eli was burdened with a disproportionate risk of developing a chronic disease.

Fifty years ago, someone like Eli was more likely to have been engaged in farming work, with high physical activity; in coming decades, people like Eli will be working in an office managing a database or answering telephones. The shifts from agricultural production to manufacturing to technological and intellectual production are leading to decreased levels of physical activity. Importantly, this transformation, already complete in high-income countries where people like Eli live, is now rapidly occurring in low- and middle-income developing countries.

Eli's neighbourhood lacked the financial resources to invest in healthy urban engineering, which would provide pedestrian- and cyclist-friendly paths and green spaces for physical activity. Indeed, the lack of safety or desirable well-lit walkways in many urban areas prevents people from leaving their homes or leads to a further reliance on the use of motor vehicles for transit.

Importantly, many people's dietary options are strongly influenced by socioeconomic factors. Fruit and vegetables are less filling and cost more than high-fat, high-sugar processed foods that are also high in salt and low in essential nutrients. Fast-food outlets provide increasing numbers of working families with a low-cost alternative to home cooking. Even if Eli wished to maintain a traditional diet of home-cooked food, his wife and family would have found that unhealthier foods and the options to eat at restaurants were the most convenient and affordable options. This transformation in where and how people eat is central to the world's changing disease profile.

Of course, Eli and his family could have made healthier choices in their lives, but they were constrained and more difficult in their community than elsewhere. This way that Eli's environment increased his risk is referred to as the 'built environment', indicating that the ways in which people have developed modern societies have produced risks of chronic disease. These risks are not just about industrialized wealthy countries. Overall, transformations of environments to create more circumstances like those facing Eli are most rapidly occurring now in low- and middle-income countries, where the burden of NCDs is also growing. We refer to these processes of how diet-related risks of NCDs have been encouraged by current models of social development as dietary dependency, as we explain in the following sections.

Clue 3: Prevailing models of societal development are creating additional risks of chronic diseases through a process of dietary dependency.

Towards a framework of chronic disease: embedded hierarchical web of causation

How can we conceptualize this understanding of the choices and circumstances that people like Eli face? One framework for understanding how large groups of individuals are exposed to high

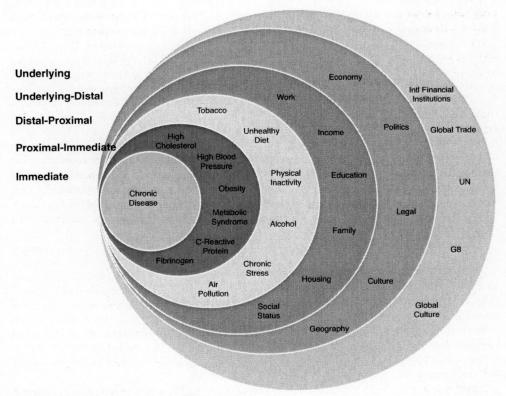

Fig. 2.4 Embedded hierarchical web of causation.

degrees of risk is through an embedded model of disease, as set out in Figure 2.4, 'Embedded hierarchical web of causation'. The framework is based on socio-ecological models of health, which situate the experience of a chronic disease, like heart disease, within a range of immediate and proximal distal factors, as discussed above. In turn, this disease experience is embedded within a range of distal factors acting on individuals, reflecting the importance of people's work, education, housing, culture, and environment to their health.

The importance of the distal factors can be seen in the strong associations of measures of social position with risk factors. There is a strong gradient in health across the socioeconomic spectrum, and in some countries inequalities in chronic diseases have widened between those in different income, educational, and occupational classes. One important observation is that chronic diseases and their risks, initially visible among the most affluent populations, slowly trickle down the social gradient, becoming embedded in the poorest populations. This process also appears to occur for entire societies. But why does this happen? It is a social, not a biological, process.

Here it is helpful to look to social and economic theory about why people make unhealthy decisions. An economic framework of individual choice can be of use in this regard. According to this framework, people make decisions according to their desires to maximize their overall well-being (a discussion picked up in the next chapter). This theory has many apparent limitations, especially when people are not fully informed about the health consequences of their decisions or when their actions affect the health of others; however, it does provide a strong model for understanding why individuals like Eli are progressively becoming sicker and making worse choices.

Many chronic disease risks involve choices; people are thought to weigh carefully the perceived costs and benefits of each decision. These costs and benefits are affected by three main things; price (including time), availability, and marketing. Getting these costs and benefits aligned with better health is an important public health goal. Figure 2.5 provides a model that traces the ultimate decision about whether to eat an unhealthy diet to these factors and how they are in turn shaped by underlying forces such as trade liberalization, urbanization, and economic growth.

1 Price—study after study finds one of the most powerful determinants of what people do is driven by its price (71). People have fixed budgets and, within them, have to provide food for their family. When money is tight, people buy cheaper foods that are richer in calories. Often these products, like fizzy drinks or crisps, are much lower in other nutrients. The same applies for products that provide little or no nutritional value, like alcohol and tobacco. As shown in Figure 2.6 the consumption of tobacco in the US matches the trends in the price of cigarettes. The importance of price to consumption can also be seen from the 'scream factor'—how much do companies get upset when taxes are proposed. As Philip Morris put it: 'Of all the concerns, there is one—taxation—that alarms us the most. While marketing restrictions and public and passive smoking [restrictions] do depress volume, in our experience taxation depresses it much more severely. Our concern for taxation is, therefore, central to our thinking' (72). Similarly, food companies have been less resistant to physical activity campaigns but have strongly opposed tax interventions to make healthier choices the economically smarter choices (73).

People's sensitivity to price depends on their income. When a person is poor, money may be a more crucial driver of dietary decisions than when people have more discretionary income. One reason for the ethnic disparities in health likely relates to the relatively lower incomes of some minority groups.

As incomes rise, people's lifestyles change. They usually start buying foods that are more enjoyable, often tending to be less rich in calories but higher in other nutrients. This phenomenon has been described as a 'nutrition transition'. However, it depends on local circumstances and the underlying level of income. For example, studies of China find that people's diets become richer

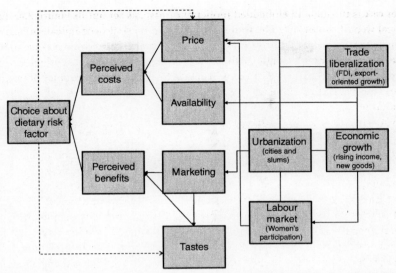

Fig. 2.5 Choice and circumstance: how market integration can lead to dietary dependency. FDI is foreign direct investment.
Notes: Reverse dashed-lines refer to feedback loops from markets responding to individual decisions to affect prices, availability, and marketing. It also reflects how tastes can respond to initial choices, such as how research has found children who eat more fatty foods begin to prefer fatty foods (and less fruits and vegetables). Price includes the opportunity costs of time in addition to monetary costs of a given dietary risk factor.

both in saturated fats (reflecting increased meat consumption) and lower in fruits and vegetables at higher levels of income (see Chapter 7.2).

Over time food is becoming cheaper, so that people eat more. Advances in technology enable companies to deliver more food to people at a lower price. Rising obesity mainly is driven by

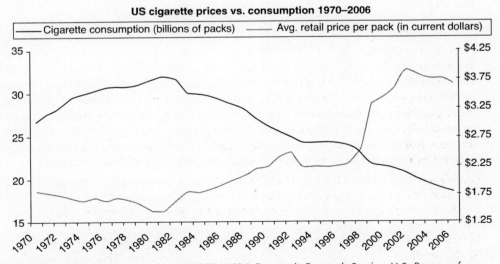

Fig. 2.6 *The Tax Burden on Tobacco*, 2007; USDA Economic Research Service; U.S. Bureau of Labor Statistics. Cited in: Campaign for Tobacco Free Kids. 2009. *Raising cigarette taxes reduces smoking, especially among kids*. Washington D.C., Tobacco Free Kids, Fact Sheet.

rising caloric intake (74). As food becomes cheaper, changes in prices make unhealthier foods relatively more affordable. In particular, snack foods are implicated in a large portion of the increasing obesity in the US (75). Portion sizes are increasing in many settings (76), which are also known to increase a person's caloric intake (77).

Clue 4: Decreasing prices of unhealthy foods make nutritionally poor choices and greater food quantities become easier and economically smarter choices.

2 Availability—places where people live matter. At the extremes, a person living in Mongolia has little option but to eat an unhealthy diet, dominated by animal fat and bereft of fresh vegetables. In contrast, an inhabitant of Crete may find it difficult to eat anything but a healthy diet. Similarly, a person living in rural Nepal has little choice but to walk, while someone in Atlanta may search in vain for a sidewalk (78).

Studies of US and European neighbourhoods consistently find that people's consumption of fruits and vegetables as well as fast food depends on their availability. These 'neighbourhood effects', albeit smaller in magnitude than individual effects, have a high PAR because so many people are affected by them. Extensive work has also documented that people living in urban settings have greater risks of chronic diseases. Similarly, people's decisions to exercise or not will depend on how desirable it appears to be. In places where parks are readily available, people exercise more. Studies find that the cost of gym memberships, as well as the opportunity cost of exercising, also influences an individual's decision to be physically active. Creating enjoyable, easily accessed sites of physically active recreation is an important public health goal. Unfortunately, many cities are developing in such a way that limits access to these spaces for being physically active (79). Much urban design centres around disability—emphasizing convenience and flexibility, not exertion and activity.

Place is also critical for influencing consumption. As McDonald's executives have emphasized, the company is less a burger chain than a company in the real estate business. They have an explicit strategy to making 'selecting McDonald's to satisfy hunger an easy decision for customers' (80). Or as one Kentucky Fried Chicken executive put it: 'Location, location, location!'. The key reason these companies focus on location is because the 'effective price' of their products depends not just on the sticker price tag, but on a broader set of costs such as time and effort a person must make to access the food (see Chapter 3 for a further discussion). In this way, when unhealthy food is more convenient, it is effectively cheaper, lowering the price—as depicted in Figure 2.5.

Clue 5: Increasing availability of unhealthy foods and declining availability of green spaces and sites of physical activity act to increase the 'effective price' of healthy choices.

3 Marketing—what people know or do not know about a risky choice also influences their decisions. It is increasingly clear that providing nutrition labels that are easy for people to understand (such as traffic light systems) can help people make better dietary choices (possibly healthier, but also not). Yet, studies find that a lack of knowledge about the health risks of products such as tobacco cannot explain why people choose to smoke. Instead, what matters most is how people perceive the overall costs and benefits of a product.

Clue 6: Marketing attempts to influence people's choices by increasing the perceived benefits and decreasing the perceived costs as part of a strategy to create demand.

Substantial misinformation exists about diets. This can be seen in the success of fad, but fraudulent, dietary strategies. Their prominence reflects a failure of the public health community to inform the public about appropriate nutrition. In part, this misinformation can be traced by to the way researchers have released study after study to the media about correlations (often conflicting) among dietary risk factors and outcomes, causing public confusion.

The role of knowledge is often hidden. Information that people acquire can slip under the radar of conscious awareness. Aggressive 'viral marketing' campaigns use strategies to encourage individuals to pass on messages to others, creating potential for exponential growth of the marketers' message and its influence (they even use infectious disease epidemiology approaches to monitor how contagious they are) (81).

These marketing campaigns typically seek to shape people's preferences, preying on people's psychological dispositions (82). Biologically, people have strong preferences for foods high in fat, salt, and sugar. These also happen to be some of the most profitable ingredients. For example, salt can make otherwise unsavoury food palatable when its concentrations reach levels of sea water; it does not create a feeling of being full (satiety), and increases thirst so that people consume more (hence the widespread sales of salty snacks, rather than, say, fruits, in bars). Tobacco companies used complex tactics to sell addiction. As their executives put it, 'We are . . . in the business of selling *nicotine*—an addictive drug effective in the release of stress mechanisms', specifically seeking to bypass people's rational thought processes and hook them biologically to their products. In the same way that tobacco companies used complex tactics to sell addiction, today food companies are experimenting with ways to enrich foods with nicotine, caffeine, and salt (the last two which commentators suggest also can have addictive properties) seeking to enhance their addictive potential (83). As one example, food companies have added caffeine to unlikely foods such as sunflower seeds, potato chips, jelly beans, and candy bars. Beverage companies have added nicotine to lollipops, bottled water, and fruit juices.

Clue 7: Sophisticated marketing strategies explicitly aim to 'slip below the radar' so that people are unaware of their influence and spread them to their friends and families.

Marketing also tends to take advantage of people's underlying dispositions and attitudes. For example, poor people also tend to have more short-term orientations; living pay day-to-pay day makes it difficult to plan for the future (economists refer to this as a high time-discount value). In general, the more people focus on the present, the more likely they are to make risky decisions, benefiting the present at the expense of NCD risks years later (75, 84, 85). Unsurprisingly, marketing tends to emphasize the immediate pleasures as well as images of pleasure and hedonism that encourage more short-term gratification (86).

Increasingly Western food companies have turned their focus to developing countries (80). As one Coca-Cola executive put it, 'Marketing creates demand' (87). Similarly, a McDonald's executive in Singapore notes, 'Two to three percent of all meals eaten outside the home are taken at McDonald's. So the market is far from being saturated . . .'(88). As PepsiCo's business strategy put it, 'our goal is to identify "untapped" thirst occasions'.

This widespread creation of demand in developing countries reflects rising interest in the potential of developing countries. One marketing director of Coke claimed, 'One hundred percent of our success is due to marketing' (89). Since 1994, Coke's marketing budget outside the US has grown from $500 million in 1994 to $2.4 billion in 2006 (90).

Clue 8: Food and tobacco companies have increasingly focused their marketing investments on low- and middle-income countries where there is the biggest potential to create demand.

Many products specifically aim at children, seeking to addict them to salty snacks that offer no feeling satiety but create thirst. As an Indian executive of Pizza Hut from put it, 'We have to build a franchise with kids now' (80); a Hungarian executive of Kentucky Fried Chicken said, 'The philosophy is, if you get them in grade school, you'll have them until they're ninety'(91). Coke's marketing aims to 'penetrate the teen psyche' (92), and PepsiCo, too, claims they are 'focused on working our way into the skin of younger people' (93). These efforts do influence children's behaviour. One study estimated that a significant proportion of rising childhood obesity in the

US could be explained by children's exposure to fast-food advertising (94). Other studies have found children's exposure to movie and television ads placed by tobacco companies increase their likelihood of initiating smoking.

Clue 9: Marketing tactics prey on people's biological predispositions toward higher sugar, fat, and salt. These tactics have the greatest effects on lower-income groups (because of a general preference for the present over the future) and on children (because they are unable to process the information to make educated choices).

Supermarkets place the most profitable items where they are most visible, often relegating healthier items to lower or higher shelving spots. Products targeting children are situated at the lower shelves, so that children will nag their parents to buy them (so-called 'pester power' in the 'parent aisles' according to marketers). At every juncture where a person can make a risky dietary decision in a supermarket, marketers have carefully analysed the psychological possibilities to increase people's spending on the most profitable products, often of low nutritional quality (95). Corporations have incentives for people to eat and drink more (as well as exercise more, a stimulant of appetite).

Clue 10: Marketing strategies aim to lower the effective price of unhealthy choices by placing them in more convenient settings.

Societal determinants of chronic disease

Rising incomes, living in cities, technological advances—what factors are driving changes in people's life patterns? We must look to the 'causes of the causes of the causes' to understand the broader societal changes giving rise, ultimately, to higher NCD risks. These are depicted in the underlying determinants of Figure 2.4. Here we describe a few of these major forces:

Trade liberalization and market integration

Trade liberalization is an economic policy of opening markets to trade, potentially resulting in both imports of foreign products and exports of domestic ones. Theoretically, each country could specialize in products that can fetch a higher value on the global marketplace (a notion referred to as comparative advantage), returning more income to countries than if the country had diversified its domestic production. A related policy has been to open developing countries' markets to foreign investment from Western companies. Between the 1940s and 1970s, the dominant model of development had reflected a strategy of protecting domestic markets referred to as 'import substitution'; instead of importing a company, such as McDonald's or Walmart, countries would develop a local version of these companies as substitutes. Whether the turn to the integrated market model and its focus on export-oriented growth and foreign direct investment has benefited economies is highly disputed within economics (96). For example, recent papers seek to understand the 'elusive gains from international financial integration' (97), with others pointing out that in the long term there appears to be, at best, no effect and at worst, risks created by economic volatility of financial crises (98).

Irrespective of this debate, it is clear that markets have become greatly integrated over the past 30 years, to an extent not seen since the period of 1880–1920s (98). People's breakfasts can consist of locally sourced grains and milk, alongside orange juice from Africa, coffee from Latin America, or fresh salmon from Nordic countries. All these goods travel long distances, yet manage to reach consumers at low cost. For example, an apple grown in the UK might be sent to South Africa to be 'waxed' (keeping it from ripening too soon), only to be shipped back to the UK and sold as a local fruit.

Opening markets to trade has had profound influences on people's diets and risky behaviours. One World Bank study found that reducing tariffs in some parts of Asia resulted in a 10% increase in smoking rates above what it would have been without trade liberalization (99). In South Korea, the observed rises were the greatest among teens, rising by 10% within 1 year. Ultimately, trade liberalization can be shown to affect the key economic forces driving people's decisions (price, availability, and marketing, see Figure 2.5).

In general, most of the flows of food and investment, aside from exotic specialty products, are 'downhill', flowing from rich countries to poor countries. (This phenomenon, too, has created a puzzle in economics—money and resources are flowing from poor countries to rich countries, the opposite of what is predicted by theories of comparative advantage (100).) These Western products tap local markets and often create new ones. These flows tend to favour items that can be easily transported, such as processed and pre-packaged items, like fizzy drinks and cigarettes. They also favour more profitable foods and beverages which, as previously noted, tend to be the least healthy.

Why is this the case? Rich countries have both economic and political advantages over poor countries. Supply chains, economies of scale, and more advanced technology enable large agricultural firms in rich countries to outcompete the more expensive domestic foods made by local farmers. This gives multinational companies a significant market advantage when countries open their markets to trade, giving rise to the large-scale entry of Western companies into developing economies.

The rich countries also have advantages for political reasons. One is that they do not play by the free-market rules (101). The case of the North American Free Trade Agreement (NAFTA), as further detailed in Chapter 7.4, is illustrative. Arguing that the economies of Mexico and the US would grow faster if trade barriers were lifted, NAFTA was introduced under President Clinton, with claims of mutual benefits to growth. But the results were devastating for many Mexican farmers. Mexico's staple product, corn, had provided subsistence for rural peasants for centuries. Yet, when the US introduced NAFTA, it did not remove its subsidies to US farmers for corn. As a result, US farmers could outcompete Mexican producers. Now Mexico imports much of its corn from the US, and many farmers have lost their livelihoods, instead seeking illegal entry into the US, creating immigration pressure (at times in response to advertisements from US farm companies). A similar case has arisen with the EU Common Agricultural Policy. This program subsidizes farmers to produce chicken; but too much was produced, creating a glut. The EU farmers then shipped the chicken across the world, to countries like Ghana, ultimately putting their farmers out of business (102).

The unhealthy aspect of these subsidies, beyond distorting markets, is that they provide the wrong financial incentives to people about nutrition (103). Money is going to making fruits and vegetables more expensive but oils, fats, and sweets cheaper in rich countries. One of the worst is palm oil, a heavily subsidized oil that increases substantially the risk of heart disease (see also Box 6.1 in Chapter 6). It is as though the agricultural subsidy structure is the complete opposite of public health dietary advice and, worse, being exported to developing countries on a massive scale. For example, the US ban on imports from Cuba protects American sugar farmers. But, as a result, the US produces excess sugar, which it subsequently 'dumps' to other countries, putting their farmers out of business (leading to waves of farmer suicides across the globe) (95), while flooding local producers with additional sugar. Because it is so cheap, filling, and desirable local cooks use more sugar in preparing food than before (95).

Clue 11: US and European countries subsidize oils, fat, and sugar, making them cheaper as well as putting farmers and small businesses in poor countries at a competitive disadvantage.

Specializing in food products for market exchange (so-called cash crops) also creates risks of starvation when markets are volatile. Instead of producing diverse crops to meet the people's food needs, countries produce large quantities of cash crops to sell on the global marketplace in exchange for other basic foodstuffs. The dangers of such a model are evident by the mass starvation that occurred as a result of the rapid commodity price fluctuations of 2008 (104). When speculative investors bet that the price of rice would continue to rise in 2006, they created a bubble in its price, reflecting demand of investors, not the demand of hungry people (105). These rapid rises in food prices pushed over 75 million to the brink of starvation in Africa and Latin America (106, 107).

Clue 12: Producing foods as cash crops increases the dependence of consumers on foods produced in other countries.

Even when farmers are successful, making vast sums exporting specialty products, diets can transform in seemingly undesirable ways. One example is the effect of trade liberalization on diets in Micronesia, a group of small Pacific islands, rich in some of the world's finest tuna (108). For centuries the islanders subsisted on the fish, but today, very little of that tuna is now eaten in Micronesia. Fishermen fetch a high price for selling tuna on the global markets, a much higher price than any of the islanders can afford. Using its earnings, the country trades its tuna for turkey tails, an extremely cheap leftover product from US agriculture that the Americans find too undesirable to eat. These turkey tails also happen to have extremely high fat and added salt content, and Micronesia suffers from one of the highest rates of diabetes in the world.

Clue 13: Opening markets to trade can increase the price of traditional, healthy foods in resource-poor countries and potentially price people out of the market, especially when there is high demand in the Global North but scarce supply from the Global South.

So far this paints a negative picture of trade liberalization. This is not entirely correct. Much good arises from integrating markets. When foreign companies enter into markets they bring advanced technology and capacity, as well as jobs and managerial skills. For this reason ministers of finance often wish to encourage this foreign direct investment, because it provides expertise and resources that may not be available at home.

However, in order to woo these companies, ministers of finance seek to integrate themselves ever more fully into the global marketplace by releasing protections on trade, leaving their people's diets every more susceptible to influence by the choices of product specialists in Western companies. This is one reason why diets are becoming 'Westernized'.

Many companies seek to tap local markets for labour because costs are lower. One example is the assembly plants in Mexico (so-called maquiladoras), employing about 60% women, which have adverse working conditions including poor ventilation, few rest periods, repetitive tasks, excessive noise, unsafe machinery, and exposure to toxic chemicals and carcinogens. This outsourcing of jobs also leads to major debates in rich countries, as lower-income groups are outcompeted by low-income countries. Another example has been the outsourcing of call centres to places like India. Such transformation in working life leads to less opportunities for physical activity; in agrarian societies physical activity is part of daily life—people are paid to exercise—but in industrialized societies, the opposite occurs, people are paid to be sedentary and have to pay to exercise (with time or gym memberships) (109).

Clue 14: Transformations of working life have increased the effective price of physical activity.

Privatization and deregulation

Another way finance ministers encourage foreign direct investment is through privatization and deregulation. When companies think the state is intervening in the economy or there is political risk, they can be reluctant to enter a country. These companies have considerable bargaining power, especially over poor countries; if one country does not offer a favourable package of tax-breaks or subsidies or union-busting measures, companies could move on to the next. A key strategy of finance ministers has been to transfer the ownership of state companies to the private sector; the rationale is that private ownership improves incentives, removes market distortions, and allows for more efficient production and delivery of foods, all of which are designed to increase economic growth.

When markets work well, people are better off. Greater competition brings lower prices and more efficiently delivers goods to populations. Foreign direct investment has lowered the prices of foods to many populations, increasing the food available to people at low cost. But, by displacing local diets, it can also constrain the range of food choices available to people.

In circumstances where people lack key information about food choices (market failures, see Chapter 3), increasing a market's competitiveness through privatization will ultimately spread risks of chronic disease. Box 2.2 shows an important example where the International Monetary Fund (IMF), a major international lender to poor countries, required tobacco privatization as a condition of its loans, in so doing greatly increasing the efficiency of a market which distributes a product that regularly kills half of its users. While tobacco and food companies are sometimes vilified in public health, there is little initiative to tackle the fiscal policies and the institutions promoting them which create conditions for those companies to flourish.

Box 2.2 International Monetary Fund and tobacco privatization

Loans from the IMF come with strings attached. Recipient governments must accept 'conditionality,' a process that can encompass rigorous qualification criteria and strict systems for monitoring their implementation. One element of these policies is frequently the privatization of state-owned enterprises, which since the mid-1980s has been included as part of both the Washington and post-Washington Consensus. The rationale is that privatized enterprises relieve governments of the burden of investment financing, increase efficiency, and bring in a new emphasis on performance-oriented commercial management. Yet the evidence for this assertion at the time the IMF began to promote privatization was largely non-existent, and for parts of the world it remains, at best, equivocal. However, the effectiveness of IMF conditionality in promoting privatization is unambiguous, with one study finding that every US$1 loaned by the IMF was associated with the subsequent privatization of 50¢ worth of state-owned enterprises. Focusing on traditional justifications for privatization, however, ignores the question of whether the enterprise in question is producing 'goods' or 'bads'. On this, as on many other issues not directly connected to its goals, the IMF is agnostic.

One area where this distinction becomes important is tobacco. Tobacco companies are unique in making and selling a legal product that, when used as intended, will kill about 50% of its users. The ethics of improving the efficiency of, and encouraging competition between, such companies, as would occur with privatization, is, to say the least, dubious. Economic theory indicates that such changes would encourage reductions in price and increases in tobacco advertising, the two factors most likely to stimulate tobacco consumption. Yet there is a growing list of countries where the IMF has promoted privatization of state-owned tobacco companies, in some instances even withholding loans when privatization was not undertaken. The IMF has also pushed for tobacco tax and tariff reductions. Its defence of privatization is that governments owning tobacco companies are less likely to enact stringent anti-smoking policies and thus, paradoxically, privatization will facilitate tobacco control. What does the evidence show?

Box 2.2 *(continued)*

While state-owned tobacco companies, as monopolies, faced little incentive to advertise, privatization has been accompanied by massive marketing campaigns by the transnational tobacco companies that bought the newly privatized companies. In particular, they aggressively targeted young people and women, who in many low- and middle-income countries had, traditionally, not smoked. In many cases, the transnationals either ignored local restrictions or redrafted laws to lift restrictions on marketing. Transnational tobacco companies have also been able to take advantage of the limited capacity in finance ministries to rewrite tax policies, leading to substantial (up to 50%) reductions in excise. Predictably, marked reductions in real cigarette prices have been seen since privatization. As price and marketing are two of the major determinants of smoking prevalence in a country, it is unsurprising that both cigarette consumption and smoking prevalence rates have increased markedly in countries where privatization has taken place. Moreover, these increases have been most marked in the population subgroups specifically targeted by the industry. Finally, as the evidence summarized above suggests, the literature from all countries in which privatization has been closely studied shows that it has led to an intensification of lobbying by the industry against the introduction of new tobacco control measures, particularly advertising restrictions and tax increases— fundamentally undermining the IMF's prediction that privatization would improve tobacco control. The adverse public health consequences of IMF-driven privatization in itself raises serious doubts about the policy. Yet it is not even clear that countries achieve the economic benefits that the IMF presumes privatization to bring. This is true of privatization in the general economy (29), but the experience with the tobacco sector suggests that the benefits may be even more illusory. The transnational tobacco companies have been able to buy state-owned enterprises at below their real market value, both by directing the smuggling of cigarettes into these countries prior to privatization, thereby undermining their value, and by obstructing competitive tenders. Once purchased, they have often succeeded in negotiating highly favourable tax regimes that allow them to maximize the share of profits that can be repatriated, and, along with their efforts to reduce cigarette excise, have substantially reduced government revenues. Finally, by investing in modern machinery, they have reduced employment in the domestic tobacco industry. The actions of the IMF contrast with those of the World Bank. The Bank has placed a high priority on tobacco control, drawing attention to the human and economic costs of smoking, and, more recently, to some of the dangers inherent in tobacco industry privatization. Yet such efforts appear to have had little influence on the IMF. It is surely not too much to ask that the IMF should acknowledge the Bank's evidence that tobacco control benefits economies and growing evidence of the adverse effects of tobacco industry privatization, and join in the struggle to reduce the toll of avoidable death and disability caused by this exceptionally dangerous product.

Source: Gilmore A, Fooks G, McKee M. The International Monetary Fund and tobacco: a product like any other? *International Journal of Health Services* 2009; **39**:789–93. Reproduced with permission

From an NCD control perspective, opening markets to trade, privatizing companies, and reducing regulations, may be hazardous strategies that spread global vices like tobacco (and, in some regions, alcohol). But these economic policies could be used to improve access to nutritious fruits and vegetables (returned to in the case of Poland described below). Many critics, however, believe that the current market environment in poor countries, where regulatory regimes are often underdeveloped and where global companies may be able to undermine efforts to strengthen regulation (110), privileges risky rather than healthy products.

Of course people are not passive in markets; they could stress a desire for markets to provide healthy, nutritious foods—a process beginning to occur in rich countries. Yet unlike in Western countries, where people buy more healthy foods and spend more time exercising as their income levels rise, in developing countries the opposite seems to happen. Why might this be the case?

Here it is relevant to revisit the sophisticated marketing strategies employed by food companies. Using tactics honed in the West, transnational companies aggressively engage in information campaigns in developing countries. In less competitive information environments, such as those in developing countries, marketing is much more powerful than people living in the West appreciate (95). One particularly effective strategy has been to confer social status or prestige on eating in restaurants, often by associating restaurant consumption with cosmopolitan Western habits. This and other effective marketing strategies raise the desirability of Western imports and outside-the-home food consumption as they become more affordable—that is, as incomes grow. In the context of deregulation, it is very difficult to prevent companies from marketing to children or abusing information. As we have already seen, misinformation is a key problem in rich countries; the situation is far worse in poorer countries with less well-educated populations.

In other words, privatization and deregulation risk weakening the capacity of governments to place limits on marketing practices, tax unhealthy products like tobacco and implement some of the most effective public health measures to shift diets in a healthy direction.

Rapid economic growth

As a population's income level increases, people's habits and consumption patterns change. Rapid growth creates many opportunities to modify a population's risk just as people's lifestyles catch up to their newfound wealth. This is particularly true for rapidly developing countries such as Brazil, India, and China, which are experiencing record economic growth rates and rapid rises in chronic disease (see Chapter 7).

What the ultimate drivers of growth are remains hotly debated. One factor is thought to be a population's health—healthier is wealthier. There is compelling evidence that foreign direct investment has boosted growth, thought to relate to the technological benefits it can provide.

However, its economic benefits are often highly unequally distributed. For example, profits from foreign direct investment often do not 'trickle-down' to stimulate the host countries economy, but flow back to rich countries (111). Some economists estimate that considerably more resources flow out of resource-rich, but low-income countries from mineral-sector foreign direct investment than these countries receive in aid (contributing to the paradox about capital flowing from poor to rich countries). Despite decades of economic growth, about the same number of people live on under $2 a day as 30 years ago—while the value of those $2 has fallen substantially in terms of buying power (112).

Urbanization and slums

The processes of economic growth in low- and middle-income countries lead people to move to cities en masse. In general, societies modernize (combining rising income and technological advance), labour shifts from agrarian to intellectual production, and workplaces become increasingly sedentary. Work becomes more centralized with technological advances driving people into cities to capitalize on the new market opportunities.

This drive toward urbanization only partly reflects new economic opportunities. In many cases, it has a dark side. One example is the devastation of rural agricultural livelihoods; farmers losing livelihoods as a result of trade liberalization and export-oriented growth strategies. Moving to the city without a job is a recipe for the growth of slums—the urbanization of poverty (113).

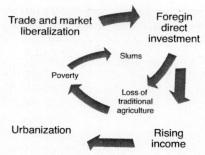

Fig. 2.7 Cycles of dietary dependence and the urbanization of poverty.

These slums are the most dangerous and toxic places in the world to live. Chronic stress, rampant crime, overcrowding, and lack of toilets and clean water, create breeding grounds for every disease imaginable, both chronic and infectious.

In urban settings, food production can be concentrated and take advantage of economies of scale, leading to lower prices and further encouraging people to eat outside the home. Urban settings in developing countries also commonly have few opportunities for safe physical activity. Figure 2.7 sets out this cycle of dietary dependence and the urbanization of poverty.

This rapid process of urbanization is often unplanned, perpetuating reliance on motorized travel rather than planning for bike lanes, green spaces, and sites of physical activity. For example, in India, new peripheral satellite cities are catering to a growing information technology industry. These suburban areas link to sites of work by motorways, locking in a pattern of development that discourages active lifestyles (79).

Clue 15: When a country's structure of price, availability, and marketing favours unhealthy diets, rising incomes and urbanization lead to significant population rises in diet-related chronic diseases.

Labour market participation

Empowering women is a major aim of development. This process is encouraged by technological development, new market opportunities in cities, and a general shift to non-agricultural forms of work. As more women begin to enter the workforce they face greater time constraints for the household production of food, and this reduction of time also acts to move food consumption away from the home. Several studies have found that maternal employment is a risk factor of childhood obesity and can explain a significant portion of rising obesity rates in high-income countries (114). Because of the market structure and incentives previously described, the net effect on society is a greater consumption of unhealthy products, especially energy-dense foods, and increasingly sedentary behaviour.

Taken together, these processes of trade liberalization, export-oriented growth, agriculture subsidies, and foreign direct investment in the food industry effectively lower the price and increase marketing of unhealthy products, leading to increases in their consumption. These processes result in the dietary choices of poor people living in poor countries becoming more dependent on the choices of producers, companies, and governments in rich countries (dietary dependence). This dependence can lead to both the convergence and divergence of diets in poor countries with those in the global North (115, 116), but tends to emphasize divergence. For example, when healthy foods are exported to rich countries in exchange for unhealthy foods being imported to poor countries, divergence occurs.

These underlying forces may seem distant from chronic disease outcomes, but they remain powerful. One study found that as much as three-quarters of the population rise in CVD could be attributed to trade liberalization, market integration, foreign direct investment, economic growth, and urbanization (21). Importantly, the study also found that whereas these processes were linked to worse chronic disease outcomes in low- and middle-income countries, they were linked to improved chronic disease outcomes among high-income countries.

Who determines the societal determinants of chronic disease? The Role of International Agencies . . .

Under the pressure of an ascendant global package of market-oriented economic policies, including significant reduction in the role of the state and levels of public spending and investment, a different development model was pursued from the 1980s. That model has been the target of a great deal of deserved criticism. Structural adjustment programmes, following the Washington consensus, had— and continue to have, in other policy and programme forms—an overreliance on markets to solve social problems that proved damaging.

World Health Organization (2009)

It is useful to pause to reflect on the model of development that has driven these policy decisions affecting population chronic disease risks. Who makes these societal decisions about trade liberalization, foreign direct investment, agricultural reform, and deregulation? Not just financial leaders of countries, but also international financial institutions are extremely influential in shaping the economies in poor countries (117). Key institutions here are the World Bank and IMF. For example, in 7 out of every 10 years finance ministers borrowing from the IMF have been obligated to implement financial reforms as a condition of receiving loans.[1] These financial institutions largely achieve this influence through a cycle of debt obligations and international aid. Ever more money is siphoned out of countries through debt repayments and mineral resource extraction than through international aid. In this way, international financial institutions have been among the leading determinants of economic policy decisions that affect risks of chronic diseases and the capacity of healthcare systems to respond (see Chapter 4).

In part through international trade agreements, such as the General Agreement on Trade in Services and the World Trade Organisation, as well as debt crises, these organizations have successfully pursued and locked-in a model of economic development called the 'Washington Consensus' (118). This consensus has been the development mantra for the past several decades. It reflected what rich people in high-income countries believed was good for development (and their own economic interests), often referred to as neoliberalism. The neoliberal economic model emphasizes trade liberalization, privatization, and deregulation as main components of economic development strategy. With regard to agriculture, it pursues export-oriented growth, based on each country specializing in a producing a particular good.

A brief historical overview of the development of the IMF helps illustrate how these international financial institutions have come to enforce the Washington Consensus, a model of development that builds societies with high risks of chronic diseases.

After World War II, the IMF was created to promote international financial cooperation, maintain economic stability, and ensure balanced and equitable growth. John Maynard Keynes, one of the IMF's main architects, hoped the Fund could help prevent another Great Depression and improve how financial crises were managed (119). To meet these goals, the Fund was given control over a pool of resources that it could lend to its member countries experiencing short-term balance of payment problems (120). The IMF provides loans to financially ailing countries, but with strict conditions, typically involving a mix of privatization, liberalization, and fiscal austerity programmes. These loan conditions have been extremely controversial. In principle, they are designed to help countries balance their books. In practice, they often translate into reductions in social spending, including spending on public health and health care delivery (121).

Toward the mid-1980s, these conditions, referred to by the IMF as 'conditionalities', began to include strict targets for privatizing state-owned enterprises, liberalizing markets to remove regulations on prices and trade, and reducing government spending on programmes in fields such as health and education. The rationale for these policies was to boost the role of private industries in poor countries, increase the influence of market forces over government intervention, reduce dependency on foreign aid, and prevent inflation. Many policymakers and investors in high-income countries argued that these policies were good for development (the Washington Consensus) (118).

This package of neoliberal policies was treated as neutral economic wisdom, but it actually was based on the ideology of the self-regulating market (122, 123). Conveniently, these policies happened to be the most suitable model of development for Western multinational food and tobacco companies. Failing to comply with the IMF's conditionalities to implement the Washington Consensus could result in a withdrawal of IMF funds and make it very difficult for countries to borrow from other sources, largely through the damage to their international credit ratings (119).

One main catalyst for spreading the Washington Consensus policies to Latin America and Africa was the so-called 'Volcker Shock'. It occurred when the US hiked interest rates to above 20% in the early 1980s, forcing many indebted countries, most which at the time held debts denominated in US currency, into bankruptcy virtually overnight. One economic historian documented that, 'Medium and long-term public debt shot up from $75.1 billion in 1970 to $634.4 billion in 1983. It was the so-called Volcker Shock . . . that ushered in the debt crisis, the neoliberal counterrevolution, and vastly changed the roles of the World Bank and IMF in Latin America, Africa, and parts of Asia'. Responding to concerns about the human suffering caused by these policies (as extensively documented by UNICEF in their volumes, *Structural Adjustment with a Human Face*), Volcker said, 'Africa was not even on my radar screen'. This is what some people mean when they talk about globalization.

Similar processes occurred in the 1990s, as the Washington Consensus policies were spread to the post-communist countries in Eastern Europe through the expedient of the region's Transformational Depression and further to East Asia in the aftermath of the East Asian financial crisis. Crisis in financial markets have become a key way to introduce these radical development models; once they are introduced, it is extremely difficult, if not impossible, to change without severe reprisals from the financial markets (124). It is in part through the decisions of these international agencies, themselves influenced by powerful vested interests, that entire societies have transformed their profiles of chronic disease risks.

In the next section we provide a few examples of just how powerful these forces can be, drawing on a series of extreme cases where societal changes resulted in major rises or falls in chronic diseases.

Selected case studies

Eastern Europe and Former Soviet Union: political choices as a risk factor

In setting out to build capitalism from state socialism's ruins, policymakers faced uncharted territory: how to proceed? While countries had moved from capitalism to socialism, few had experience the other way around, with the notable exception of China.

Many Soviet politicians (and many in the West) wished to seize the opportunity of the 1989 disintegration of the Soviet bloc to enable the socialist countries to make the leap to capitalism in one jump. There were fears that, if they did not, the Communists would return to power. The debate centred on what was the appropriate pace of transformation. One side of the debate argued for a policy platform, referred to as 'Shock Therapy', which called for the rapid privatization, liberalization, and stabilization of Communist institutions. Box 2.3 describes the logic behind these programmes.

How would risks of chronic diseases be affected? These programmes were expected to have at least two major impacts on health: one by increasing job insecurity and job losses, with their known consequences for health, and second, by dismantling the Soviet-era cradle-to-grave welfare system at a time when people were suffering the most. As one World Bank economist put it, 'The central premise is that before long-run gains in health status are realized, the transition towards a market economy and adoption of democratic forms of government should lead to short-run deterioration' (128). In other words, people would die.

Indeed, these rapid free-market reforms on health triggered a devastating rise in psychosocial stress, insecure unemployment, and hazardous drinking, which resulted in a rise in death rates especially among working-age men in Russia of about 80%. A severely weakened Russian state had little capacity to respond to these rapidly emerging threats, such as the increasing production of highly toxic surrogate alcohols, typically drunk from aftershaves or perfume bottles which were marketed not by their scent but by their flavour.

Poland provides an alternative scenario. The country delayed privatization, but did rapidly open its market to trade with Western Europe. This led to a beneficial influx of counter-seasonal fruits and vegetables, as well as a shift from saturated fats from animals to an increased uptake of oils with lower saturated fats (rich in both omega-6 and omega-3 fatty acids). As a result, Poland has experienced remarkable success in reducing rates of CVD and diet-related chronic diseases (129).

Belarus provides a third scenario. The country, largely similar to Russia, defied international advice, being critiqued as a 'Soviet theme park' for delaying its privatization reforms. While it did not benefit from market integration as Poland did, Belarus did avoid the short-term rises in heart disease and alcohol-related mortality strongly linked to social upheaval and stress.

Radical and rapid restructuring to people's ways of living in the former Soviet Union led to a devastating rise in chronic diseases, resulting in over 3 million excess deaths—the worst peacetime mortality crisis in the past half-century.

Box 2.3 Political arguments for shock therapy

As one Western advisor argued, 'The need to accelerate privatisation is the paramount economic policy issue facing Eastern Europe. If there is no breakthrough in the privatization of large enterprises in the near future, the entire process could be stalled for years to come. Privatization is urgent and politically vulnerable' (125). As the World Bank's head of mass privatization implementation wrote, 'There was a concern by Russian reformers, above all, that the communists might soon take control again; their desire, therefore was to move as rapidly as possible, i.e., to create "facts on the ground" that made a market economy irreversible' (126). Although the logic was mainly political, there was remarkable consensus among economists. As Lawrence Summers put it, 'Despite economists' reputation for never being able to agree on anything, there is a striking degree of unanimity in the advice that has been provided to the nations of Eastern Europe and the former Soviet Union. The legions of economists who have descended on the formerly Communist economists have provided advice very similar . . . the three "ations"—privatization, stabilization, and liberalization—must all be completed as soon as possible' (127, pp. 252–3).

Clue 16: Radical disruptions to people's societal conditions increase the risks of chronic disease.

Case of Japan, Finland, and Cuba: economic recession as a protective factor

Finland was strongly tied to the Soviet Union through international trade. When the Soviet Union collapsed, Finland's GDP dropped by one-third. Widely expected to lead to worse health, as experienced in many of the Eastern European countries, a surprising thing happened: health in Finland improved substantially (130). In fact, all-cause mortality diminished more during the recession than the subsequent economic boom of the 1980s. Mortality due to alcohol-related causes dropped considerably, as alcohol consumption declined by more than 10% as people's incomes fell. Road traffic injuries also dropped, plausibly because people drove less, a pattern consistent with evidence from other parts of Europe during recessions (131).

A similar experience occurred in Cuba, during its 'Special Period'. Incomes were cut in half virtually overnight as the Soviet Union, Cuba's major trading partner, collapsed. People would have been brought to the brink of starvation were it not for a return to traditional diets, consisting largely of rice, fruits, vegetables, and beans, which maintained levels of protein while reducing consumption of red meat and saturated fats. (Nonetheless it is still considered impolite in some quarters to ask Cubans about their pets, because some people had to resort to eating them to survive.) As people could no longer afford oil or expensive imports of cars, motorized transit ground to a halt, leading to a situation where many people relied almost exclusively on bicycles (lugging them up many flights of stairs to their work) and walking. Other risks such as tobacco use fell sharply, although consumption of rum was maintained to some degree through state rations and local production. This remarkable natural experiment led to precipitous declines in diet-related chronic diseases, particularly CVD, during the 1990s (132).

A final case, Japan, which has the highest life expectancy in the world, points to a similar scenario. During the 1990s it experienced a prolonged recession as a result of a glut in manufacturing output; efforts to adjust government spending led to a series of setbacks, when budgets were cut in 1995, the economy was plunged into a second wave. Throughout the 1990s Japan's population experienced a faster pace of reductions in chronic diseases than in preceding years of rapid growth, as one study found that CVD, liver disease, and accidents dropped substantially (133).

While no one would wish a recession upon a country, it appears recessions could be a protective factor against chronic diseases, especially when they result in people returning to traditional, healthy diets—taming global markets. Finland, Japan, and Cuba also stand out for being more egalitarian societies (1). Rather than implementing doses of strict austerity, their leaders chose to put in place social protections that help people in times of hardship (134).

Such cases point to how even a negative event like recession can be made healthy if society is organized to promote health rather than focus on economic growth.

Clue 17: When recessions reverse the trend towards unhealthier diets and less physical inactivity, there is potential for reductions in chronic diseases, especially when governments implement social supports to protect populations from economic shocks.

Nauru—a Western Pacific island: rapid economic growth as a risk factor?

Nauru is a small Pacific island, containing about 9000 people. It had long been one of the poorest countries in the region; isolated from other countries, and subsisting on locally produced foods, a basic diet comprising legumes and fruits.

This all changed rapidly when it was discovered that the centuries of droppings of sea birds had built up valuable mineral deposits deep within the island's limestone rocks. Suddenly Nauru was whirled into the centre of the global economy, turning Nauru into one of the richest countries per capita overnight—the highest income per capita in the world in 1968.

Traditional diets gave way to imported foods rich in saturated fats, especially red meat, resulting in a massive rise in diabetes and heart disease. Nauru's population today has the world's highest level of type 2 diabetes—prevalence of more than 30% (135). Ninety per cent of the population have a higher BMI than the world average (136). Life expectancy at birth in Nauru ranked in the bottom third of the countries in this region, calculated at 42.6 years in 1995–1996 (137), as bad as countries facing perpetual civil war and famine in Africa, such as Sierra Leone. As shown in Figure 1.6 of Chapter 1, Nauru has, overall, one of the highest mortality rates due to chronic diseases, of about 1100 deaths per 100,000 population, which is more than three times the rate in the US. Clearly, wealth is no guarantee for better health.

But the story does not end here. Nauru's resources ran out sooner than anyone anticipated, in the early 1980s, a result of aggressive strip mining by foreign companies. Completing a vicious cycle, Nauru's income per capita fell back to what it was before the discovery of phosphates. Now the country, railing from an epidemic of chronic diseases, lacks the money to fund care for its population. Youth are emigrating from the island; unemployment is 90%; and the way of life and culture of the people of Nauru is disappearing. In 2006 it became isolated from the world when its only airline, Air Nauru, foundered. Now it relies on aid from Australia in exchange for providing an immigration detention centre that processes illegal immigrants.

Of course, growth does not have to lead to worse chronic diseases—and in most cases it does not (see Chapter 7). Increasingly, there is evidence that the magnitude of economic change poses greater risk to health than its direction (138).

In Nauru, hasty pursuit of wealth, dietary dependence, and resulting chronic diseases combined to undermine sustainable development.

Clue 18: Rising economic growth is not sufficient for reducing chronic diseases and, in the context of poorly performing markets, could threaten a rise in chronic diseases.

These three case studies reveal the potential for remarkable gains in health if understanding these broader societal forces can be harnessed to positively change the risks of chronic diseases borne in environments in which people work, eat, and play. On the other hand, they also provide a note of caution that failing to identify and act on potential adverse influences could threaten the sustainability of an entire society.

Strategy 3: Re-engineering societies to promote healthier diets could lead to major health gains.

Transition theories—revisiting common explanations of rising chronic disease

So far we have covered how societies in which people live greatly influence their risk of NCDs. But we skipped a couple important things—namely, nearly all of the leading explanations of population chronic diseases talked about in the literature.

The main theory of changing population health is called "epidemiologic transition", also labelled at times as health transition. It refers to the change in the burden of disease from infectious to chronic causes over time. Described as a sequence of stages, the model predicts drops in mortality and decreases in its variability as societies advance (see Box 2.4). Usually it is thought to be spurred by a combination of causes, including modernization, improvements in hygiene and sanitation (including access to vaccines and clean water); education among women; strengthened health system performance and public health capacity; and general economic development and modernization. Debates about the relative strength of these factors are ongoing, not in public health, but mainly among Nobel Prize-winning demographers and economic historians (see, for example, work by McKeown, Fishback, and Fogel).

Box 2.4. Epidemiologic transition: a theory of population health and development

1 Stage 1: *The age of pestilence and famine* when mortality is high and fluctuating, thus precluding sustained population growth. In this stage the average life expectancy at birth is low and variable, vacillating between 20 and 40 years . . . In this stage the major determinants of death are Malthusian 'positive checks', namely, epidemics, famines, and wars. Graunt's study of London's Bills of Mortality in the mid-17th century shows, for example, that nearly three-quarters of all deaths were attributed to infectious diseases, malnutrition, and maternity complications.

2 Stage 2: *The age of receding pandemics* when mortality declines progressively; and the rate of decline accelerates as epidemic peaks become less frequent or disappear. The average life expectancy at birth increases steadily from about 30 to about 50 years. Population growth is sustained and begins to describe an exponential curve.

3 Stage 3: *The age of degenerative and man-made diseases* when mortality continues to decline and eventually approaches stability as a relatively low level. The average life expectancy at birth rises gradually until it exceeds 50 years. It is during this stage that fertility becomes the crucial factor in population growth.

Source: Omran A. The epidemiologic transition: a theory of the epidemiology of population change. *Milbank Quarterly* 1971; **49**(4):509–38.

One leading idea is that chronic diseases rise because infectious diseases fall, reflecting a belief that 'if you cut out one disease, something else will take its place'. The other leading explanation relates to population ageing. The logic is simple. As child mortality declines, largely owing to infectious causes, a greater fraction of the population survives to adulthood so that crude adult mortality rates (and thereby chronic diseases rates) begins to rise. Because older individuals have high risk of chronic diseases, older populations have greater rates of chronic diseases. This has already been shown to be false in Chapter 1, but as additional evidence in Figure 2.8 we show the correlation of chronic disease and infectious disease mortality rates. Using crude data, lower infectious disease rates do appear to correlate with greater chronic diseases; after infectious disease death rates fall below about 500 per 100,000 population, chronic disease rates begin to rise extremely rapidly. But once age is accounted for, greater infectious disease rates correlate with higher chronic disease rates—the *opposite* relationship (see Chapter 1 for biological explanations).

Despite the common observation that the reductions in infectious diseases coincide with rises in chronic diseases, there appears to be no simple causal link. Risks of poor health, be they infectious or chronic in nature, are interconnected. The other main explain for rising chronic diseases, ageing of populations, has the basic analytical problem of correlation is not causation and cannot explain rising youth incidence of chronic diseases and associated risks (see Box 2.5).

Falling infectious diseases and population ageing obviously cannot account for situations like those in Eastern Europe in the 1990s. So an extension to the theory of health transition is made to account for risk factors, explaining epidemiologic changes. Here theories, such as 'nutrition transition' or 'risk-factor transition' or 'Westernization of lifestyles', fill the gap. In understanding why these transition occur rise, concepts like globalization are invoked, often referring to how the 'world is flat', space becoming compressed, and flows of information, people and products have increased massively (144).

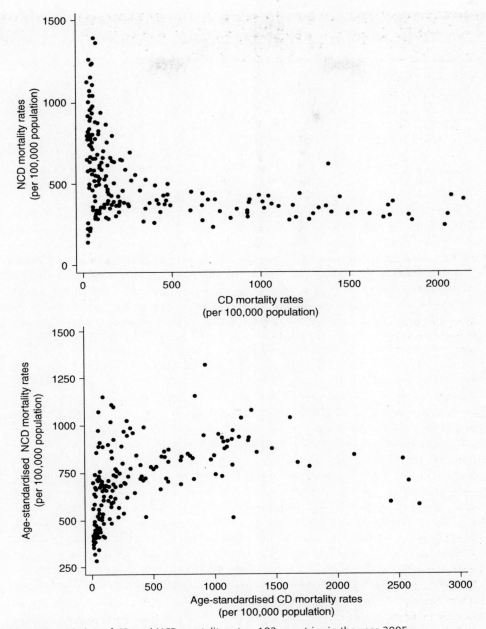

Fig. 2.8 Association of CD and NCD mortality rates, 192 countries in the year 2005.

The flimsiness of these overarching concepts is apparent in light of the preceding discussions. Boxes 2.6 and 2.7 provide common examples of how people in public health talk about the causes of chronic diseases. Later in this book we will see more examples of how people think about these causes in descriptions of chronic disease burdens in a series of case studies (see Chapter 7).

Returning to examples covered in this chapter, we can assess what these transitions mean in terms of the embedded hierarchical framework set out in Figure 2.4. Risk factor transition in

Box 2.5 Population ageing—correlation or causation?

Many studies cite the ageing of the population as the principal driver of the rise in crude population chronic disease rates (10, 48, 139–141). With regard to diabetes, scholars note, 'age is the single most important determinant of mortality' (141, p. 34); the WHO Burden of Disease Project notes that the 'ageing of the population will result in significantly increasing total deaths due to [NCDs] over the next thirty years' (140, p. 65). Strong, Mathers, and Bonita note that 'these countries have experienced a rise in the burden of chronic diseases, to almost 50 percent of total disease burden over the past decade. This increase can be attributed to population ageing and [risk factors]' (142, p. 182). Finally Marks and McQueen observe that the 'aging of the population in the first quarter of the twenty-first century will be *the* major force in the further tremendous increase in the burden of chronic diseases' (139, p. 119).

How do these authors draw their conclusions? It relates, principally, to a method used in the Global Burden of Disease project for decomposing population health changes into epidemiologic and demographic components. This method works as follows: first the analysts use a statistical model to assess the effects of income, income-squared, a human capital index (including education), smoking and time-trends on age-specific mortality rates using data from 1950 to 2002. When chronic disease data are missing, a combination of interpolation and imputation approaches are used to estimate adult mortality from child mortality and chronic disease burdens from mortality levels (see Chapter 1). Then, using a series of forecasts for these predictor variables, the model estimates mortality in 2030. Finally, the researchers make two calculations: the expected number of deaths in 2030 if the population structure stayed the same, labelling this demographic change, and the expected number of deaths in 2030 if the age-specific mortality rates stayed the same. They take the difference between the total deaths and these two values to calculate demographic and epidemiologic change, respectively. The logic is appealing: hold mortality rates constant and vary the population to determine the mortality attributable to demographic change; similarly, hold constant the population's composition and size to determine the mortality attributable to epidemiologic change.

Should the WHO forecasts suggest that chronic disease growth is being fuelled entirely by the ageing of a population? Several aspects of chronic disease epidemiology suggest otherwise.

First, population ageing cannot account for why the incidence of chronic disease is dropping within various groups faster in some countries than in others and at different speeds in different age groups. At most, about half the variation in population chronic disease experience relates to ageing; to see this, one can examine the population differences in chronic disease experiences based on crude chronic disease rates, then correct for population age-structure, observing that about half the variation remains. In other words, once differences in chronic disease burdens due to age are accounted for, there is at least 50% of population differences left to explain.

Second, the explanatory variables that are used to capture changes in age-specific mortality rates do not include chronic disease promoting factors, such as obesity. This is a common misspecification issue; while the total deaths projected may be reasonably accurate (questionable given high degrees of error in estimating diabetes, which exceed the pessimistic scenario in regions such as Latin America), the omitted variables will falsely be branded as attributable to ageing (which is the unexplained portion of the model, or the error). The dependent variables, age-specific chronic disease rates, are lacking in the majority of low-income countries. Unsurprisingly, these models have failed to account for rising incidence of chronic diseases among youth populations in these settings.

Box 2.5 *(continued)*

Third, trends in population ageing do not directly track with country-specific changes in the rate of chronic disease. For example, the ageing population appears to be growing faster in rich than in poor countries (depending on the age-cutoff used). According to Center for Disease Control estimates, the percentage of the population over age 65 is rising faster in developed than in developing countries, even though the absolute numbers of persons ageing is much higher in developing countries (143). Only by means of an interaction with other factors, such as the healthcare system, behavioural risk factors, or socioecological determinants can a population's ageing be connected to the observed trends.

Fourth, an issue with this explanation is that ageing is not biological process per se. It does relate to telomeric shortening and other biological factors still being investigated. Ageing is also itself determined by other chronic disease factors, such as economic growth, reducing fertility, and other factors that also could affect chronic diseases.

Lastly, it is highly misleading to decompose epidemiologic and demographic change as though the former were tractable and the latter intractable. Such a determination can have important policy implications, for if chronic diseases are driven principally by population ageing, as the WHO models imply, there will be little rationale for intervention (see 48, 140). The World Bank notes that 'an overemphasis on ageing . . . could result in a mistaken belief that policy cannot make a difference' (48, p. xxiv). But it is also inaccurate. According to these models, rising tuberculosis mortality is driven, not by epidemiology, but almost entirely by population ageing. Would anyone in the tuberculosis community believe this to be the case?

tobacco happens because of tobacco companies operating in a deregulated environment where private companies make (or prevent) government intervention. Nutrition transition happens because of a complex combination of trade liberalization, transformation of agriculture, rising incomes, urbanization, and Western marketing. It is better conceived of as a process of 'dietary dependency'.

But in using these inadequate concepts, we must point the finger at the authors of this chapter. We, too, have put forward a notion of a 'social transition', to describe how risks of chronic disease progressively become embedded in the poorest populations (see, for example, Figure 2.9 depicting shifts in the social gradient of obesity risk). Reality is far more complex and specific (see Chapter 7). These theories, at best, provide a set of clues and puzzles for public health to explore as part of its quest to heed Geoffrey's Rose call that motivated this chapter—to understand the causes of sick individuals and sick populations.

Summary

This chapter has shown how the societies in which people are born, live, work, and age create risks of chronic diseases. About half of all deaths due to chronic diseases relate to tobacco, physical inactivity, or alcohol. However, these risk factors are in turn determined by powerful social and economic forces (such as trade liberalization, foreign direct investment, deregulation, and urbanization), which are driving rises in chronic disease burdens and risks.

The rise of heart disease in the global South, and the welcome decline in the global North, has often been attributed to changes in smoking, cholesterol level, high consumption diet, physical inactivity, and obesity. However, as shown by evidence reviewed in this chapter, all these factors are socially patterned or strongly influenced by societal factors and economic development.

Box 2.6 Risk factor and nutrition transitions

Risk factor transition

The world is currently experiencing a 'risk factor' transition, with developed countries characterized by high disease burden from tobacco, suboptimal blood pressure, alcohol, cholesterol, and overweight. Disease burden in the poorest countries, on the other hand, is primarily caused by underweight, unsafe sex, unsafe water and sanitation, indoor air pollution and micronutrient deficiencies (zinc, iron, vitamin A). This juxtaposition of what might be termed 'new' and 'old' risk factors strongly suggests that health policy in developing countries must increasingly address risks such as tobacco and blood pressure that have often mistakenly been labelled, and treated, as conditions of affluence.

Nutrition transition

The nutrition transition addresses a broad range of socioeconomic and demographic shifts that bring rapid changes in diet and physical activity levels to most regions of the world. The changes are occurring most rapidly as is shown by the shifts in the distribution of the population, income, and occupation patterns. The diet changes, most specifically the shifts towards the higher fat and meat/reduced carbohydrate and fibre diet, is also a shift towards a more diverse and pleasurable diet. The activity patterns also represent a shift away from onerous, difficult labour-intensive activities. Thus, these dietary and physical activity shifts are desirable in many ways. Yet they carry with them many onerous nutritional and health effects.

Sources: top section: Lopez AD. The evolution of the Global Burden of Disease framework for disease, injury and risk factor quantification: developing the evidence base for national, regional and global public health action. *Globalization and Health* 2005; **1**(5). Bottom section: Popkin BM. The nutrition transition and its health implications in lower-income countries. *Public Health Nutrition* 1997; **1**:5–21.

Box 2.7 Common explanations of causes of rising population NCDs

Example 1: this 'epidemiological transition' reflects the higher proportion of adults in the population (due to declines in both fertility rates and infant mortality) who, over time, age and become ill from diseases that disproportionately affect adults. In addition, it reflects the rapid rise in behavioural risk factors including smoking and high-sugar, high-fat diets. The 'nutrition transition' towards diets that are richer in saturated fats and poorer in complex carbohydrates and dietary fibre, fruit, and vegetables; the growth of urban lifestyles involving less physical exertion; and the promotion and rising consumption of tobacco and alcohol, have set the scene for 'lifestyle epidemics' to become the greatest health challenge of the 21st century.

Example 2: the ageing of populations, mainly due to falling fertility rates and increasing child survival, are an underlying determinant of NCD epidemics. Additionally, global trade and marketing developments are driving the nutrition transition towards diets with a high proportion of saturated fat and sugars. This diet, in combination with tobacco use and little physical activity, leads to population-wide atherosclerosis and the widespread distribution of NCD.

Sources: example 1: Magnusson RS. Non-communicable diseases and global health governance: enhancing global processes to improve health development. *Globalization and Health* 2007; **3**:1–16. Example 2: Beaglehole R, Yach D. Globalisation and the prevention and control of non-communicable disease. *The Lancet* 2003; **362**:903–8.

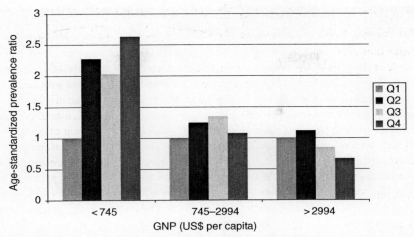

Fig. 2.9 Age-standardized prevalence ratio for women's obesity by quartiles (Q) of years of education in low-, lower-middle-, and upper-middle-income economies (1992–2000). *Source:* Data from Monteiro CA, et al. *International Journal of Obesity*, 2004; **28**:1181–6.

The sum of this evidence reveals that choices about risky lifestyles depend strongly on social circumstances. As outlined in the final report of the WHO Commission on Social Determinants of Health, 'heart disease is caused not by a lack of coronary care units but by the lives people lead, which are shaped by the environments in which they live . . . the main action on social determinants of health must therefore come from outside the health sector' (1). Increasingly, these social circumstances have been driven by the priorities of global financial institutions such as the World Bank and IMF, and the vested interests whom their economic policies serve (145).

These global macroeconomic processes lead to what we term 'dietary dependence':

1 Trade liberalization leads to greater intercountry dietary dependence.

2 Foreign direct investment in foods and beverages in developing economies favours less healthy products.

3 Export-oriented agriculture and trade specialization models increase the dependence on western dietary goods and products of foreign food and beverage companies; technological change speeds up this process.

4 Transnational companies' marketing strategies influence persons in poor countries to prefer Western products as their incomes rise.

5 Urbanization, partially driven by agricultural reforms, leads to less physically active lifestyles and shifts food consumption away from the home.

In other words, dietary dependency is a process by which food choices come to depend on choices by governments, farmers, and transnational companies. It is fostered by models of economic development emphasizing trade liberalization, export-oriented agriculture, foreign direct investment in foods and beverage sectors, especially in the context of unregulated marketing and government agricultural subsidies. Such dependency has tended to be beneficial in rich countries although governments continue to subsidize sugar, salts, and fats. Among poor countries, however, it has tended to increase risks of chronic disease as traditional diets are replaced by Western multinational foods.

Such processes of dietary dependency are most visible in small islands, such as Micronesia and Nauru, but they also have transformed diets in subtle, yet profound, ways in Brazil, China,

Box 2.8 Critiques of methods used in NCD epidemiology

When we talk about our epidemiological frameworks to study chronic disease epidemiology, it is worth clarifying why the field has adopted the approaches it has, and what further must be done to improve our methods. Chronic disease epidemiology has been accused at various times of reductionism, determinism, or individualism. First, it is overly simplistic to reduce NCD risks to a few common, proximal risk factors. In a series of seminal studies, called the 'Framingham heart study', a statistical analysis of a cohort of 5209 men and women aged 30–62 years followed since 1948 revealed the substantial contribution of a few core risk factors to CVD risk, including fibrinogen, high-density lipoprotein cholesterol, obesity, and diabetes. In ongoing work, however, the field has shrunk the scope of its inquiries into this small subset of the potential causes of poor chronic disease outcomes. Surveys and instruments have abounded to quantify this narrow set of factors, to the exclusion of others, ultimately shrinking the scope of inquiry for PhD students and researchers to those variables which were available from standardized datasets whose mining became the basis for academic careers and, in some cases, entire institutes. According to philosophers of science, this is bad science, in the respect that this research programme does not achieve truly novel findings or ideas that enable the field to grow.

Another critique is that the focus on risk factors makes chronic disease risk appear inevitable, or deterministic, characterizing individuals as having little ability to construct, negotiate, or reduce risk. For example, studying the effects of cigarettes on lung health makes it appear as though the cigarette rather than the tobacco company was the cause of lung cancer. This approach also does not give rise to intervention strategies. Rarely does it go beyond description to explanation, let alone the identification of effective interventions. Researchers have undertaken countless studies on common proximal risk factors and diagnoses, both individually and in combination: obesity and breast cancer; obesity and diabetes; tobacco and diabetes; diabetes and heart disease.

A related problem is the tendency of chronic disease epidemiology to work in the absence of theory or to rely on so-called 'low-level' theories commonly referred to as the 'black box' approach to chronic disease epidemiology. It is quantitative, probabilistic, and usually incomplete. Like the rest of the social policy sciences (including social work and criminology), this approach has come to dominate approaches to studying chronic disease risks and patterns. (Incidentally, the failure to elucidate new biochemical mechanisms is also argued to be the main reason why Doll and Peto—the two most prominent chronic disease epidemiologists— were not recognized with a Nobel Prize for their work showing the link between tobacco and lung cancer, even though these findings led to many more lives saved than other prize-winning findings.)

Finally, chronic disease epidemiology, similar to infectious disease epidemiology, tends to zoom in on individual experience, especially 'lifestyles', to the neglect of the roles of meso- or macro-level forces that determine them. The field implicitly views populations as an aggregate of representative individuals, rather than as a social unit characterized by structured interactions that modulate which people become sick and how (147). This analytical approach is commonly referred to as 'methodological individualism'. It pervades not just epidemiology but the entirety of the social sciences. It results, in part, from scepticism about the scientific validity of population-level analysis, which began to emerge in the 1930s. Concerns about the analysis of group-level factors can be traced to Durkheim's seminal study of suicide (148), pointing out the potential for spurious associations of religion and suicide at both individual

Box 2.8 (continued)

and ecological levels. Subsequently, Robinson's seminal paper on illiteracy and black ethnicity in the US (149) revealed bias between investigations at individual and societal levels. These developments in the field ultimately led to Selvin's coining of the term 'ecologic fallacy' in the 1950s (150)—methodological concerns that subsequently filled epidemiology textbooks (but not Durkheim's original point about individualistic fallacies). Yet, as Geoffrey Rose pointed out, to study sick populations requires the study of risks that act at both individual and population levels (9). This calls for the development of a range of new theories that can specify how social context influences individual NCD risks and outcomes. Important interactions can arise between social context and individual choices (151), necessitating both multilevel theories and analysis of NCDs. Just as ecological fallacy has the potential to obscure mechanisms acting at individual levels, an individualistic fallacy can obscure mechanisms acting at societal levels (148). Researchers are now using innovative methods to describe the ways in which health is shaped by the environments in which people live, invoking measures such as the 'obesogenicity' of neighbourhoods in which a combination of lack of attractive open spaces and fear of crime deter walking and where the cheapest and most accessible form of nutrition is energy-dense fast food (70).

Mexico, India, and South Africa (as documented further in the case studies of each of these countries in Chapter 7).

People's ways of living have also been transformed in ways that discourage physical activity. Patterns of urbanization have locked in a reliance on motorized transit, especially in resource-deprived countries where planning has been haphazard. This is worse in those states which have lacked resources to steer urban development in a healthier direction, especially those weakened by extensive privatization and deregulation. These risks of physical inactivity are compounded by economic transformations to centralized work, which typically involve people sitting at desks for many hours without much physical activity.

As emphasized by Geoffrey Rose, individual and population approaches to control chronic diseases are not incompatible, however, in order to effectively reduce them in a society, the focus should always be to discover and act upon the ultimate causes of incidence at the population level (146). Consequently, the dominant focus in epidemiology on continued studies of individual risks have low value-added to understanding why populations are sick and others healthy. These studies also could divert attention from the major risks causing people to die prematurely from chronic diseases in resource-deprived settings. In the future, two kinds of additional studies are needed: those that identify and understand the specific biological hazards of the risk factors and those that identify the underlying societal causes of rising population exposure to the main risk factors.

To address such profound transformations in the risk of entire societies, public health experts must move beyond the proximal individual risk factors to identify and address what is driving unhealthy urbanization, ageing, and growth processes—the 'causes of the causes', the 'risk factors of the risk factors'. In the next chapter we assess the social and economic consequences of the poor health being caused by these environmental transformations.

Endnote

1 Of course, countries do not always implement these conditions placed on loans and, at times, use the IMF as a bargaining chip to do what they want to do anyhow but with the political advantage of being able to blame the IMF if things go wrong (see references 117 and 119 for more details).

Chapter 3

Social and economic consequences of chronic diseases

♦ What are the social and economic consequences of chronic diseases?
♦ Who suffers from the costs of these diseases?
♦ Is there a case for governments to act to reduce the social harms caused by chronic diseases?

David Stuckler and Marc Suhrcke

Key policy points

1 Rising costs of chronic diseases threaten to overwhelm resource-poor health systems.

2 Chronic diseases put households at risk of poverty.

3 People with chronic disease suffer in the labour market, working fewer hours, missing more days of work, being less productive on the job, and retiring at much younger ages.

4 Not paying for chronic disease care delays and ultimately increases downstream expenditures as chronic diseases become more difficult to manage and produce expensive consequences when unaddressed early.

5 Left unchecked, rising chronic diseases are likely to slow economic growth.

6 Chronic diseases impede progress toward the health and poverty Millennium Development Goals.

7 Some economists view obesity as a market success, rather than failure, or a type of collateral damage that we can live with. Market failures can contribute to the spread of chronic diseases, and can worsen their social harms.

Key practice points

1 Economic perspectives focus on overall well-being, or 'utility', not just money.

2 Specific types of health and labour market protection programmes can reduce the social harms caused by chronic diseases; when these supports are absent or weak, families have greater risks of being driven into poverty by the economic and social consequences of chronic diseases.

3 Evidence of market failures provides a powerful rebuttal to those who argue that 'individual choice' drives risks of chronic disease.

Understanding the social and economic consequences of chronic disease

Health is about more than physiology. People want to lead fulfilled, meaningful lives. Without health people cannot achieve their most basic desires. Good health—and being healthy—is both a means to other desires and an end in itself.

In view of this broader importance of health, considerable effort has gone into understanding not just the health consequences of chronic diseases, as summarized in Chapter 1, but also the social effects of these diseases on individuals, families, and their societies.

The payoff from identifying these effects is twofold. It can help find appropriate ways to mitigate the suffering that accompanies illness, a major aim of public health policy. This is especially important for diseases where medical treatments cannot offer a readily available cure, such as with type 1 diabetes, Alzheimer's dementia, or non-small cell lung cancer.

The second benefit is political. Once the social consequences of disease have been identified, making an epidemiologic case to prevent the diseases that are particularly debilitating can provide clear directions for improving society. In the case of chronic disease research, investigations into the consequences of chronic disease help dispel common fallacies. There is a prevailing view among policymakers that healthcare is simply an economic cost to be contained. Others believe that if we first take care of the economy, health will improve, viewing health as an effect, not a cause, of better society. Yet these ways of thinking ignore the bi-directional relationship between health and wealth: people are healthy because they are rich; people are richer because they are healthy (see Figure 3.1). Evidence about the social consequences of illness can enable policymakers to envision a richer, happier society, should they choose to invest in a society's health.

Starting as early as the 1920s and 1930s, public health practitioners sought evidence about the costs of diseases to increase the resources available to public health. For example, during the early history of the automobile, public health experts argued, 'The economic loss [due to road deaths] every year according to reliable figures is $2,500,000,000. This loss is greater than the annual sum spent on the public school system of the United States . . .' (152). In a period when public health faced significant budget cuts, William Welch, president of American Medical Association, wrote

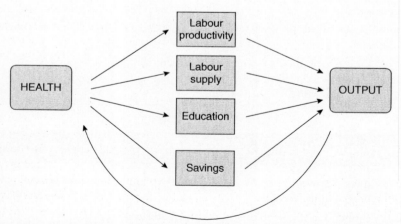

Fig. 3.1 Mechanisms linking health and wealth. Notes: the reverse arrow from output to health reflects the bi-directional health–wealth relationship, showing that the economy affects health. *Source:* Adapted from: Bloom DE, Canning D. The health and wealth of nations. *Science* 2000; **287**:1207–9.

to *The New York Times*, 'Any undue retrenchment in health work is bound to be paid for in dollars and cents as well as in the impairment of the people's health generally. We can demonstrate convincingly that returns in economic and social welfare from expenditures for public health service are far in excess of their cost' (153).

More recently, two major UN reports—the World Bank *Investing in Health* report (154) and the WHO's *Commission on Macroeconomics and Health* (155)—helped shift the culture of thinking about healthcare away from the 'cost-containment' paradigm to viewing health spending as a vital investment for reducing poverty and increasing economic growth.

Paradoxically, this change in the culture of thinking about health appears not to have extended to chronic diseases. Both UN reports almost entirely ignored chronic diseases, focusing mainly on the costs of malaria, TB, and HIV/AIDS. Yet poor health—be it chronic or infectious in nature— carries a similar set of social harms. And, as shown in Chapter 1, when incomes exceed about $3500 GDP, NCDs become leading causes of death and disability. Because chronic diseases are highly prevalent—owing to rising incidence and their long-term duration—they could cause even greater healthcare costs than acute diseases. That chronic diseases account for over two-fifths of deaths among working ages, the productive base of economies, suggests they could have even greater impacts on the workforce in resource-poor countries (8, 17).

The rest of this chapter will detail how economic perspectives can enlighten us on how best to respond to chronic diseases. As we will show, such economic tools are powerful, but they have ethical, policy, and technical limitations. Hence, first we set out what we mean by an 'economic perspective' and address its important drawbacks. We then focus our discussion on four key questions: What are the social and economic costs of chronic disease? Who carries the burden of these costs? How do we measure them? Can these social harms caused by chronic diseases be avoided at low cost? In considering the final question, we will assess whether in a 'no-change' scenario the harm caused by chronic diseases can be expected to 'take care of itself' through market forces, evaluating the economic case for government support of broader public health interventions.

What is an economic perspective on NCDs?

The field of economics provides a rigorous set of methods to help allocate scarce resources. Often, health economics focuses on estimating the cost-effectiveness of healthcare interventions as a way to decide which approaches could save the most lives at the lowest cost (see Chapter 4). This is just one narrow aspect of economics and, for that matter, of public health. Health is about much more than healthcare.

Contemporary economic approaches recognize the importance of health to society as one of several desirable goals. Economics focuses on maximizing 'utility', defined as a person's overall, subjective well-being. This concept covers the full range of social harms. Albeit often expressed in narrow financial terms, it can be usefully and flexibly extended. Costs and benefits, in economic terms, are not just about money. Sadness, for example, is a cost, and happiness is a benefit.

In order to create a 'fair' comparison between health and other socially valued investments, such as education, the economic approach tried to convert poor health into a common base unit, usually denominated in money. The approach could be reversed so that life-years served as the common currency, or any arbitrary representative unit can be used to represent how much a person values something such as their health; the end results would be the same mathematically (but requires quantification, a disadvantage).

At times, this can lead to clashing opinions between economists and public health experts. It is important to bear in mind that health is not the only thing people want. People can make unhealthy choices, at times knowing fully that their health could suffer. An economic perspective—seeking to maximizing utility—is unlikely to yield the same priorities as a public health perspective—seeking to maximize health. While public health experts might like to see zero tobacco use as the objective of policy, some economists might view the optimal social level of tobacco use as above zero, in view of the pleasure that tobacco can provide to some persons who value it more than the potential risk it represents to them (although there are disputes, as we return to in the discussion about time-preferences below).

Economic perspectives can help public health practitioners to understand the importance of people's priorities as they relate to public health goals. We will return to this at the end of the chapter, but for now it is sufficient to note this economic approach is very important for building a case about whether it is appropriate for the government to intervene to support public health policy interventions.

Several additional concerns have been raised about applying an economic perspective to health, including relying on a narrow ethical approach, turning health into a commodity like any other by putting a price on human life, and deciding health policy through simple financial calculus. These important limitations will be examined in turn.

One key concern is that economic perspectives 'commodify' health; they reduce what is valuable about human health to money. How do we put a price on human life? Treating health as a commodity like any other, it is argued, reflects a set of misguided approaches to value and improve global health. It is at odds with, for example, rights-based and social justice approaches to health, which emphasize equality and fairness, or that investing in health is 'the right thing to do'(1). Yet, economic approaches are based on principles to 'do the greatest good for the most people'—utilitarian principles—an ethic that many persons support. Similarly, the way people think about health is as both a means and an end, such that it can be thought of in economic terms as health being both an 'investment' and used for 'consumption' (or something people enjoy). 'Cost-of-illness' studies evaluate the effects of NCDs on financial outcomes, calculating how much diseases cost health systems. But these studies can be applied to poverty, education, gender-gaps, and other key social measures, like happiness. In fact, an economic perspective would emphasize fundamental social welfare objectives, like improving health and well-being, over mere financial goals.

Yet, even in narrow financial terms, cost of illness analysis can contribute to policy debate by seeking to answer a range of questions that reflect priorities of people in power making decisions, such as: Will investing in health reduce healthcare spending in the future? Will society be happier if more resources are invested in health? Can the money we have available to us create greater good if it is spent on education or employment instead of healthcare? Often, public health assumes prevention is better than the cure, but is it true that the costs will also be lower?

Their answers can have a dark side. In the early 1950s, after evidence emerged about tobacco's lung-cancer risks, several groups provided evidence that tobacco saved the health system money, because people died early. At the time, the famous tobacco control specialist Sir Richard Doll, suggested that this somewhat cynical view might explain the failure of the government to act resolutely against it. People claimed that they were 'doing society a great service by dying young'. These arguments continue today in various forms, especially in low- and middle-income countries. One recent report commissioned by Philip Morris suggested that that smoking benefited the Czech Republic's government spending surplus because smokers died before they became old, unproductive, and costly through extended illness (156).

Some public health leaders argue that if the chronic disease community wishes to get more attention, they—along with other health constituencies—should present arguments that chronic diseases can be commodified. These leaders claim that a rights-based approach, however agreeable from an ethical perspective, is unlikely to compel policymakers to action who do not already view NCDs as a priority. As discussed in Chapters 2 and 5, powerful global institutions such as the World Bank and IMF have oriented their development agendas toward the pursuit of growth, stability, and efficiency. Making economic calculations can 'instrumentalize' NCDs, showing people in power how reducing NCDs can help them achieve their objectives—the 'co-benefits' to intervention.

The economic approach also recognizes that people value health very highly—no one would trade their life for money.[1] But beyond a minimal level of health, how important is better health compared with education or a better house? Many persons, for example, sacrifice good nutrition in order to work in jobs that require poor eating habits in exchange for remuneration from long working hours. Just like approaches to measuring the suffering associated with poor health (using disability-adjusted life years) predicate on the notion, 'it is not how many years of life but how much life is in those years', economics seeks to understand what people value. This puts a price on values—even when those values are not for sale—developing a so-called 'shadow price'. This is extremely challenging. The famous economist, John Maynard Keynes, said that, when it comes to understanding what determines price, 'We are one equation short'. We simply don't know enough about how to relate price to value (usually resorting to market value)—a fundamental challenge in market economics.

One way to value disease is to ask people how much they would be willing to pay to avoid it. Asking people directly can produce bias, but furthermore it begs the question of who really knows how bad a disease is until they have experienced it? To overcome this challenge, economists use an approach in which they observe what people actually do as a way to infer how much they value health (so-called 'revealed preference'). This method obviously has limitations; if people do not have full knowledge about the extent of social harms arising from disease, they would actually be happier if they made different decisions that prioritized their health. People also may not think about health in similar ways, because having a health condition alters people's states of being and combinations of diseases can be much worse than a single disease. This is especially the case with NCDs, where people are likely to have multiple diseases in the course of a lifetime and experience periods with co-morbidities arising from interactions between diseases.[2] Adding to this difficulty, the values people place on different states of health (as well as their perceptions of suffering) can depend on the social context, such as the state of existing care, so whatever value is calculated is by no means universal.

Finally, economic analysis seeks to inform policy makers about the likely financial consequences of their decisions. While economists pride themselves on assessing overall welfare of individuals and societies, this is very difficult to do in practice. The critics are correct to observe that financial considerations dominate the discussions about economic costs, relating both to methodological ease of analysing the financial dimension of costs and, importantly, because money is often of greater interest to those in power. When this happens, unfortunately, evaluations tend to understate the true economic benefits of health policies that do not directly produce revenue but act in a distributed way throughout society, because the latter do not factor how much people value health.

Estimating the full costs of a disease or risk factor to society and individuals at different times under alternative future scenarios is methodologically challenging and highly uncertain. Only after decades of research by some of the world's leading economists were widely held views that tobacco use saved taxpayers money overturned (157) (and indeed some might argue that debate is far from settled). Like epidemiological studies of the health consequences of risk factors, these economic investigations of costs and benefits were complicated by 'confounder' studies put forward by the industry, often through paid researchers or fraudulent pseudo-scientific front NGO groups, as has been extensively documented (158, 159). Nonetheless, investigations concerning the costs of smoking continue today in the US—and the debates are just getting underway in tobacco-growing countries where misleading arguments about tobacco production's benefits to the economy strike a chord with ministers of finance and agriculture.

Clue 1: Estimating the full costs of a disease or risk factor to society and individuals at different times under alternative future scenarios is methodologically challenging and highly uncertain.

Strategy 1: Economic perspectives can help public health practitioners to understand the importance of people's priorities as they relate to public health goals. They can also help show people working outside of public health the benefits of reducing chronic diseases to the economy, education, environment and other desirable societal goals.

In the next section, we summarize the types of social and economic costs caused by NCDs, then we assess the methods used to assess the magnitude of these costs.

What are the costs of chronic diseases?

Let's return to the scenario about Eli Peterson, the middle-aged factory worker introduced in Chapter 2. What happened to him? The story continues a few years later, when Eli is diagnosed with type 2 diabetes.

Up until this point, Eli was performing reasonably well at his job and had a healthy family life. Soon after being diagnosed with type 2 diabetes his health started deteriorating. Fortunately, Eli's health insurance covered medical procedures, which over the next several years became increasingly frequent and disabling. Kidney failure required regular dialysis, leading to major changes in his lifestyle. It became harder for Eli to pick his kids up from school. His circulation grew worse, impeding blood flow, ultimately leading to the amputation of several toes. But these harms were minor compared with what was to come. Over the next 5 years Eli began progressively losing his sight. This was a major blow. It took away his ability to work and his independence. Eli's health insurance covered medical procedures but not long-term care. Eli's wife had to scale back her working hours in order to care for Eli, placing pressure on Eli's teenagers to study less in order to work to help make up for the financial shortfall.

How can we think about the costs of Eli's case? Clearly, Eli's diabetes came with a set of medical complications, such as painful medical procedures, disfiguring amputations, growing disability, as well as social complications, such as loss of work, status, identity, and control over life. His costs also went beyond his experience, affecting his wife and children.

Evaluating such a broad range of costs requires using a causal framework, much like that set out in Chapter 1 to describe epidemiology of NCDs. For example, economic costs were progressively increased as risk factors gave rise to clinical illness. These could be located at differing points on the chain of disease, and be attributed with varying degrees of certainty to differing causal factors. As in Chapter 1, whichever framework we adopt will inevitably oversimplify the full picture.

One common approach is to divide costs into three categories: healthcare costs, involving treatments, medical procedures, doctor visits, hospitalizations and drug expenses; labour market (or work-related) costs, involving losses of earnings, early retirement, and missed work days; and overall well-being costs, including feelings of pain, disability, and suffering. Sometimes these components are referred to as 'direct', 'indirect', and 'intangible' costs, respectively (such as shown in Figure 3.2); however, it is unclear why healthcare costs are more or less direct than, say, the loss of earnings.

In Eli's case, healthcare costs were provoked by his medical needs, including insulin, testing equipment, routine dialysis, invasive surgeries, and long-term follow-up, to name a few.

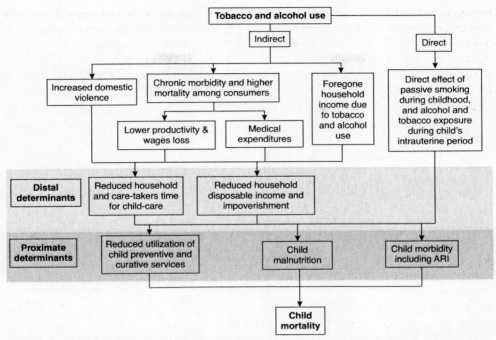

Fig. 3.2 Direct and indirect cost model of tobacco and alcohol use risks to child health.
Bonu S, Rani, M, Jha, P, Peters, DH, Nguyen, SN. Household tobacco and alcohol use and child health: an exploratory study from India. *Health Policy and Planning*. 2004; **70**:67–83.

The expense is high and lifelong. His employment costs included reduced performance while working, sometimes (referred to as 'presenteeism') and missed days of work (referred to as 'absenteeism'). They also included consequences for his family, who had to make major life changes to compensate for Eli's lost earnings and need for ongoing care (referred to as 'consumption smoothing'). His wife left the labour market, while his daughter lost study time—working instead of preparing for college. These, too, are long-term costs, and typically they are larger than healthcare costs. The final set of well-being costs is the hardest to measure, but potentially are the greatest, as they subsume the previous two categories. Eli's shame, loss of friends and identity all contribute to the overall suffering, or 'disutility', caused by diabetes. As noted above, it is this harm that economic approaches seek to reduce.

Not just individuals but households, firms, and entire societies shoulder the costs of chronic diseases. For example, Eli lost wages, displacing funding that would have gone to his daughter's education. Meanwhile his firm lost productivity. Sick employees like Eli are less likely to show up to work and, when they do, they produce less in the same amount of time. When workers retire early or die too young, firms bear higher costs for replacing them.

Entire economies can be slowed down by a high chronic disease burden. This happens in several ways, as summarized in Figure 3.1, affecting the supply of labour, the productivity of labour, education (affecting the productivity of labour), and savings (affecting a society's investment in productive capital). As firms are the engine of a society's productivity, their underperformance can diminish economic growth. When there are many Eli's of working-age who become sick, society's supply of labour is reduced and becomes less productive. Greater spending on healthcare can also prevent people from investing in productive equipment and machinery or saving money (allowing the government to invest in physical infrastructure), leading to less output than would have occurred without spending on medications. High premature death rates from chronic diseases also lead people to plan for the shorter-term. In a situation where people expect to live 50 additional years versus 20, they are more likely to plan for their future. That means they are less willing to forego immediate pleasure in order to save money (so providing investment for economic growth) or invest in education, which could potentially yield great dividends over the long-run.

Clue 2: Chronic diseases can have a significant negative impact on the economy by reducing a person's productivity and time spent working as well as his/her desire to seek education and save money.

How do we measure these costs?

Are the costs of NCDs large or small? How do they compare with other diseases?

Our discussion structures around the healthcare and work costs, as they relate to the pathways affecting economic growth. In analysing economic costs of chronic diseases, it is important to avoid double-counting. For example, adding up his firm's productivity and his individual earnings losses would be duplicating the consequences of Eli's foregone work. Costs can be evaluated at the individual, household, or firm levels ('microeconomic approach') or population level ('macroeconomic approach'). We begin with the data of costs to individuals and households. In each case, we summarize how these types of costs relate to a society's economic potential and conclude with an analysis of societal costs that extend beyond the economy.

Individual-level costs

Healthcare costs (reducing savings)

What does it cost to purchase medical care for persons who have NCDs in resource-poor countries? Can this reduce the resources that would have otherwise gone into more productive uses?

Lifelong treatment of NCDs drains income. Substantial evidence shows that people who have an NCD in resource-poor countries, especially those lacking health insurance, spend considerable portions of their incomes on the costs of care. The case of diabetes is illustrative: in Tanzania, as but one example, paying for diabetes care costs 25% of the minimum wage (160), roughly $156 for a 1-month supply—well beyond the means of the majority of the Tanzanian population. Not surprisingly, people in developing countries report experiencing financial difficulties as a result of chronic diseases, and many avoid some medical treatment because of financial constraints.

These costs create a lethal dilemma—forego care or risk financial ruin. One study notes that 'if African patients with diabetes have to pay for their treatment, most will be unable to do so and will die' (161). In many cases, when essential medicines are not available, there is no choice. Surveys of 25 countries in Africa found that insulin was frequently unavailable in large city hospitals and the situation was far worse in rural areas (162).

There is strong evidence that, for those families choosing to finance care for a member suffering from a chronic illness, the costs of care for NCDs can be the cause of poverty. Research from countries as diverse as Burkina Faso (163) and Thailand (164) find that the presence of a chronic illness in a family is one of the most important determinants of whether the household will incur 'catastrophic health expenditure'. The notion of 'catastrophic expenditures' can be used to study when healthcare costs endanger a household's ability to survive (usually based on a threshold of household income of between 5% and 20% is defined as 'catastrophic', although whether healthcare costs are catastrophic depends on the healthcare financing system) (165). WHO studies of two countries found that when a family member becomes sick between 2% and 3% face catastrophic health care expenditures and, in about half of these cases, the costs push households into poverty (165). One World Bank study of catastrophic spending in India found that men with CVD were 20% more likely to have catastrophic spending and 8% greater risk of impoverishment. Translated into numbers of people, this corresponds to at least 1.4–2.0 million people incurring catastrophic spending and at least 0.6–0.8 million people impoverished.

Clue 3: High costs of treating chronic diseases can deplete people's savings and, in extreme cases, cause people to choose between poverty or a slow, painful death.

Labour market costs (decreasing labour supply and productivity)

People who are diagnosed with NCDs describe the experience as a lifelong change. Does long-term illness provoke such changes to a person's life—both social and biological in nature—that can affect the way people work?

There is strong evidence that people who have NCDs work and produce less. They tend to earn significantly less money, work fewer hours, miss more days of work, be at high risk of job loss, leave the workforce early, and retire at younger ages.

These topics have been most extensively studied in the US (perhaps because employers there have a financial incentive to understand how health relates to work activity). As one example, people living in the US who have chronic diseases were found to earn lower wages (men, about 5.6% lower; women 8.9% lower) (166). There is clear evidence showing how chronic diseases and their risks result in worse job performance, fewer hours worked, greater missed days, higher risks of unemployment, premature retirement, and social stigma.

Relatively few studies investigate the labour market consequences of NCDs in low- and middle-income countries. Unsurprisingly, they find similar patterns as in high-income countries. As a couple of examples, in Indonesia, tobacco use was estimated to result in US$115 lost individual income per year (167). In Taiwan, the probability of being in the labour force was estimated to be reduced by 27% by CVD and 19% by diabetes (168).

While the precise reasons why people with NCDs fare worse in the labour market remain unclear, resulting from a combination of the performance of sick persons and perceptions of managers, there is no doubt that NCDs, beyond the clearly high medical costs, can reduce the financial resources available to a family.

Clue 4: People who have chronic diseases or engage in their risks tend to earn less money and have a greater risk of being unemployed. In this way, chronic diseases reduce the amount of money available to families and children.

Reduced education (decreasing labour productivity)

When a family member loses money due to poor health, especially those on the brink of poverty, other members of the family often attempt to compensate in a variety of ways to enable to the household to survive financially.[3] These reactions typically counteract the costs of care, making them overestimates, at least in the short-term. For example, when a male head of household gets sick and loses work, his wife may begin to work more than before. Or, depending on whether care is available, she may have to provide care for him at home, while instead her children leave school to work (169).

These household responses to sickness, while potentially offsetting healthcare or financial costs, can create a set of additional costs that are borne many years down the road. Figure 3.3 shows how a household's response to illness vary based on the household's lines of defence, such as using emergency savings or pulling children out of school to work.

One study of rural households in southwest Ethiopia identified three main strategies families used to cope with the financial costs of adult illness (170): seeking to have medical costs waived due to financial hardship (16.8%), selling valuable household assets (13.3%), and using up

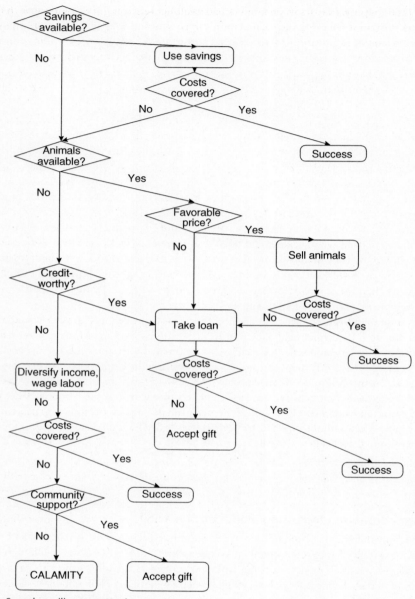

Fig. 3.3 Sample resilience strategies.
Sauerborn R, Adams, A, Hien, M. Household strategies to cope with the economic costs of illness. *Soc Sci Med*. 1996; **43**(3):291-301.

savings (13.1%). Sick individuals lost an average of 9 days of work per month; their carers lost about 7 days of work per month. To compensate for this loss of work, healthy household members increased their working hours. Another study interviewed people living in urban slums in Dhaka, Bangladesh, finding that rural-to-urban migration or vice versa was a common strategy (171). When illness affected the woman in charge of the household families joined together with other households in the city. In cases when families had wealthier relatives, they would move to the city to join them, or, in some cases, they would return to rural homes and join extended families.

When a parent dies too young, their children's education suffers (169). A study in Indonesia found that a child whose parent has recently died is about twice as likely to drop out of school as children whose parents are alive. Youth who face key decisions about whether to continue to junior secondary from primary school or senior secondary from junior secondary school face the greatest risks.

Clue 5: When a parent is sick or dies prematurely, there is a risk that a child will be forced to leave school early to work in order to help the family survive.

Health and work-related costs of caring for family members with chronic diseases—even in settings where healthcare is unavailable—are expensive. These costs can add up to significant declines in an economy's overall productivity.

Clue 6: Even in settings where healthcare is unavailable, the costs of caring family members who have chronic diseases are expensive.

We will return to this point shortly, when we examine the population-level impacts of chronic diseases, but first we address some of the broader societal costs, including those to the environment, women and other health issues.

Broader societal costs (full-welfare)

People care about health for reasons far beyond their biological needs. It is usually a precondition for people to do other things in life they enjoy. How much does health reduce people's overall well-being?

Unfortunately, few studies, to our knowledge, have investigated these full social welfare consequences explicitly, although overall subjective well-being does factor as one component into calculations of quality-adjusted life years (see Chapter 1). Clearly, the consequences can be devastating, often fatal, especially for the poor. The precise magnitude in relation to other diseases, however, is not well-understood. One study suggested that the self-reported quality of life among children who were overweight or obese was on par with children suffering from terminal cancer. The authors attributed this to social stigma and teasing at school (171a).

Some social harms can be difficult to assess and quantify in financial terms. For example, hazardous drinking is a major cause of domestic violence, road-traffic accidents, and weakened social cohesion (when people fear going into the city because of drunken teens). Tobacco use in public places like restaurants or parks can also deter non-smokers from using those areas. Litter from tobacco butts on beaches and streets also make cities unsightly, deterring people from walking. These are just a few examples of broader costs that do not easily fit within in a narrow view of financial costs.

As described in Chapter 1, chronic diseases can increase the risks of poor child health and the spread of infectious diseases. A few examples are tobacco and indoor pollution as key risks of TB spread and HIV infection (172), to name a few. In other words, chronic diseases create an additional and indirect set of costs by causing poor health due to non-chronic diseases which have in turn been found to be costly (173).

There are also social consequences of chronic diseases that create additional health risks. Spending money on chronic disease care or risk factors can reduce money available for healthcare, education, capital or savings—thereby affecting the economy—but also food, clothing, and shelter—thereby affecting people's overall quality of life. The case of tobacco illustrates these 'opportunity costs'. One study found households in Bangladesh spent more than twice as much on cigarettes as on housing, clothing, health, and education combined in the 1990s (174); the poorest households spent close to 10 times as much on tobacco as on education. One researcher estimated that, 'The average amounts spent on tobacco each day would generally be enough to make the difference between at least one family member having just enough to eat to keep from being malnourished' (175).

Rising incidence of chronic disease risk factors among children, as described in Chapter 1, also poses risks to education and cognitive development, for both social and biological reasons. For example, smoking during pregnancy can impair cognitive and behavioural development. Overweight or obese children were found to be more likely to miss school or suffer from lower self-esteem, greater shame and perceive themselves being teased compared with their peers (stigmatization). However, this stigma may be less prominent in settings where obesity is a marker of social status (especially the case in countries with a high burden of infectious diseases; see Chapter 7.5 for the example of South Africa).

Overall, the social and biological risks of chronic diseases experienced by households can combine to put children at significantly greater risk of illness. One study in India found that children living in households with smokers were 21% less likely to be immunized, 15% more like to have acute respiratory infection, and 21% more likely to be underweight. The researchers estimated that, overall, parental smoking increased the risk of infant mortality in India by 7% (176, 177).

The impacts of NCD on other health outcomes is far from trivial. One study estimated that high burdens of NCDs were a significant cause of slow progress in reducing child mortality and TB rates, key targets of the Millennium Development Goals (2). The study estimated that each 10% higher burden of NCDs was associated with about 5% slower progress towards the child health target and about 7% slower progress towards the TB goal. This was estimated to be equivalent to more than a several decades worth of progress in increasing income. In other words, a high burden of NCDs undermines progress to the world's top global health goals to increase child survival and stop the spread of TB.

Thus, we have found another set of key clues about the societal costs of chronic disease:

Clue 6: When parents spend money on tobacco, alcohol, or chronic care, they use money that could have otherwise been used to provide food and clothing to their children.

Clue 7: Chronic diseases create biological and social risks of poor child health and the spread of infectious diseases.

Clue 8: Chronic diseases can cause considerable social suffering, such as teasing and stigma caused by disfigurement, which can greatly reduce people's quality of life.

Population-level costs

Focusing on the individual level offers several advantages over the population approach. First, the evidence is generally easier to relate to than evidence that describes relationships at the comparatively abstract macro-level. It clearly sets out who bears the costs and why. Second, relationships observed at the individual level overcome critiques about potential for ecological fallacy. They also identify mechanisms of impact and who bears costs, providing policymakers with key information about how to mitigate social harms of NCDs. Third, it is easier to construct a counterfactual at the individual level, as the intervening social resilience mechanisms are less operative. Nonetheless, the highest quality studies have attempted to construct scenarios of 'what if' the NCD or risk factor had not been present. Fourth, the individual-level evidence provides support to the population-level evidence, corroborating the pathways set out in Figure 3.1.

But the individual level may not attract the same level attention from policymakers who are concerned with the 'big picture'. Estimates of population costs can help alert policymakers to the severity of a given illness. Given that our preceding evidence suggests that it is plausible that NCDs could have major population-level consequences, we can ask: do these individual-level costs add up to a significant figure at the societal level?

Descriptive approaches

One way to calculate population-level costs draws on the epidemiologic notion of population attributable risk, ascertaining costs as:

Population attributable costs = Individual costs of NCD × the population prevalence of NCDs

This method is straightforward. First assess the average healthcare costs for a certain disease (first term of the equation), then multiply them by the number of persons with the disease (second term of the equation). Costs can be thought of broadly, assessing, for example, labour market costs by adding up the total time lost through premature death and illness (such as self-reported missed days of work multiplied by the worker's earnings). Such estimates provide a first glimpse of the scale of the economic burden of disease, often yielding alarming figures—for example, reporting that in 2002 CVD cost the US $352 billion (50).

What should we make of such numbers? Is spending out of control? Putting these data in perspective can help people understand their meaning. For concerned individuals they should be presented in terms of per head of population. For healthcare planners they should be shown as a fraction of society's overall health spending. For financial planners they should be scaled to society's overall economic product (gross domestic product, GDP). Table 3.1 summarizes some estimates of the healthcare and employment costs of chronic diseases as a fraction of GDP in high-income countries. To illustrate the magnitude, healthcare and labour market costs ranged between 0.8% and 7% of GDP.

The case of the US demonstrates the potential for costs of obesity and diabetes to rise. In the span of 5 years, medical costs due to diabetes more than doubled, from $44 billion to $92 billion, reaching $123 billion by 2001 (more than 1% of GDP). Much of the rise in diabetes costs reflected rising levels of obesity, which were estimated to impose health-system costs roughly equivalent to 20 years of natural ageing.

While the US may seem like an exceptional case in view of its heavy reliance on expensive drugs and technology, costs of a similarly high magnitude have been observed throughout the developed world, where obesity-related costs ranged between 2% and 7% of total healthcare costs and more than 0.5% of GDP. Tobacco-related medical costs account for between 6% and 8% of total health expenditure in the US.

Clue 9: Among high-income populations, the economic costs of chronic diseases and their risks amount to a significant fraction of a country's overall spending, suggesting the potential for freeing up considerable resources if their healthcare burden could be reduced.

Relatively fewer studies have been done of healthcare and work-related costs in developing countries, but they indicate that chronic diseases and their risk factors can be as expensive as in developed countries. As a few examples, costs of treating diabetes ranged between 1.8% of GDP in Venezuela and 5.9% of GDP in Barbados in Latin America (178), a region where nearly one out of every three hospital bed-days were occupied for diabetes-related causes, with costs averaging about $550 per person.

Clue 10: The economic burden in terms of a country's overall wealth is often as high, if not greater, in low-income countries than in high-income ones.

Simple descriptive approaches such as these have significant limitations. First, substantial differences in methodologies and data used prevent accurate comparisons of the magnitudes of costs

Table 3.1 Estimated costs of selected chronic diseases and risk factors

Country	Condition	Year of estimate	Total cost (% of GDP)	Percentage of costs indirect
United States	Tobacco use	1997–2001	1.71	55.09
Canada	Tobacco use	1991, 1992	1.39–2.20	–
Australia	Tobacco use	1992	3.40	48.7
France	Tobacco use	1997	1.10	49.87
Finland	Tobacco use	1995	0.80	–
Hungary	Tobacco use	1998, 2002	3.2–4.0	–
Peru	Tobacco use	1997	0.77	–
Venezuela	Tobacco use	1997	0.30	–
Myanmar	Tobacco use	1999	0.14	–
China	Tobacco use	1989	1.50	74.4
Taiwan	Tobacco use	2001	0.50	77.8
India	Tobacco use	1990–91	0.02	–
South Korea	Tobacco use	1993–98	0.59–1.19	–
United States	Obesity	2000	1.20	47.86
Canada	Obesity	2001	0.73	69.81
Switzerland	Obesity	2002	0.64	–
Germany	Obesity	1998	0.20	48.2
India	Obesity	1995	1.10	67.3
China	Obesity	1995	2.10	23.8
Germany	Alcohol use	1995	1.13	–
France	Alcohol use	1997	1.42	56.51
Switzerland	Alcohol use	2001	0.14	n/a
United States	Depression	2000	0.85	68.6

Source: Suhrcke M., Nugent R, Stuckler D, et al. *Chronic disease: An economic perspective.* London: Oxford Health Alliance, 2006.

of chronic diseases across diseases, in different countries and over time. Second, many of these costs are likely to be underestimates, especially in resource-poor countries, because National Health Accounts do not always capture all treatment and surveillance systems underdiagnose the burden of chronic diseases used in these calculations of economic costs. Third some economists argue these methodological approaches represent a public health view of economic 'costs', not an actual economic perspective. They do not consider 'alternative futures', such as whether these costs could actually be reduced. Fourth, in relation to this lack of a counterfactual, these studies often narrowly focus on the financial consequences of health, usually on healthcare, and not on overall well-being or utility. These methods risk understating the true costs of chronic diseases, as people intrinsically put a high value on health. But they also could also overstate the costs, especially if people are knowingly choosing to eat, drink, and smoke despite the risks. Provocatively, one economist calls chronic disease deaths 'rational suicides', because people are fully aware that they are trading off health risks for the pleasure, or utility, they bring (179).

Finally, and importantly, in the presence of high social costs, societies find ways to adapt, as described in summarizing the household level evidence above. People are resilient—a concept used to define how individuals, families, communities, and societies positively adapt to major changes in their environment, or 'shocks' like a financial crisis or sickness. For example, climate change sceptics suggest that the economic costs of global warming will be low because humans can mitigate the potential social harms. As one example, in low-skill labour markets of developing countries, where there is often a surplus pool of workers, one person losing a job will be quickly replaced by another, leading to little change in the society's output. But, at the household level, the responses to disease could compensate initially to maintain a family's income but greatly add to the costs, especially ones that accrue many years later (economists identify 'income' and 'substitution' effects—where the latter refer to how the household can compensate to lost income by substituting labour). Evidence from Ethiopia in coffee-growing districts indicates that healthy household members worked more hours to compensate for the loss of working time by the sick adult and to provide care for the sick household member (170). Firms also attempt to counteract costs. Walmart, for example, has been accused of selectively employing workers who appeared to be healthier to minimize healthcare expenses. The company also at times has purchased life insurance policies on its workers. Mining companies in South Africa, concerned about HIV rates affecting its workforce, have been encouraged by consulting firms to create financial derivatives to offset potential losses to productivity in case an epidemic occurs at the mine.

Thus, there can be marked differences in how societies respond to illness, depending on the structure of labour markets and available social protections. These differences impede our ability to generalize the evidence about economic impacts of poor health and to predict the potential consequences in the future based on experiences of the past.

Clue 11: *Ways in which people, households and firms respond to the social consequences of chronic disease can either increase or decrease their costs to the economy, but also could risk greater social and economic consequences in the long run.*

In attempting to account for people's resilience and ways of coping with illness, we next turn to methods that can be used to either estimate economic impacts on the basis of historical experiences or to simulate economic impacts based on theoretical models of economic growth.

Mathematical models—neoclassical models of economic growth

One way to estimate the full effect of chronic diseases on social outcomes, accounting for how people have responded to sickness, is to use statistical models. This approach essentially assesses whether rates of economic growth were higher, lower or about the same when chronic diseases rates change. However, chronic diseases are not the only factor involved in determining whether countries grow or not; there could be many confounding factors (education, other diseases, savings, capital, etc.). In other words, the model has to be built on a foundation of strong theory about what causes growth.

The most widely used model of economic growth is called the 'neoclassical growth model', referred sometimes to as the Solow–Swan model after the economists who developed it. Consistent with the pathways set out in Figure 3.1, in the neoclassical growth model two key parameters determine whether a country grows: capital (K) and labour (L). In terms of L, greater health increases both supply and productivity. Better health also increases education, which further increases labour supply and productive. In terms of K, lower healthcare costs provide more money to be invested in physical capital, like machinery or productive equipment, that create additional goods and services. Better health also increases savings, as people spend less on healthcare, which can further add to a society's investments in its means of production.

Despite a strong theoretical basis, the neoclassical growth model is a relatively poor predictor of economies' actual growth experiences. In other words, they cannot account well for why some countries are growing faster or slower than others. This does not mean that the model is wrong; every model is wrong to some degree, the challenge is to choose the least wrong one. Doing so is, however, important.

Many development agencies focus on growth to lift countries out of poverty. But with about half of the variation in growth rates unexplained, there is clearly much to learn. Usually, the large unexplained component of growth (called the residual) is attributed to factors that are difficult to observe, such as technological change, which increases labour's productivity, referred to as 'total factor productivity'. Alternatively, the model's predictions could be inaccurate because the data used to generate them are measured with a lot of error. These inaccuracies could also relate to limitations of cross-national studies, which tend to rely on fewer data points and observations from which to draw inferences. One review found very few economic variables consistently to be significant predictors of economic growth (180). Others have pointed out that the results can vary substantially based on the researcher's choices about what to include or exclude from the model as control variables, which data sources are being used to estimate variables in the model (such as health or education or even which measure of GDP is chosen), and the potential for confounding (181).

Or could unexplained growth, at least in part, be caused by poor health?

Health status—measured as life expectancy or adult mortality—is a robust and strong predictor of economic growth rates according to the two major UN reports on this topic (154, 173). One study estimated that a 5-year increase in life expectancy will give a country a 0.3–0.5% higher annual GDP growth rate in subsequent years, a result that could in principle be used to infer a relationship between chronic disease mortality and growth. Other studies have assessed the impact of specific diseases—such as malaria, HIV/AIDS, malnutrition, height, and TB—on growth, controlling for a set of other standard determinants of growth. Nobel Prize-winning work by Fogel identified that as much as 30% of Britain's contemporary wealth related to progress in improving human health, and that, in part, health gains played a crucial role in Britain's faster industrialization in the 19th and early 20th century than its western European counterparts such as France and Germany.

Clue 12: There is strong historical evidence that health improvements have contributed to increasing economic performance.

Because chronic diseases make up a major portion of the global disease burden, especially of adult mortality, like other diseases they could be expected to affect growth adversely. However, there are a couple of reasons to argue that they might not. The long-term nature of chronic diseases might lead to less costly coping strategies (although HIV has been found to have high economic costs). Or the communicable nature of infectious diseases elicits high costs (although malaria does not spread from one person to another). Both explanations seem unlikely. In view of evidence found in individual-level studies, it is highly plausible that chronic diseases slow down economic growth. Yet, ultimately, ascertaining whether chronic diseases significantly affect economic growth is an empirical question.

Only a handful of studies have assessed the effects of chronic diseases on rates of economic growth. One study analysed the long-term effects of crude CVD rates among working-age population on growth rates in 26 rich countries over 5-year intervals covering the period 1960 to 2000 (109). Their model included a set of standard controls (such as initial income, openness to trade [sum of exports and imports as a fraction of GDP], and secondary schooling rates). To the extent that education rates, or returns to education, were significantly affected by CVD, these results would conservatively estimate the effects of CVD on growth. The researchers found that each 10% reduction in cardiovascular mortality rates was associated with 1% higher per capita growth. This seems like a small amount, but it adds up in the long run to a large figure.

A second study evaluated the long-term effects of crude NCD mortality rates over the period 1960–2002 in 23 high-income OECD countries (20). The model adjusted for inflation and education, shown in Table 3.2. It found both NCD and CVD mortality rates were associated with reduced economic growth rates. When savings rates were added to the model, this association was attenuated by about 15%, suggesting decreasing savings rates may have been an important pathway of chronic disease's economic effects.

The results from these two studies have to be interpreted with caution. First, both studies measured NCDs based on crude mortality rates, because they better reflect the healthcare costs arising from high rates of chronic diseases. Alternatively, the age-standardized rate could better capture broader social consequences of a high risk of chronic diseases among the poor, such as how high chronic disease risks influence individual decisions about whether to invest in education, save money, or seek jobs. Second, the data are of poor quality, as described in Chapter 1. Where there are no adult mortality or cause-specific data, especially true of low- and middle-income countries, NCDs rates are estimated from the country's level of income. This circularity in the data can make it difficult to detect a potentially causal relationship between NCDs and growth. Third, as the crude chronic disease burden has yet to develop (following an inverse U-shaped trajectory with rising income), the economic costs of chronic diseases may only become substantial in future years.

Clue 13: There is strong evidence that chronic diseases reduce economic growth.

Table 3.2 Effect of chronic noncommunicable disease working-age mortality rates on economic growth

Dependent variable: real GDP per capital change			
Covariate	Fixed-effects model, 1972–2000	Fixed-effects model, 1960–2002	Fixed-effects AR(1), 1960–2002
Log male CNCD working-age mortality rate	−5.11** (1.43)	−4.67*** (1.63)	−5.10*** (1.80)
Log inflation	−1.73** (0.37)	−0.74 (0.49)	−1.12*** (0.30)
Openness	0.01 (0.02)	0.06*** (0.02)	0.04* (0.02)
Secondary education levels	−0.02 (0.03)	0.03 (0.04)	0.01 (0.02)
Savings rate	0.23** (0.07)	0.07 (0.05)	0.06 (0.04)
Number of country years	532	758	758
Number of countries	20	23	23

Notes: Robust standard errors are in parentheses, clustered by country to reflect nonindependence of sampling and for robustness to serial correlation. AR(1) model uses panel-corrected standard errors (Beck and Katz 1995). Models include country-and time-fixed effects.

Significance at $*p < 0.05$, $**p < 0.01$, $***p < 0.001$.

Countries included: Australia, Austria, Belgium, Canada, Denmark, Finland, France, Germany, Greece, Ireland, Iceland, Italy, Japan, Mexico, Netherlands, New Zealand, Norway, Portugal, Spain, Sweden, Switzerland, United Kingdom, United States.

Given the lack of data in low-income countries, the authors of the two studies suggested that the chronic disease costs identified in high-income countries provides a model of what would be expected in low-income countries. Thus one study provided an out-of-sample estimate of the consequences of projected rises in chronic diseases for economic growth over the next 30 years (20). They estimated, for example, a 50% rise in chronic diseases—the amount expected in Latin America from 2002 to 2030—would be predicted to result in more than a 2% slowdown in economic growth each year. This is indeed a sizeable effect: by comparison, the US economy grows an average of about 2% every year.

A third WHO study analysed a similar economic growth model of 23 low-income countries with high NCD burdens (182). Instead of attempting to estimate the associations of chronic diseases with growth statistically, the researchers applied a mathematical model based on the neoclassical growth model, taking parameters from existing databases. This included treatment costs from the WHO-CHOICE methods and database (183). Limitations of these data have been described elsewhere; but, briefly, they lack comparability across countries and over time. The WHO model was highly conservative because it did not take into account labour productivity channels. On the other hand, its estimates of the impact of healthcare spending on economic output could be overstated because they failed to account for the principle that countries converge to a long-term growth equilibrium, such that any short-term change in capital is compensated for in subsequent periods. Nonetheless, the researchers did consider that higher mortality rates would reduce a population's labour supply and that higher consumption of healthcare could reduce savings rates (but failed to capture how shorter anticipated lifespans and higher time-discount rates could affect savings). Overall, they estimated that US $84 billion of economic output would be foregone between 2006 and 2015 as a result of the chronic disease burden in the 23 countries studied. However, this assumed a theoretical minimum of zero chronic disease death rates. Hence, they further estimated that *The Lancet*'s feasible goal of a 2% yearly reduction in death rates could save $8 billion, or about 10% of the total projected losses.

Another framework could draw on micro-level estimates of the consequences of chronic disease for worker's productivity and likelihood of employment to estimate L costs. This would apply demographic methods, drawing on life table techniques, to create a 'worktable', constructed using age-specific employment rates, available from the International Labour Organization. Like a mortality life table, these age-specific employment rates can be used to calculate 'worklife expectancy', a measure of L assuming employment conditions remain consistent in the future (the same assumption used in calculating life expectancy). Then, a 2% reduction in deaths due to chronic diseases at each age-band can be calculated and removed for age-specific workrates, giving rise to a new estimate of worklife expectancy. This method can also be used to identify the historical contribution of changes in mortality patterns to an economy's overall labour supply. Further refinements can improve the validity of this approach, such as accounting for differing productivity by age-group and the fact that those persons at risk of premature deaths were more likely to have been inactive.

Yet, controversially, several recent economic studies dismiss the preceding evidence that health affects the economy, arguing on the basis of the predictions of the underlying neoclassical growth model (the Solow–Swan model as described above). According to this model, technological advance is the only factor that can improve an economy's growth in the long run (184). The model predicts that over time countries will converge to a balanced growth path: a sustainable rate of growth given the country's supply of labour and capital. New investments in labour or capital simply speed up the rate of a country's convergence to this balanced growth path. Drawing on this prediction, a recent critique suggested that health (including NCDs) could lead to short-run growth, but not translate into higher long-run growth. Any short-run increase in growth that exceeds the long-run balanced growth path will be compensated for by medium-term reductions, as part of the process of convergence.

In supporting this theoretical prediction, the authors provide evidence that greater life expectancy is associated over the medium-term with reduced living standards, as increasing population size lowers GDP per capita (because the denominator grows) (185). Further the authors criticized findings suggesting that confounding was a problem, because the institutions associated with better life expectancy could in turn be the ultimate drivers of growth; however, what those institutions could be have not been specified and it remains plausible that health is an important pathway by which institutional development delivers economic benefits. It also remains to be determined whether or not these additional short-run periods of growth, even if they do not achieve longer-run higher growth rates, can lead to greater income levels.

Another common notion is that entire populations are caught in poverty traps. They lack labour supply to convert capital into production, and they lack production to create capital. Health is at the centre of this vicious cycle of poverty and illness. Short-run boosts in growth, according to this theory, could 'break the cycle', unleashing economic potential. However, precise evidence in support of this process is lacking.

No study, to our knowledge, has assessed the full welfare implications of health at the population level. An initial study has attempted to quantify how much well-being gains in life expectancy have achieved in Europe (186). To do this the authors had to estimate how much utility people derived from better health, ultimately drawing on estimates of how health related to utility by Nobel Prize-winning economist Gary Becker and colleagues (a so-called utility function) (187). The research team estimated, using Becker's estimates of the quantitative health-utility relationship, that the value of life expectancy gains in Western Europe between 1970 and 2003 were worth about 29–38% of GDP. In the Eastern European countries, where comparable data were available only for 1990–2003, the variation was even greater. Countries suffering declines in life expectancy (see Chapter 2 for a brief case study) incurred a welfare loss of 16–31%, whereas those gaining life expectancy, mainly central and Eastern European countries, realized benefits of 12–31% of GDP.

Clue 14: Investing in strategies to lessen the burden of chronic diseases could substantially help improve economic performance and people's overall quality of life.

Who suffers from these costs? Governments, firms, households, individuals . . .

So far we have documented high economic costs of chronic diseases, evident at both individual and population levels. A key question about resilience remains in understanding the social harm they cause: Who bears these costs—the individual or society?

Ultimately the answer is 'it depends'—mainly on whether social welfare systems are in place to protect people from the social consequences of NCDs. Without these safety nets, the burden tends to fall onto individuals, both in terms of healthcare and employment costs. For example, heavier reliance on private sources of funding, or out-of-pocket expenditure, shifts the burden of direct treatment costs onto the individual. On the other hand, systems such as the National Health Service in the UK pool risks of poor health, spreading the costs onto society. Because poor people are sicker than rich people (see Chapters 1 and 2), universal healthcare systems redistribute society's resources from the rich to the poor, acting as an equalizing force in society. While in the UK individuals ultimately pay for their healthcare in the form of higher taxes or lower wages, the overall cost is lower than systems lacking a mechanism to share health risks (as seen in comparing US healthcare spending, about 15% of GDP, versus Western Europe, about 8% of GDP).

Two issues arise from relying on individuals and families to pay for care themselves. First, a society's overall spending on health may be used less efficiently (that is, achieving lower health improvements for the same amount of money invested). Second, the broader social costs of NCDs may be much greater. There is evidence for both possibilities. For example, in settings where individuals pay for care out of their pockets, they tend to consume a greater portion of expensive, tertiary inpatient care, and less primary, preventive care (lowering efficiency). In other words, private-based systems of financing can lead people to wait until it is too late to seek care. They may use costly emergency care as a substitute for affordable primary care. In general, this situation is worse in poor countries, as a well-known observation is that the poorer a country, the greater the fraction of costs paid by sick people themselves.

Conversely, it has been argued that investing more resources in healthcare is unlikely to be cost saving. It is argued that chronic disease healthcare costs could be lower in countries that do not provide effective care because people die more quickly. In the design of Seguro Popular, the Popular Health Insurance scheme in Mexico, a burden of disease analysis found an 'advanced transition' to chronic diseases in the poorer segments of the population and an 'unmet demand [for chronic disease care which] has been serviced by the mostly unregulated private sector, with more than half of total spending on health paid out of pocket' (188). In such circumstances, the World Bank suggests 'improving health status is unlikely to be cost saving relative to a status quo in which only a few dollars per person are spent annually on chronic disease care'.

Yet if such a premature death occurs, as documented in the preceding sections, it is likely to come with significant medium- and longer-term costs that fall outside the healthcare system.

In cases where health infrastructure does not exist, the health systems spend excess sums providing treatment abroad. As one unique example (but one that applies in other remedial secessionist situations), in 2005, more than 31,000 patients in the occupied Palestinian territory were referred for treatment outside the Palestinian Ministry of Health facilities, both within the occupied Palestinian territory or in neighbouring countries. The total cost was about US$60 million (189).

Similarly, in the absence of employee protection systems, employment costs shift to the individual and can be greater overall. For example, if a person loses a job because a heart attack causes many lost work days, there are fewer cash benefits or worker reintegration programmes to help. This can lead to worse consequences to the worker's family than in the context of a social welfare system which provides financial support to the unemployed and services quickly to find gainful employment.

Other social welfare systems can spread costs to different groups, depending on how they are organized. In the US the employer-based insurance system means that sick workers add costs to running a company, because the firm pays higher healthcare premiums. This has become a significant operating cost to US firms, diminishing the US economy's global competitiveness and leading some firms to relocate to other countries. Several top US CEOs cite poor health as their top operating cost and concern about future viability of their business (190, 191). As a further example, the World Economic Forum, surveying the landscape of global risks for 2009, ranked NCDs as the third most likely risk to occur and the fourth most severe in its impact (192).

Ultimately, whether providing chronic disease care creates higher or lower costs overall is an empirical question. Careful analysis is needed to account for both the healthcare and employment costs. In general, there is evidence to support the notion that failing to provide NCD care could both delay and increase the overall expense to society.

Clue 15: Failing to provide care for persons living with chronic diseases could both delay and increase the overall expense to society.

Will the problem take care of itself? The evidence about failing markets . . .

Simply because failing to prevent chronic diseases will be expensive is not enough to justify broader public-policy intervention. People could be happier when they smoke, fully knowing the risks to their health. It would be unfair for policymakers to try to change their choices. Further, many economists view risks of chronic diseases like obesity as a sign of market success—an indication that the 'developing countries' are catching up with the 'developed countries' as markets spread goods and services. As one author of the World Bank World Development report put it, 'Isn't obesity a sign of progress?' It is sometimes argued by economists that, at worst, obesity is a collateral damage of development that we can live with.

In the prevailing view of public policy 'markets are always best'. The idea, drawing from Adam Smith, is that competitive markets will set prices to be in line with people's values. In doing so the market brings the most well-being to everyone involved. Any interference by the government would make people worse off and should be avoided—except under special circumstances.

These exceptions are called 'market failures'. In such cases the market will fail to bring about the greatest good for everyone involved. Simply put, this goes wrong when people don't take account of the harm they cause themselves or others. Let's examine how this can happen more closely.

Suppose you go to the store to buy cigarettes. The price is $3. Eager to smoke, you step out of the store, quickly light up, creating a cloud of smoke around you. People passing by you cough as they walk by, grumbling to themselves about the noxious smell.

This is a classic case of an 'externality'. This happens when one person takes part in a market, but creates costs for others who were not involved. The market will not account for these other people's interests. How could markets take into account the full price so that the smoker is a bit more considerate of the discomfort his tobacco use causes others?

One way is for one of the disgruntled customers to get upset, yank the cigarette from you, and stamp it out. Another customer might simply decide to kick you pretty hard instead. These reactions could go too far or not go far enough. If they could be factored in as costs, they would raise the price of the cigarette pack, perhaps to as high as $40 (as one group of economists estimated the true price of smoking), although unless the smoker was a trained economist, they may not be apparent. The usual approach to correcting these costs involves strategies like smoking bans, confining the smoker to places where no harm is caused, or putting in place taxes that try to estimate how much people suffer, so that smoking is reduced.

The basic idea of the policy is to try to correct the market failure, making the market work to keep everyone as happy as possible.

Leading institutions uphold this view of public policy. For example, the World Bank explicitly states that its Poverty Reduction programmes are not actually about poverty, but correcting these market failings. Before the US Office of Management and Budget office assess the costs and benefits of regulation, they require a detailed analysis of potential market failures. Yet sometimes externalities are invisible to policymakers—especially those afflicting the poor who may be excluded from markets (and political processes needed to correct these markets, see Chapter 5) that ultimately affect them in hidden ways.

Several other important types of market failures are worth flagging. Continuing with the example of tobacco, people may choose to smoke, fully knowing the risks. But these choices are compromised when people are incapable of informed decisions or the information they have has been manipulated. Children are commonly regarded as being unable to choose; hence age restrictions are in place. Tobacco companies were discovered to have falsely advertised health benefits of cigarettes; hence warning labels notifying users of the risks are introduced. Market failures of this kind are referred to as 'asymmetric information', where one group in the market exchange (in this case the tobacco company) has more information than the other, and 'imperfect information', when someone simply lacks necessary information or cannot use it properly, like children.

A final type of market failure is more controversial within economics. It relates to addiction. Do people become addicted knowingly (so-called rational addiction) (193)? Or do people inherently have predispositions to get 'sucked in' to addiction, preyed upon by highly professional marketing tactics? Clearly both can play a role. One aspect of addiction is common in tobacco. Return to the scene where you rushed into the store to buy cigarettes. Two days ago, you told yourself, 'no more smoking'. Yet each new day brings another personal failure. This is sometimes called 'time-inconsistent preferences'—acting as though you changed your mind one day to the next. A surprising finding has been that people report being happier when governments tax tobacco because it helped them achieve what they could not do on their own (194). Observing this puzzle, some argue that a key aim of a welfare state is to compress the time of decisions (i.e. convert longitudinal decisions into cross-sectional ones). When uncertainty and future planning enters the equation, people make mistakes, and government can help people make healthy choices they truly desire the easier choices (195).

Many examples of market failures exist, such as nutrition labelling and obesity (lack of information and imperfect information), environmental tobacco smoke and lung cancer (externality), alcohol and cirrhosis (time-inconsistent preferences) (4, 48, 109). Signs that market interventions can improve health and markets have been found. One example is that smoking bans led to increased use of bars in New York City. Further cases will be described in the next chapter summarizing social policy interventions.

Clue 16: In the presence of inadequate or imperfect information (an 'internality' whereby a person's market choice does not reflect their best outcome) and external consequences of decisions (an 'externality' whereby one person's market choice affects another person's well-being), markets for alcohol, food, and tobacco will be risk factors for chronic diseases

As made clear in Chapter 2, the societies in which people live are transforming rapidly. These changes are increasing risks of chronic disease. Foreign investment changes the scope of markets for goods and services. Viral Western marketing provides a narrow set of information about these products. These economic transformations can aggravate market failures. How does this change the appropriate roles for individuals and their governments to take care of rising chronic diseases? Do these transformations lead to better or worse market failures?

Trying to correct a market failure can make matters worse, especially when multiple market failures happen at the same time. For example, a market for tobacco in Moldova used to be run by inefficient, state-owned companies. To improve the economy, the IMF urged Moldova to privatize its company, opening up competition in the tobacco industry, as a condition on its loan to the country (196). When this happened, one market failure was solved—more competition lowered tobacco prices, making people happier. But the externalities of tobacco use grew much worse, making more people sick and unhappy (197). This is precisely the process at play in how many macroeconomic forces, however favourable to corporate interests, can create risks of chronic disease, as documented Chapter 2.

Clue 17: Correcting one market failure can exacerbate another market failure so to increase the risk of chronic disease.

This case illustrates why showing evidence of a market failure is not enough. It must further be shown that i) causes of chronic diseases contribute to these failures and that ii) society would be better off if the state intervened (rather than doing nothing). The case that market failures are giving rise to chronic diseases is becoming increasingly clear (109). The race is now on to see what will be done and by whom. Will the private sector correct these failures by becoming more responsive, or governments will be forced to step in?—A debate taken up in the next two chapters.

Clue 18: Failing markets will continue to spread chronic diseases.

Strategy 2: Public health experts can make a strong case for government intervention to reduce chronic diseases by showing that market failures increase risks of chronic diseases and showing that state intervention can correct these failures so to improve health outcomes.

Summary

Health is not the only thing people value in life. Economic perspectives can account for this basic fact. In doing so, they can create a powerful set of arguments to raise the importance of health to decision-makers.

But these perspectives can have a dark side. Debates about the economic costs of tobacco, thought to be resolved in rich countries, continue in resource-poor countries. Obesity and alcohol are going through the same, lengthy process of marshalling evidence about their economic costs in rich countries. It is a challenging process, at times confounded by the sophisticated economic arguments produced by vested interests to counter effective public health interventions.

Despite the evidence lacking detail for some poor countries, a large body of work about the economic costs reaches a central conclusion: caring for people with chronic diseases is expensive. However, there is an important second point. Not caring for people with chronic diseases could be even more expensive, because of the costly complications of untreated NCDs and the negative impacts on the labour market.

Much of the extensive work that has gone into identifying the economic costs of HIV, TB, and malaria apply directly to NCDs. In fact, the costs of NCDs may be even greater because they are so highly prevalent—rising in incidence and lasting lifetimes.

Policymakers should anticipate rising healthcare costs due to NCDs. These rises threaten to overwhelm resource-deprived health systems which are already struggling to control infectious disease burdens, such as HIV and TB.

Not paying for chronic disease care can delay and increase the expense. In situations where there is no healthcare, the consequences of NCDs are devastating—leading to a slow, painful death. In situations where there is no health insurance, the costs of care can be catastrophic and lead to impoverishment—trapping households in cycles of illness and poverty. In situations where there is health insurance, entire societies must still finance lifetimes of care for the sickest (and usually poorest) populations.

Living with a chronic disease also diminishes a person's opportunities to lead to a fully productive life. People with chronic disease work fewer hours, are less productive when they work, take more sick days, and are more likely to retire at a younger age. This adds up to a significant burden to a society's economic potential.

Chronic diseases, left unchecked, will slow down emerging economies, like Brazil and India. As rises in chronic diseases will be concentrated in poor countries, chronic diseases will contribute to a widening economic gap between the global North and South.

We conclude with a question: who will take action? Will it be governments, through concerted social policy, or the private sector and individuals, through personal and voluntary choices? In the following chapters, we contrast two views about the appropriate roles of each group and explore alternative strategies for preventing and managing chronic disease.

Endnotes

1 There are argued to be exceptions, such as in rational-choice models explaining the decision to participate in suicide bombing

2 A key principle in economics is that if a person prefers *a* to *b* and *b* to *c*, the person also prefers *a* to *c*. This is a property known as transitivity. However, this principle becomes complicated in the context of co-morbidities. For example, looked at individually, a person might believe heart disease is worse than diabetes is worse than lung cancer. Yet when diseases interact, such as when diabetes and heart disease together create much worse suffering than either disease alone, a person might believe heart disease and diabetes is worse than lung cancer but heart disease and lung cancer worse than diabetes. Such interactions greatly complicate the techniques needed to ascertain the value of avoiding disease.

3 Similarly, firms can try to compensate for high economic costs.

Chapter 4

Comprehensive strategies to reduce the burden of chronic diseases

◆ What are the best ways to reduce the burden of chronic disease?

David Stuckler, Karen Siegel, Kathleen O'Connor Duffany, Sandeep Kishore, Denise Stevens, and Sanjay Basu

Part 1

Management of chronic disease

Key policy points

1 Systems of chronic disease care in high-income countries are largely uncoordinated and fragmented, as many patients receive treatment that fails to meet recommended standards and results in high rates of medical errors; the situation is far worse in low-income countries.

2 There is a need to reorient healthcare delivery from acute, episodic care to long-term, patient-centred management.

3 There are dangers in transposing current models of care in high-income countries, especially the US model, to resource-poor settings.

4 The emphasis on narrow, vertical and highly biomedical models of intervention is a barrier to scaling up prevention and treatment interventions. More focus is needed on interconnected health risks and outcomes, such as tobacco use and the spread of tuberculosis.

5 Practical approaches to scaling up chronic disease treatment and access can build on existing logistic routes and facilities used to deliver and monitor antiretroviral therapy for HIV and directly observed therapy for tuberculosis.

6 Market forces alone are unlikely to transform health systems into models of care that are appropriate for helping people with long-term illness.

Key practice points

1 There is a need to rethink how we train and learn medicine and public health in order to break out of the smallpox paradigm that focuses on a limited set of magic-bullet interventions.

2 Until the 1960s medical care had little effect on chronic disease, as the greatest health gains came about as a consequence of improvements in housing, sanitation, safe water, improved nutrition, employment, wages, and education. The future scope of personal care to contribute to extend human life, in the absence of a major unanticipated breakthrough, is likely to be limited. The main healthcare challenge is to ensure that those who can benefit from existing knowledge are able to do so.

3 We should be critical of unproven strategies to shift health service planning from need to demand, turning patients into consumers, and transforming health into a private market good.

Caring for persons with chronic disease: the role of the healthcare system

Let's flash back to the story of one of public health's biggest successes: the campaign to eradicate smallpox. A contagious disease, causing painful fluid-filled blisters, smallpox killed about one out of every four victims. Those who survived were never the same; most had severe scarring, blindness, or deformed limbs. No effective treatment was ever developed, but in 1796 the microbiologist Edward Jenner found that an injection of a similar disease, cowpox, could provide immunity. Providing this effective vaccine, together with improving living conditions, enabled several European countries and the US to eliminate smallpox by the early 1900s. Nevertheless, throughout the 20th century, smallpox killed more than 300 million people, mainly in low-income countries (198).

Recognizing the gross unfairness of avoidable deaths due to smallpox when cheap, preventative strategies were available, in 1958 the Russian health minister, Viktor Zhakov, called on the World Health Assembly to launch a major initiative to eradicate smallpox. A global plan was approved the next year, but little action was taken for another decade. In the 1960s smallpox continued to infect 10–15 million people and cause about 2 million deaths each year, until 1967, when WHO invested $2 million per year to set up an international Smallpox Eradication Unit. The Smallpox Eradication team, led by American physician Donald Henderson, had a global mandate to implement a comprehensive strategy to identify cases aggressively, isolate infected patients, and mass vaccinate close relatives (estimated to cost about $0.14 per person) (199). Within a decade smallpox was eradicated (200).

Such a heroic scenario will never work for chronic diseases. Beyond the obvious point that no single treatment exists that can prevent or cure all chronic diseases, the daily realities of managing chronic diseases are far more complex. Doctors alone cannot solve chronic diseases, but have to work with patients to manage chronic diseases together so that the disease does not lead to painful complications like amputations or blindness. Not just the patients but entire communities are the scope of treatment, as the causes of chronic diseases are deeply embedded in the current and unhealthy way that modern societies are being engineered (see Chapter 2).

So far, however, the global responses to rising chronic diseases have continued to perpetuate what has been called a 'smallpox paradigm': a focus on seeking to eradicate diseases using drugs and medical technology (201). In the smallpox paradigm, well-functioning healthcare systems to care for patients are not needed, because teams of Western scientists can administer a few key, low-cost technological interventions that can save millions of lives. To date, smallpox is the only infectious disease to have been conquered using this approach, as other eradicable infections (such as polio, measles, malaria, and TB) continue to kill. Yet the smallpox vision and its ambition to get rid of human disease using a medical approach continues to dominate global health thinking (an imperialist discourse that has links to the colonial mantra that Europeans had a moral duty to conquer and enlighten people from their primitive darkness) (201). Shortly after the last case of smallpox occurred in 1977 in Somalia, WHO launched its major 'Health for All' strategy, declaring boldly that 90% of all human disease could be prevented through a series of low-cost interventions.

These health fantasies are inappropriate models for building health systems. Their focus, principally on acute, medically-oriented care, has been perpetuated by a private-sector focused model of health system development relying on donor funding (in the case of the world's most deprived countries), markets, and a lingering quest for magic bullet solutions. In practice, this paradigm has meant that real healthcare system needs have fallen by the wayside, including basic things like training people, paying them, organizing an administrative and logistical system for delivering drugs and care, and establishing health centres and hospitals in deprived areas.

Box 4.1 State of chronic disease management in Africa

How are chronic diseases currently managed in the routine healthcare settings of African countries? In brief, badly. Anecdotal reviews point to poorly managed healthcare systems with frequent stock interruptions of essential drugs. Untreated hypertension is blamed for high rates of stroke morbidity and mortality in urban and rural Tanzania and rural South Africa. Only a small proportion of patients with epilepsy receive drug treatment at any one time, mainly due to poor healthcare delivery systems and unavailability of drugs. Even in specialist centres, asthma patients are given substandard care and have poor access to essential medications. There is a growing burden of diabetes mellitus and its associated complications, and many patients with type 1 diabetes mellitus have extremely short life expectancies. Some of us know from personal experience of running routine diabetes and hypertension clinics in African hospitals that there are no formalized systems of recording how many patients have been diagnosed and started on therapy, how many are retained on therapy, or what proportion have died or developed complications. We treat patients with whatever drugs are available, and consider that our mission is accomplished. In summary, unstructured and unmonitored clinical care and little information about morbidity or mortality from chronic diseases are mostly the norm in sub-Saharan Africa.

Source: http://www.plosmedicine.org/article/info:doi/10.1371/journal.pmed.0050124.

Reflecting decades of neglecting the health system's needs, the current state of chronic disease care in resource-poor settings is, for lack of a better phrase, appalling. Doctors scrap together chronic disease medicines, at least when they are available, often making up care regimens on the fly for patients who they may see only once or twice, typically when it is already too late to make a difference (see Box 4.1). Patients, when they think doctors can actually help them (which at times is questionable), are often stuck paying for costly care themselves. In many cases the patients, rather than waiting in long lines for affordable public care, choose to take matters into their own hands, seeking care outside the healthcare system, such as herbal remedies (in richer countries) or traditional healers (in poorer countries).

Indeed, the challenge is not just among resource-poor countries. In the US, where money is plenty, technology is the most advanced in the world, and the government has made improving chronic disease care its top healthcare priority, chronic care has been described as 'severely under-developed', 'underfunded', and 'fragmented' (202, 203). The majority of people who live with chronic diseases receives care that fails to meet basic medical guidelines. Surveys of chronic disease patients indicated that over one-third were unable to afford a necessary service, one-fifth found that those necessary services were simply unavailable, and another 13% felt the quality of chronic disease services was so poor that they were not worthwhile. Only about 3% of US state health budgets actually is used to address what made people sick from chronic diseases in the first place. As the Centers for Disease Control and Prevention (CDC) put it: 'the nation's public health system framework is severely underdeveloped to address the tremendous burden of chronic disease . . . Coordinated and comprehensive national chronic disease prevention efforts have not been nearly adequately or systematically applied' (202) (see Figure 4.1).

The challenge of designing societies and care systems that meet current health demands is therefore substantial in all regions of the world. Neither rich nor poor countries can afford to continue along the path they have followed. But the most intractable problems are in resource-deprived settings: the countries with the worst burdens of disease have the fewest resources to address them. It is a paradox known as the 'inverse care law', as displayed in Figure 4.2 plotting

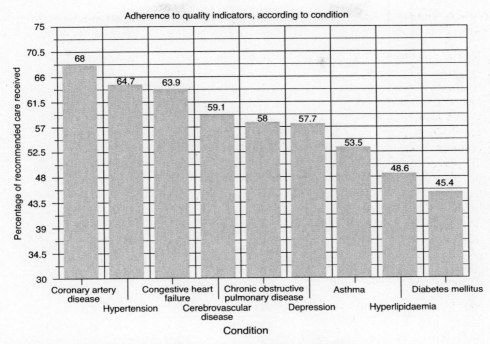

Fig. 4.1 The quality of healthcare delivered to adults in the United States.
Source: Data from McGlynn EA, Asch SM, Adams J, et al. The quality of healthcare delivered to adults in the United States. *New England Journal of Medicine* 2003; **348**:2635–45.

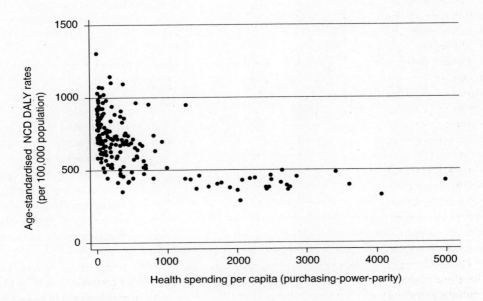

Fig. 4.2 Inverse care law and chronic diseases, 164 countries, 2004. Each dot represents one country's value for the year 2004.

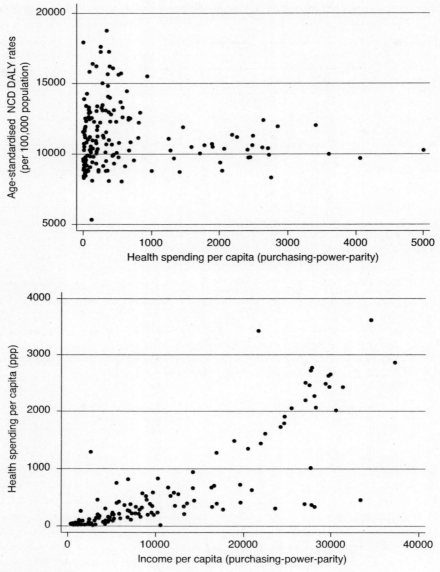

Fig. 4.2 (Continued)

health spending per capita against the age-standardized burden of chronic diseases (r = −0.61, p <0.001, 191 countries).

What can we do to adapt existing care systems to be more appropriate for dealing with society's increasingly chronic needs?

The rest of this chapter addresses this question in two parts. The first half discusses the approaches to caring for persons with chronic diseases. The second half assesses the potential to prevent people from getting sick in the first place by acting on the underlying social determinants of chronic diseases. In the first half of the chapter, we provide a brief historical overview of how medical care systems came to focus on a narrow set of medical challenges, relying on curative approaches to infectious diseases (the smallpox paradigm). Then, we set out an alternative chronic care model of healthcare that is better designed for people living with chronic diseases, what we call liberatory medicine. After reviewing the context of health system development, namely the debate between Primary Health Care and the interim Selective Primary Health Care strategy, the rest of the section discusses ways of transforming existing systems to the chronic care model. We also consider how to deliver chronic care to people in real-life clinical settings as well as to find the money to pay for it. We conclude with a note of caution about relying too heavily on market-driven healthcare and medical interventions in attempts to extend human life and alleviate suffering.

A brief history of the development of healthcare systems: the focus on acute care . . .

Healthcare systems grew out of informal systems of social protection at the turn of the 19th century. It was a period of major social and economic transformations—the Industrial Revolution—that created 'winners' and 'losers'; as documented by authors like Charles Dickens, it was the best of times for a few and the worst of times for the rest. Among those for whom it was the worst, life was short, brutal, and sickly, with a life expectancy of less than 40 years of age. Both rich and poor had only about a 50/50 chance of their health improving after an encounter with a doctor, yet significant inequalities in health existed, as the rich were able to avoid infectious diseases through patterns of geographic segregation, for example, by living at higher altitudes and less densely populated settings, limiting rates of contact with pathogens such as cholera. Medical care, if it could be called that, was provided through private, voluntary philanthropy, often bundled with other social services, such as financial relief or food rations. In the US, churches and non-governmental organizations (NGOs), like the American Red Cross, delivered these welfare services. In places like the UK, these services were state-sponsored, legally mandated by Poor Laws, and provided through so-called workhouses for paupers (then a legal term describing impoverished, jobless people). These informal systems began to give way as the welfare state, including the National Health Service, was introduced in the UK in 1948.

Infectious diseases were the dominant threat to public health during this period. Appropriately, healthcare systems were designed to focus on acute events, requiring advanced, but episodic, clinical care. With the discovery of sulfonamides in the 1930s, and its strongly protective effects on bacterial infections such as streptococci, and subsequently penicillin (by accident) in 1928, medicine could begin to aim to cure disease. Driven by a combination of scientific progress (especially laboratory science, imaging, asepsis, and pharmacology, including anaesthesia), healthcare systems rapidly expanded. The early 20th century also marked a transition from guilds to professions; doctors emerged as one of the most powerful professions, setting up the American Medical Association and basing their social standing on their command of the biological and pharmacological sciences (204). These forces came together in the development of hospitals as the epicentre of care, where doctors were 'captains of the ship', commanding teams of nurses, caretakers, and even secretaries. In this system patients played a minor role, bringing little to the clinic other than their illness.

An alternative model was experimented with in Russia, which, shortly after the October Revolution to communism, adopted the first universal healthcare system in 1918, the so-called 'Semashko' system. Its basic principles were government responsibility for health; universal access to free services; a preventive approach to social diseases; quality professional care; a close relation between science and medical practice; and continuity of care between health promotion, treatment, and rehabilitation. Despite rhetoric prioritizing healthcare, such as Lenin's statements about typhus that 'if communism does not destroy the louse, the louse will destroy communism', the system was grossly underfunded. Health was allocated money according to the principle of 'leftovers', as defence and military sectors took the first major cut of state spending and whatever remained went to health (205). In practice, the system also emphasized specialist care (all doctors were specialists) in hospitals (like other sectors of the economy there was a tendency towards gigantism). Although the Semashko system had remarkable success, being one of the first countries to eradicate smallpox and maintaining very low rates of tuberculosis until the 1990s, it failed to keep pace with the West in addressing heart disease in the 1960s (206).

These healthcare systems, with their focus on infectious diseases, were spread to the Latin American, Africa, and Asian countries by major European colonizers, Britain and France. Referred to as systems of 'imperial medicine', they imported the basic features of Western models, centring on acute care, but with an added emphasis on maintaining the health of troops (who would soon leave) against indigenous seasonal threats like mlaria and hookworm. Those countries with stronger ties to the Soviet Union, such as Ethiopia, incorporated the Semashko principles to a greater extent; reflected in Ethiopia's decision to provide free medical care to the needy in 1977 (albeit less than half the population were found to have access in the year 2000).

Clue 1: Historically, healthcare systems have been set up in a period when acute, infectious diseases were dominant. This has resulted in a focus on the smallpox paradigm.

Breaking down the acute, infectious disease care paradigm

Each of these historical systems of care for infectious diseases, as put in practice, is poorly suited to the challenges of chronic diseases, for three reasons. First, the medical approach to caring for people with chronic diseases is not curative, but instead aims to halt the progressive degeneration that chronic diseases cause, a strategy referred to as maintenance management. For example, type 2 diabetes patients who need renal dialysis will require a lifetime of services, which are often to be provided in accessible, local settings and outside of hospitals. We may not be able to cure chronic diseases, but may be able to prevent, postpone, and lessen avoidable suffering.

Second, chronic diseases come with extensive complications and co-morbidities, requiring extensive coordination and management. During a person's lifetime, most people will experience more than one chronic disease, especially for people living in rich countries. For example, most men who live to average life expectancy will experience prostate cancer, but are more likely to succumb to CVD. In cases when morbidities coexist, the patient does not simply have diabetes and slight allergy or increased susceptibility to colds, but a combination of major conditions that require unique treatments to be coordinated by healthcare providers. Such interrelated conditions can leave patients to be 'ping-ponged' from one specialist to another, receiving treatments that can potentially compromise care of other conditions, often with little coordination or oversight. It is not uncommon for persons over the age of 65 to be taking more than 20 different medications in a complicated sequence on a daily basis, creating risks of adverse interactions and risks of medically-induced causes of illness (iatrogenic causes).

Third, the marked differences in each patient's biological circumstances require treatment regimens that are tailored to their specific needs. Such differences can also be social in nature. Ethnic minority and low socioeconomic status patients are known to adhere less well to treatment, increasing their risk of debilitating complications and morbidities. Strategies, to be successful, also have to consider how to address not just the patient's biology but environmental circumstances that lead to what doctors call a 'revolving door', whereby patients cycle in and out of the doctor's office for seemingly avoidable health problems and complications of chronic diseases.

Clue 2: Current healthcare systems are inappropriate for caring for people living with chronic diseases.

What is an appropriate alternative system of care that could be implemented in daily medical practice?

Restructuring toward chronic disease care models: liberatory medicine

When a patient visits a doctor, the encounter traditionally plays out as follows: the patient describes a set of symptoms, often involving pain or discomfort; then the doctor evaluates the patient's symptoms, making a final diagnosis and prescribing medication, procedures, or additional diagnostic tests. It is analogous to what sociologist Paolo Freire called a 'banking system' approach to education: students open their mouths, and teachers deposit information (207).

Dealing with chronic diseases, however, requires a new model that puts patients at the centre. This reflects the importance of the patient's day-to-day management of their condition and the need for adhering to treatment standards. Chronic diseases shift the burden of achieving successful treatment from residing squarely with doctors to also including their patients. Continuing with the example of education, Freire alternatively called for a broader model of education, what he termed 'liberatory education', envisioning an exchange of information between teacher and student that put them on equal footing. In its broadest sense, education is 'any act or experience that has a formative effect on the mind, character or physical ability of an individual'. In other words, the best kind of chronic disease care can be viewed as an education.

Clue 3: The best kind of chronic care is an education.

This vision is commonly referred to as a 'chronic disease care' model (CCM) (208). While the specific components of CCM vary (for example, the International Chronic Care Model), it is generally designed to offer a holistic treatment of patient needs. The main model, developed by Edward Wagner, emphasizes the following aspects (Figure 4.3):

1 Continuity of care;

2 Preventing unnecessary hospitalization;

3 Coordinating and integrating care services;

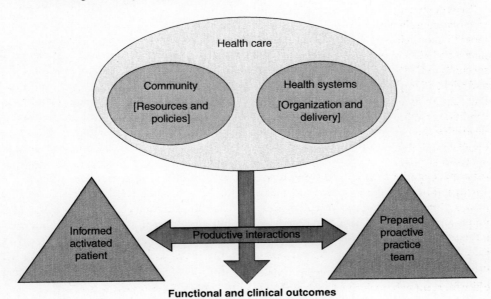

Fig. 4.3 Model for improvement of chronic illness care.
Source: Adapted from Wagner EH. Chronic disease management: What will it take to improve care for chronic illness? *Effective Clinical Practice* 1998; **1**:2–4.

4 Empowering patients to know about and manage their conditions (self-care); and

5 Joint decision-making between doctors and patients (collaborative care).

A more compact way of viewing the model emphasizes the three 'C's of the CCM: Continuity, Coordination, and Collaboration. We regard the CCM as a model of liberatory medicine,[1] because, much like liberatory education, it empowers patients to play active roles in defining their care needs and establishes a reciprocal relationship between doctor and patients.

Strategy 1: On the supplier-side, chronic care models emphasize continuity of care, preventing hospitalizations, and coordinating and integrating care services. On the patient-side, these models give patients and their families a greater voice in defining their care needs and finding appropriate solutions.

Implementing this approach requires a substantial change to the status quo (209).

Doctors, rather than playing the role of the expert, caring for patients sick in hospitals beds, would operate more like managers, coordinating a range of care services for multiple conditions. Similar to how a financial planner might help a family plan ahead for a healthy retirement, doctors would help their patients plan for a long, healthy life. In fact, doctors may be overqualified for the skill-set required; relying on a team-based approach, including nurse practitioners or physicians assistants, could provide more personnel needed to invest time and care for helping patients manage a lifetime of chronic disease.

Clinical consultations, traditionally a one-on-one encounter with a doctor, might be with nurses, dieticians, or counsellors, or even possibly all three at the same time. On the patient side, they would involve an entire family, so to identify the barriers to appropriate, long-term management of household chronic disease risks.

Instead of a medical clinic, the doctor's office would aim to create a kind of 'medical home', a place where families can see one main doctor who coordinates the patient's care (usually clinics are constructed in architectural ways that reinforce divides between patients and practitioners). For most doctors, especially those in training, the hospital is the starting point, where all the action occurs. But for people working in public health, the hospital is the end point, the sign of a failure to prevent sickness.

Strategy 2: Changing the status quo involves changing roles for doctors to manage long-term care, a team-based approach, and creating a medical home.

However desirable the CCM may sound, a note of caution is in order. First, the CCM in its entirety has not been tested. We cannot point to any clear-cut success stories of large-scale implementation of all components of the CCM in practice (although some successes in establishing medical homes for children with genetic defects have been reported). Yet, as Wagner and Groves put it, 'the efficacy of coordinated and patient centred care is established, but now is the time to test its effectiveness' (208). Second, relying more heavily on knowledge in care can also disadvantage people with less education or who are illiterate or have disabilities or language barriers; people can also be flawed in their self-assessments and management approaches. Third, shifting more duties of care onto patients without providing support or health education could lead to unintended harms. One example is the shift from providing mental healthcare in institutions to community settings in the 1980s. It was indeed an agreed upon measure, but, unfortunately, the resources for providing community care were not provided. In the US, deinstitutionalization of mental health hospitals in a period of rising social inequality under President Reagan led to a rising number of homeless persons and stigma of persons who have mental disorders (210). Fourth, there are those who oppose such an approach on ethical grounds; just as the 'nanny state' should not interfere with people's lifestyle choices, so do some doctors argue that they should similarly avoid attempting to promote health through lifestyle modification relating to physical activity or unhealthy diet (211).

Even if there was robust evidence that the CCM would improve chronic disease outcomes, major social, political, economic, and cultural barriers exist to transforming health systems. One contemporary example is the major political challenge in the US simply to put in place a healthcare system that provides insurance for the majority of its population. In terms of achieving reform towards a CCM model, the greatest barrier to change is funding. Current reimbursement structures have been designed with interests of doctors, not patients (212). Often they reward doctors based on numbers of physician–patient encounters and pay higher salaries for specialty care. The second barrier is the conservative values in the medical profession. Doctors cherish their salaries and their professional autonomy; there are fears among them that the CCM could reduce both. A third barrier is technological. Considerable research, supported by pharmaceutical companies, has been invested in finding expensive (and profitable) medical technologies for treating chronic diseases. Few, if any, of these expensive kinds of medical care and technologies being developed are appropriate or can simply be transposed to resource-poor settings. A fourth barrier is administrative capacity. Re-orienting an entire system requires resources; who will be assigned the role to develop the blueprints for re-engineering the systems of medical care?

Another key barrier is cultural: it is difficult to change the way people do things, changing their habits. Doctors are not prepared, and often not interested, in the daily, more pedestrian realities of coordinating chronic disease care. In managing chronic diseases, there are no medical heroes who save lives on the operating table. A related barrier is that many medical professionals have focused their entire lives on treating patients who are already sick (i.e. pulling bodies out of the river), often at the expense of an understanding of the factors that operate upstream. Of those doctors who obtain public health perspectives, most acquire them through professional channels linked to infectious disease control, perpetuating an acute-care model of public health. Similarly, patients are not taught to manage their illnesses, and, in the context of brief doctor visits, it is difficult to factor time in for such learning. One strategy for overcoming these barriers draws inspiration from models of community-based care, outlined in the case study in the introduction to Chapter 1.

Public Health Theorem: current systems of care cannot be changed without making someone worse off.

Clue 4: *There are substantial professional, institutional, and commercial barriers to transforming healthcare systems to focus on preventative and chronic care models.*

A final barrier, the system's current organization and resources, is one of the most substantial. It determines who pays, who delivers, and, ultimately, who gets chronic disease care, so it is worth addressing it in greater detail—as expressed in the debate between Primary and Selective Health Care.

The context of chronic disease care: primary health care and selective primary healthcare

In Figure 4.2 we showed that the poorer a country is, the fewer public resources it has available for public health. An important corollary is that the poorer a country is, the greater the burden of paying for care is placed on the poor (with high degrees of out-of-pocket spending).

These two challenges have been an overarching struggle for the field of public health. As Nobel economist Gunnar Myrdal famously noted in the 1950s, 'people are sick because they are poor, and people are poor because they are sick'. In short, poor people are almost always the sickest, have the fewest resources, and are expected to pay the most for their care. How can we design more equitable systems of public health so that poor people do not face the dual disadvantage of poverty and a lifetime of disease?

Restructuring health systems into chronic care models is part of this struggle. The debate centres on how to address poor health in resource-poor settings. One model calls for providing universal access to a comprehensive set of sanitation, hygiene, education, and broader public health interventions (a horizontal model). An alternative model disputes this approach, arguing it is far too expensive, instead recommending a limited set of technical interventions that could yield the greatest health gains at low cost for the populations at greatest risk of specific diseases (a vertical model). The former model, backed by WHO in the 1970s, came against powerful (albeit indirect) opposition from the World Bank.

In 1978, the WHO's *Declaration of the Alma-Ata* outlined its Primary Health Care (PHC) model, building on a predecessor WHO-UNICEF report, *Alternative Approaches to Meeting Basic Health Needs in Developing Countries* (1975). By 'alternative', the report meant a shift from narrow disease-specific interventions to a focus on building health systems:

> Primary health care is essential health care based on practical, scientifically sound and socially acceptable methods and technology made universally accessible to individuals and families in the community through their full participation and at a cost the community and country can afford to maintain at every stage of their development in the spirit of self-reliance and self-determination. It forms an integral part both of the country's health system, of which it is the central function and main focus, and of the overall social and economic development of the community. It is the first level of contact of individuals, the family and community with the national health system bringing health care as close as possible to where people live and work, and constitutes the first element of a continuing health care process.

Like the CCM, the PHC model envisioned a coordinated approach to healthcare, focusing on preventing hospitalizations, resisting overspecialization, empowering patients, and sharing decision-making between doctors and patients. PHC drew on examples of successful primary healthcare experiences in Bangladesh, China, Cuba, India, Niger, Nigeria, Tanzania, Venezuela, and Yugoslavia (213). With the slogan 'Health for All by the Year 2000', PHC developed into WHO's *Health for All* platform, set out at the first international conference of health promotion in the *Ottawa Charter* (WHO 1986). At the original Alma-Ata conference, H. Mahler of WHO cast the challenge in bold terms:

> Are you ready to introduce, if necessary, radical changes in the existing health delivery system so that it properly supports [primary health care] as the overriding health priority? Are you ready to fight the political and technical battles required to overcome any social and economic obstacles and professional resistance to the universal introduction of primary health care?

Ultimately, the PHC model was endorsed by all 134 countries and 67 international organizations attending the conference at Alma-Ata, USSR.

The delegates may have been ready and willing, but were unable to implement PHC. By the 1990s, the Structural Adjustment policies of the World Bank and IMF were fully in place (see Chapter 2 for more details), and countries were obligated to follow the macroeconomic advice of these institutions, as they were mired in debt after the Volcker Shock of the 1980s. At the time the World Bank's economic model focused heavily on privatization and low inflation targets, approaches that were inconsistent with the expanded role of the state required to deliver the WHO's Primary Health Care model. Instead, the World Bank invented an alternative model focusing on market principles, which came to be known as Selective Primary Health Care (154), regarding health as individual responsibility and healthcare as a private good. Responding to WHO, the World Bank wrote: 'The goal set at Alma Ata is above reproach, yet its very scope makes it unattainable because of the cost and numbers of trained personnel required. Indeed, the World Bank has estimated that it would cost billions of dollars to provide minimal, basic (not comprehensive health services) by the year 2000 for all the poor in developing countries'. The World Bank concluded that comprehensive PHC 'in the near future remains unlikely'; the effectiveness of basic PHC 'has not been clearly established'; and that the financial investment for sanitation and clean water 'is enormous' (214); and as such, it instead proposed that market principles and choosing interventions based on cost-effectiveness criteria could bring about more efficient delivery of health services. In general, it would focus on magic-bullet style solutions to infectious diseases. As the authors explained in their seminal paper 'Selective Primary Health Care: An interim strategy for disease control' (215):

> Faced with the vast number of health problems of mankind, one immediately becomes aware that all of them cannot be attacked simultaneously. In many regions priorities for instituting control measures must be assigned. And measures that use the limited human and financial resources available most effectively and efficiently must be chosen. Health planning for the developing world thus requires two essential steps: selection of diseases for control and evaluation of different levels of medical intervention from the most comprehensive to the most selective . . .

The World Bank's original set of recommended 'best-buy' approaches was eventually reduced to four interventions, known as GOBI, which stood for Growth monitoring, Oral rehydration techniques, Breast feeding, and Immunization. These were easy to monitor and evaluate, and had clear, measurable targets.

Powerful groups, doctors, UNICEF and the US, backed the World Bank's Selective Health Care Model and its vertical principles, contributing to WHO's ultimate defeat, as Selective Primary Health Care prevailed (see Chapter 5.2). Box 4.2 describes some of its implications for health system reform in the Philippines.

Clue 5: Transforming care systems to be more appropriate for delivering chronic care is part of a broader struggle to implement Primary Health Care. Over the past three decades the dominant global health institutions have sought to maintain a focus on quick-fix, magic bullet solutions, using an Alternative Selective Primary Health Care model.

Finding ways to deliver and pay for chronic disease care

Even though 'Health for All by the Year 2000' failed, to many people working in public health PHC (and, within it, CCM) remains a major public health goal. In 1997 the Pan American Health Organization (PAHO) revived calls for 'Health for All for the 21st Century' (216), echoed more recently by the call of the WHO Commission on the Social Determinants of Health to return to the principles of the Alma Ata (1).

Principles of PHC are represented in prevailing approaches to scaling-up treatment of HIV and TB. Previously an acute death sentence, HIV is now a chronic disease; requiring approaches for clinical management similar to the CCM. Both HIV/AIDS and chronic diseases have long-term and potentially debilitating clinical manifestations that result in physical and mental disability. Both require systems of long-term care and management, with patients playing greater roles in the success of treatment. Hence, it is worth briefly reviewing the approach to HIV management, as those models set the groundwork for improving chronic disease care in resource-deprived communities.

Adapting existing HIV and tuberculosis clinics to meet chronic care needs

In the 1980s and 1990s, as part of Selective Primary Health Care, approaches to HIV intervention, guided by cost-effectiveness criteria, focused on the lowest cost, easiest to implement interventions

Box 4.2 From Primary Health Care to Selective Primary Health Care: the case of the Philippines

In 1981 the Philippines was one of the first countries to adopt PHC. International publications heralded the 'impressive achievements [that] have been attained in this sector by contrast with reversals in many other sectors of the economy' (Philips 1986).

This situation began to change with the transition to democracy in 1986 and indebtedness to western financial institutions. Concerns about another dictator contributed to privatization and decentralization reforms that greatly shrunk the role of the state in financing and providing healthcare. Between 1980 and 1999, the Philippines underwent continual Structural Adjustment, receiving more than nine loans with extensive conditionalities (Bello 1999). Tariffs were nearly cut in half, resulting in a rapid drop in Gross National Product; firms went bankrupt and costs of living became more expensive. By 1987, over half of the government's budget went to repaying its $26 billion debt. Families living under the poverty line reached 46.5% and inequalities rose.

To save money in a period of austerity, PHC was discarded in favour of Selective Primary Health Care. Services were devolved to the local level to relieve state budget pressure. Overall public funding shrank; in 1991 healthcare was 2.7% of GNP, and private funds accounted for about three-fifths of all spending.

Coordination of health services collapsed. Legally, they were delegated from provincial to the municipal level, but no one told the municipalities this had happened or what to do. For example, several years after malaria-control was devolved to the local level, the local officials were still under the impression that provinces were responsible for the programmes.

After provincial governments stopped asking rural health units for the plans, the rural health units stopped planning. As one scholar put it, the rural health planning system 'withered away' (Espino 2004). A multi-agency UN study found that no funds were budgeted locally for TB control, concluding 'The role of the state had been reduced to a situation where it neither pursued the interest of the public nor protected the individual against harm caused by the behaviours of others. Effective disease control cannot be implemented without strong and functioning health systems and health system performance cannot be improved without considering which purpose the system is to serve'.

The health system has yet to fully recover. In 2004 at the World Social Forum, Filipino participants noted 'Public health is becoming a commodity. "Cost effectiveness" is becoming the criteria for determining who gets health care'. Yet, today, grassroots organizing is forming to resist the inequitable developments over the past two decades. As one director of community health education in Northern Philippines put it, 'We are organizing on the grassroots level, establishing community health programmes that include traditional medicines. What we are seeing is a global policy, a worldwide effort to privatize healthcare. It's important, therefore, to build a global response'.

Sources: Bello W. Should developing countries push to decommission the IMF? *Far Eastern Economic Review* 1999; December; Diokno B. *A Policymaker's Guide for the Use of Central-Local Transfers: The Philippine Case.* Manila: University of the Philippines Economics Foundation, 1995; Espino F, Beltran M, Carisma B. Malaria control through municipalities in the Philippines: struggling with the mandate of decentralized health programme management. *International Journal of Health Planning and Management* 2004; **19**:S1; Lakshminarayaran R. Decentralization and its implications for reproductive health: the Philippines Experience. *Reproductive Health Matters* 2003; **11**(21): 96–107; Lim J, Montes M. Structure of employment and structural adjustment in the Philippines. *Journal of Development Studies* 2000; **36**:149–181; Perez J. Health worker benefits in a period of broad civil service reform: The Philippine experience. Philippine Department of Health: Director, Health Intelligence and Local Government Assistance and Monitoring Services, 2004; Phillips DR. Primary health care in the Philippines: banking on the barangays? *Social Science and Medicine* 1986; **23**(10):1105–17.

(including condom distribution, abstinence programmes, and information interventions). Treatment was regarded as too expensive. Many HIV control advocates, concerned about the apparent failures of these preventative approaches, instead argued that HIV treatment was a basic human right and the best means of prevention. Public health doctors, like Paul Farmer, launched radical programmes of providing treatment to all patients, irrespective of the cost, in clinics in Haiti. Its model was largely a success, spreading to other parts of the world. It challenged the prevailing views in WHO, ultimately gaining prominence and leading to WHO's 3×5 Initiative (to treat 3 million people by 2005, a goal ultimately achieved after the target date).

The antiretroviral (ART) treatment model is successfully being applied in many communities. In poor countries, such as Malawi where incomes average less than US $200 per year, more than 145,000 HIV-positive patients have successfully initiated ART. Box 4.3 describes the major components: training personnel to run ART facilities; monitoring at local facilities, support by national supervision to maintain quality standards and track patient outcomes; and engagement with the private sector (217), and summarizes how they can be adapted to providing effective chronic care in deprived settings.

A second model is the WHO directly observed therapy (directly observed short-course therapy, DOTS) framework used to control TB and prevent drug-resistance. It is called DOTS because a care practitioner watches the patient take the medicine to ensure they adhere to treatment for at least 8–10 months (although there is evidence that patients, especially prison populations, find ways to fool the doctors). Unlike ART, treatment is not lifelong, but there is a need for long-term monitoring and special follow-ups, because patients are at lifelong risk of reactivation of disease (similar to chronic disease patients who live with behavioural or clinical risk factors). TB management requires continuity of care, coordination, and collaboration with patients, especially in order to avoid developing drug-resistance strains. Between 1995 and 2005 DOTS expanded to 190 countries, and 26 million people, most of them impoverished, were successfully treated with standardized anti-tuberculosis drug regimens (218).

Importantly, unlike the original vertical GOBI interventions of Selective Primary Health Care, DOTS and ART have built significant capacity, infrastructure, and delivery channels for medications. These networks can be expanded on to deliver medications like insulin to diabetes patients. Unfortunately, this is not yet happening. For example, in Liberia's government-run HIV hospitals, patients now have access to top-of-the-line HIV care (medicines, monitoring equipment, and diagnostics), but lack access to even the most basic primary care medications for diabetes such as insulin (leading some patients to wish they had HIV instead of diabetes).

Such initiatives could tap opportunities to take advantage of synergies in controlling coexisting epidemics, like HIV/AIDS and CVD or diabetes and TB. They could also emphasize the underlying social causes of illness, such as tobacco in the case of TB, HIV, COPD, and CVD. Joined up approaches have historical precedents, reflected in, for example, the 1950s specialized clinics in the UK which were established for dual treatment of 'tuberculous diabetics' (2, 219).

Strategy 3: Chronic disease care models can be built on the foundations of chronic infectious disease care clinics, such as antiretroviral and directly-observed therapy clinics for HIV/AIDS and TB.

How to pay for care: the role of markets and states

Efforts to improve access to medicines and transform systems to the CCM will not occur spontaneously. They will require concerted, organized efforts by doctors, hospitals, and health ministers, supported by political commitments at the highest level. Yet, today, there are two main settings where there is an implicit expectation that healthcare consumers, choosing health through markets, will themselves bring about these desirable changes. This heavy reliance on market forces to

Box 4.3 How to extend existing system capacity to deliver effective chronic care: the case of ART clinics in Malawi

Train personnel to run chronic care facilities

All clinicians, nurses, community health workers who work in ART clinics receive formal training through government courses or NGO courses (http://model.pih.org/accompagnateurs_curriculum). Community health workers, empowered with the ability to survey smoking status, blood pressure, and body-mass index in local communities, help identify people with NCD risks and connect them patients to cost-effective healthcare services (see WHO community health worker guidelines).

Provide access to low-cost medicines

Provision of generic medicines can help drive down these costs. Generic ART is nearly 11 times cheaper than brand name drugs. These medicines, including those listed on the National Essential Medicines List, tend to be stocked in more places than those that are not on the list. Currently, one month of secondary prevention (aspirin, beta-blocker, ACE inhibitor, and statin) for patients with established CVD could cost as much as 18 days' wages in Malawi. Learning from the ART experience, the public sector should strive to supply generic NCD medicines on National Essential Medicines List. Private sector also can play a role, as seen from the ART experience, through i) free drug donation schemes and ii) donation of reduced retail of diagnostics for case-detection and monitoring. The cost of medicines remains a barrier to effective NCD care.

Monitor patient outcomes at local clinics

Medical records are made for patients who receive treatment at the facility where they have been registered. Community health workers provide the first-line of detection for secondary outcomes such as ambulatory status, work capability, adverse effects, and drug adherence measured by pill counts. The master card (for the patient) and the register (for the clinic) make it easier to follow-up patient outcomes (i.e. 12 months, 24 months, 36 months, and so on) facile and provide a chronological record. Education and awareness on the defined outcomes and side effects are a vital component of the programme. It is important to have good inclusion criteria and define the 'basic minimum package' as a key set of interventions that are a high standard and enforce equity.

National supervision of local clinics to maintain quality and monitor national outcomes

Evaluating local programmes and clinics is an important part of chronic care. In Malawi, the HIV Unit of the Ministry of Health and its partners supervise and monitor ART facilities every quarter. Using a structured supervision and monitoring form, the supervising teams check the accuracy of the quarterly and cumulative data, the quality of registers and master cards, and drug stocks in pharmacies. The data is fed back to the Ministry of Health so as to identify gaps where they occur and reduce variations in treatment performance across clinics.

Source: Adapted from Mendis S, Fukino K, Cameron A, et al. The availability and affordability of selected essential medicines for chronic diseases in six low- and middle-income countries. *Bulletin of the World Health Organization* 2007; **85:** 279–88.

provide healthcare occurs in one case by design, the other from a lack of resources. These groups are, respectively, the US and low-income countries.

The US system relies extensively on market elements such as 'consumer choice', managed care, and diagnosis-related groups. It often boasts of having the 'best healthcare in the world'. Indeed, the US does have the best healthcare technology for those who can access it. After age 65, when patients become eligible for Medicare (a universal health system for the elderly), cancer survival rates out-perform Europe. Thus, that part of the American health system which is publicly funded, and at a significantly higher level of funding than in Europe, does deliver high-quality care. There are, alternatively, few positive things to say about chronic disease systems in low-income countries, as summarized in Box 4.1 earlier in the chapter. Medical care is inefficient, inequitable, of poor quality, and generally unresponsive to patient and community needs. Costs of care are a leading cause of impoverishment, causing patients to face routinely a lethal dilemma: face bankruptcy or forego life.

Yet the worst features of this system apply not only to these low-income countries. In the US healthcare costs are a source of catastrophic expenditure, accounting for one out of every two bankruptcies. The US consistently lags behind Europe in amenable mortality (220) and outcomes for those too young to receive Medicare coverage are significantly worse than in Europe (221). It is also a clear outlier in terms of overall spending—spending the most, while getting the least. WHO rankings, albeit contentious, put the US among the middle-income countries in terms of health system equity (222). Furthermore, several impoverished communities in the US experience higher rates of infectious disease, psychosis, and premature births than sub-Saharan Africa (20, 223).

These results are not surprising. In a seminal paper from 1963, the Nobel Laureate economist Kenneth Arrow had demonstrated that free markets do not work for healthcare because the need for medical treatments and services is unpredictable (requiring insurance systems) while at the same time, informed and rational individuals face difficulties in making decisions in their own best interests, instead requiring expert advice (preventing experiential comparison shopping for prices of services of the same quality) (224). As stated by another Nobel Laureate economist Paul Krugman, 'there are no examples of successful healthcare based on the principles of the free market' (225). Otherwise, marketization is likely to produce unintended and undesired consequences' (226).

Thus, there are dangers not just to importing Western lifestyles, but also Western medical and health system solutions. The risks can be seen in the US model's emphasis on high-price, specialist care to cope with rising diabetes (4). In the span of 5 years, the medical costs of diabetes more than doubled, from $44 billion to $92 billion. Despite this outpouring of resources, individual receive only a fraction of the chronic disease care they need. The largest fraction of diabetes expenditures covered hospital admissions for the treatment of long-term complications, such as heart disease, stroke, blindness, renal failure, and lower-limb amputations. At least 7% of these diabetes-related hospitalizations were estimated to have been avoidable (227). Only a small fraction of the resources devoted to the care of diabetes-related complications are spent for strategies that can help avoid obesity and diabetes in the first place (4).

Clue 6: There is danger in exporting US models of market-driven, acute-oriented medical care.

In the context of such high spending in the US, there are constant debates about whether healthcare money is going down the drain or even being counterproductive. Remarkable variations in spending on the elderly have been observed across the US, by as much as a factor of two across Texas cities, such as McAllen and El Paso (228). However, this additional money appears to be unrelated to quality: people living in the high-cost regions of the US get more tests, see more specialists, and spend more time in hospitals and intensive care units, yet these people do not display better health outcomes (229). Patients report having no desire for this 'excess' care (230), and about 20–30% receive bad care (i.e., contraindicated) (231). Such practices could be fatal: 'iatrogenic' causes of deaths—medical errors—are one of the top five causes of death in the US, estimated to kill about 225,000 people each year (232–236).

Many of the high-priced tertiary and specialist-care treatments driving growth of medical spending in the US are poorly suited for developing health systems. The race is on for the pill to control obesity, with pharmaceutical companies betting heavily on potential market prospects (237). While this occurs, bariatric surgery is seen by many as the only proven means of reducing the impact of severe obesity (238). Evidence of how this view is spreading worldwide can be seen in the recent formation of the Asia-Pacific Bariatric Surgery group by surgeons from 11 Asian countries (239). Driven by pharmaceutical companies and commercial interests, research funding agencies favour medical and surgical solutions over health promotion and health system interventions and policies. It is therefore not surprising that relatively few large-scale, community-based and systems-oriented approaches to address chronic disease risk factors have been undertaken.

Avoiding the mistakes of the US will also mean finding ways to open generic markets for a range of pharmaceuticals instead of sinking considerable economic resources into expensive forms of care. The patent-based US pharmaceutical industry, among the most profitable industries in the world at three times the profit as a percentage of revenue as the Fortune 500, spends 27% of its revenues on marketing and only 11% on research and development (240). Most pharmaceutical research is taxpayer-funded, developed in public universities through national grants, but then privatized by industry for two decades of patent protection. One pharmaceutical company executive noted that poor countries constitute so little of the revenue market that the entire African marketplace amounts to 'three days' fluctuation in exchange rates'. If this is true, then supplying essential medicines by generic companies (as demonstrated by the HIV antiretroviral case) will not affect these companies revenues and could even benefit them in the long run by opening new markets.

The overemphasis on expensive medical cures rather than prevention is also evident in our research priorities. Billions of dollars have poured into genetic research, yet even the world's top geneticists predict it will have limited impact on a very limited number of diseases. Most other medical research is designed to mitigate the impact of already-existing disease, such as chemotherapy, rather than avert its incidence. The research on truly preventative initiatives demonstrates that they have limited efficacy at the individual level, particularly among the poor who have the greatest burden of disease. It is often noted that the pharmaceutical industry focuses most of its research on chronic disease related care; however, little, if any, of this development is appropriate for resource-poor countries.

Despite its obvious shortcomings, the inefficient, market-driven and acute-care focused health system model of the US is being spread by global health financing mechanisms that deliver most health funding to resource-poor countries from Western donors. In low-income countries as much as half of all healthcare spending comes from aid from other countries, NGOs, or global institutions like WHO or the World Bank. For example, in Bhutan 48% and in Tanzania 35% of health system spending came from donors (20). The vast majority of this funding goes to infectious diseases, focusing on technical quick-fix, GOBI-style interventions—impeding the necessary transformation of health systems to a CCM approach (see Chapter 5). The emphasis tends to be on private, market-based solutions to global health problems. In both rich and poor countries, there is need to be critical of unproven strategies to shift health service planning from need to demand, turning patients into consumers, and transforming health into a private market good.

Strategy 4: Markets work well for delivering cans of tuna (itself questionable given overfishing), but not chronic healthcare. Relying on markets alone is unlikely to transform health systems to models of care that are appropriate for caring for people with long-term illness.

A note of scepticism about the effect of healthcare on population health

So far we have operated under an assumption that improving systems of chronic disease care could make a significant difference to a population's chronic disease burden. However, this is by no means a foregone conclusion.

Historically there has been scepticism about its contribution to population health. Writing in the 1960s, McKeown argued that most of the improvements in mortality over the previous century and a half had preceded the introduction of effective medical care and were instead attributable to improved living conditions, in particular nutrition (241). In the 1970s, Cochrane and colleagues attempted to evaluate the impact of health spending on health outcomes, finding little or no effect of medical care on mortality rates across countries (242). There is considerable historical evidence that the major declines in infectious diseases predated the development of effective medicines and were instead due to a combination of improved living conditions and public health measures such as improved sanitation. It was only in the late 1940s and 1950s that effective and safe drugs became available to prolong life for those suffering from many common diseases. Initially antibiotics, followed by a growing list of treatments for chronic diseases, such as hypertension and chronic obstructive airways disease, as well as others that, while less obviously life saving, greatly improved quality of life, such as non-steroidal anti-inflammatory drugs for arthritis and neuroleptics and antidepressants for severe mental illness. At the same time, the development of new and safe vaccines greatly reduced the risk of a number of potentially life-threatening or disabling diseases, such as measles and polio. However, until the 1960s, the greatest health gains came about as a consequence of factors outside the health system, and in particular from improvements in housing, sanitation, safe water and food supplies, improved nutrition, employment, wages, and education, which caused a steady improvement in living standards.

Consequently, it was only from the mid-1960s onward that healthcare really began to make a difference to overall mortality rates: a phenomenon observable from a comparison of the UK, where modern healthcare was being introduced, and the Soviet Union, where it was not. By the 1980s, it became possible to estimate its actual contribution to mortality, using the new concept of avoidable mortality (that is, mortality that should not occur in the presence of timely and effective healthcare). Conceived in the US, it identified that portion of mortality that should be amenable to medical intervention. This was subsequently adapted by researchers in Europe and is now used widely in comparisons of healthcare performance. Deaths from these causes have fallen markedly in recent decades in European countries, to a substantially greater degree than other causes of death, and much faster than in the US. Consequently, they now account for only 7–10% of all deaths across Europe. In the rest of the world avoidable mortality due to chronic diseases contributes to a higher proportion of deaths, albeit rarely beyond 20%.

Nonetheless, considerable variations remain in mortality amenable to medical care and, in general, the countries of Central and Eastern Europe, and especially the countries of the former Soviet Union, still lag far behind. The implication is that while future developments in personal care may be able to contribute more to the relief of disability, the scope of contribution to longevity by curing disease, in the absence of some major unanticipated breakthrough, is likely to be limited and the main challenge must be to ensure that those who can benefit from existing knowledge are able to do so.

Clue 7: Only a small fraction of differences in population chronic disease experience can be explained by healthcare. It is unlikely that improving healthcare alone will be sufficient to address rising chronic diseases.

Summary

Returning to the challenge at the beginning of this chapter: how can chronic disease care be improved in resource-poor settings if standards are inadequate in rich countries?

In this first half of the chapter, we briefly reviewed the history of healthcare systems, identifying how they were set up in a period dominated by acute, infectious care needs.

These models are inappropriate for caring for people with chronic diseases, for several reasons. First, people who live with chronic diseases are not simply passive bodies requiring medical intervention, but individuals whose disease and risk are products of their environment. Most people will have not one but multiple chronic diseases in their lifetime, requiring flexible regimens of care that can be tailored to each patient's differing biological and social circumstances. Second, many doctors find the common cycle of failed treatments and recurring illness extremely frustrating—a point we return to in the next section about upstream and downstream causes of poor health and intervention. Finally, doctors alone cannot solve chronic diseases through medical cures; patients have to play a greater role in sharing knowledge about their conditions and the challenges in managing them—engaging in collaborative care.

How might an alternative, exchange-based care model play out in practice? Instead of a traditional medical scenario where the doctor examines the patient and determines what to do, a more reciprocal encounter would play out as follows: the patient describes a series of complaints and symptoms; the doctor evaluates the patient's symptoms and makes a diagnosis. The patient asks about what the diagnosis means for day-to-day life. The doctor explains and sets out a series of treatment options as well as the potential long-term, debilitating risks of various courses of action. The patient takes time to think about the preferred strategy, possibly returning for a future consultation. Then the patient discusses again with the doctor what he/she has decided, when the doctor asks the patient to identify what obstacles he/she might face in trying to follow the treatment plan. They jointly decide ways of monitoring the patient's progress so that the doctor will know if the patient has been unable to follow the agreed upon care strategy.

These alternative models of chronic care emphasize continuity, coordination, and collaboration. The best kind of chronic care is an education. Such 'liberatory care' models of can empower patients to play a more active role in defining their care needs while doctors play a supportive role, helping patients and their families plan effectively for managing illness throughout the life course.

Achieving the chronic care model is a major change to the status quo. Both rich and poor countries face significant challenges in restructuring their healthcare systems. Currently, systems of chronic disease care in high-income countries are uncoordinated and fragmented. Many patients receive treatment that fails to meet recommended standards, resulting in high rates of medical errors; the situation is far worse in low-income countries.

Change will not be easy. One of the major barriers to restructuring has been resistance of the medical profession and the influence of pharmaceutical companies. Especially in the US, there is an overemphasis on expensive, medical care rather than interventions that could prevent people from becoming sick in the first place. Despite its limitations, this model continues to be exported to resource-poor countries through systems of global health aid and pressures from the financial community to keep health spending low.

It is especially unlikely that change will be forthcoming without directed action by public health leaders. Yet, by following the US model, there has been an excessive reliance on markets to achieve these public health goals. It is as though the global health community has learned the wrong lessons from the obvious shortcomings of the US systems. Markets work well for cans of tuna, but not healthcare. Relying on markets alone is unlikely to transform health systems to models of care that are appropriate for caring for people with long-term illness. Unfortunately, in the context of the privatization of global health and decades of continual Structural Adjustment programmes, as described in Chapter 2, the public sector has been deprived of the necessary resources.

All of these challenges are embedded in a broader debate about how health systems in resource-poor countries should develop. In the 1970s to 1980s, WHO set out a model of health system development known as Primary Health Care which focused on providing universal access to a comprehensive set of preventative and treatment services to populations (a horizontal model). Its key values were equity, community empowerment and prevention. Disputing this approach, economists as the World Bank proposed a Selective PHC model, arguing the WHO's PHC model would be far too expensive. They drew upon the successes of the campaign to eradicate smallpox, instead recommending a limited set of technical interventions that could yield the greatest health gains at low cost for the populations at greatest risk (a vertical model). Its core elements were efficiency, cost-effectiveness, and medical and technical intervention (as returned to in the next half of the chapter). From the outset the World Bank's Selective PHC was pitched as an alternative, interim model of global health. Three decades later, the vertical, low-cost, technical model continues to be the dominant paradigm guiding the development of public health systems.

Of course, neither model is perfect. A truly comprehensive public health system would likely incorporate both horizontal and vertical components. Each aspect can reinforce the other. For example, the infrastructure built up through a horizontal, system-wide approach will make it easier to deliver effective vertical interventions when needed in response to short-term health threats such as disease outbreaks.

Combining elements of both systems, the dominant minimalist and vertical models of public health have been recently challenged by long-term conditions, such as HIV/AIDS and episodic diseases, such as TB, that require coordinated care. In response to pressure from advocates (as described in Chapter 5), substantial capacity has been set up in resource-deprived settings to deliver antiretroviral and directly observed short-course therapy. These clinics and health staff provide the key entry points for building health systems that can care for persons living with chronic care needs, including chronic diseases.

In closing, we note that it would be unrealistic to expect that improving chronic care alone would achieve substantial health gains. Until the 1960s medical care had little effect on chronic disease, as the greatest health gains came about as a consequence of improvements in housing, sanitation, safe water, improved nutrition, employment, wages, and education. In the future, the scope of personal medical care to extend human life, in the absence of a major unanticipated breakthrough, is likely to be limited. The main challenge of chronic care systems is to ensure that those who can benefit from existing knowledge are able to do so.

Alternatively, in line with Geoffrey Rose's principles of public health, much greater gains could be achieved by acting on societal determinants. Reducing the avoidable inequalities in chronic disease outcomes would improve longevity and quality of life much more than giving people access to all the best medications in the world. What some of these strategies are and how they could be implemented is the topic of the next half of this chapter.

Prevention of chronic diseases

Key policy points

1 The most promising (and low-cost) interventions require reverse-engineering of some of the changes in society that have led more people to become ill. Structural interventions that address unhealthy environments can help make it easy for people to be healthy.

2 There tends to be an overemphasis on individual medical and education interventions, attempting to reshape people's bodies and minds to fit increasingly toxic societies.

3 The key magic bullets that exist for reducing chronic disease include: medicines such as the polypill (a potentially effective combination of low-dose drugs to lower blood pressure and cholesterol and provide a protective vitamin, folic acid); regulations to lower salt, sugar, and fat content of food; and fiscal interventions such as tobacco, alcohol, and food taxes. These interventions can be viewed as 'best-buys' because they are highly cost-effective and, in the cases of taxes, can be cost-saving.

4 Interventions will never be simple to do when vested interests stand to lose profits from them. Even the most basic interventions, such as tobacco control, have proven to be extremely challenging.

5 Analogous to the chronic care model, participatory, community-based approaches aim to achieve a balance of power among experts and patients and their communities in sharing values and setting priorities. Community-led interventions offer one possible way to tailor the management of chronic diseases to individual communities.

Key practice points

1 Public health practitioners often falsely leap to the conclusion that the prevention of chronic diseases is largely a matter of education. This assumes a great deal of agency and choice among the affected population. When designing interventions for a community, we must recognize the constraints to human behaviour. The limited effectiveness of education interventions relates to the fact that they fail to address the circumstances that lead people to choose unhealthy options.

2 In spite of evidence from randomized controlled trials that individual interventions can reduce individual consumption of salt, sugar, and fats and increase physical activity, it cannot simply be assumed that scaling up these approaches to the population level will achieve health gains. Even the simplest interventions are highly contested from a medical and logistical standpoint.

3 Many low-cost pharmacological interventions could be delivered more widely at low cost, including blood glucose monitoring, antihypertensives, lipid control, aspirin use, and regular screening for some chronic conditions.

Key practice points *(continued)*

4 Gaps in evidence should not stop us from starting the process of joining with communities to decide key priorities, identify risks, and search for appropriate strategies for intervention, as experts help set up experiments, replicate them, and learn from their successes and failures while building the evidence base.

Preventing chronic disease: the role of broader society

A good doctor working in South Africa went for a summer walk down the river, when suddenly he noticed a man in the water, gasping for breath on the verge of drowning. Alarmed, the good doctor, who had sworn his life to the Hippocratic oath, reached out to pull the dying man from the river. The doctor knew what to do, using his emergency care skills to resuscitate the patient, and after a few minutes the man was regaining consciousness. Relieved, the doctor called his colleagues back at the clinic to get the man to the hospital for diagnostic tests, and then continued on his walk.

After carrying on his walk about 5 minutes, to his surprise, the doctor saw yet another man floating down the river, nearing death. Again, fulfilling his moral duty, the doctor stopped to rescue the man. This time, as the man came back to his senses, he tried to explain something to the doctor, but the good doctor could not understand what the man was saying. Clearly, he needed to get to the hospital, so the doctor once again sent for help.

The doctor continued on his riverside walk, turning a corner, when this time he saw two men and a woman drowning. What could he do! Rushing to save the woman, he knew the two other men would likely die. Just about this time the doctor spotted a villager nearby and began calling for help. Fortunately, the villager spoke the same language, and soon the doctor was explaining to him how he could save one of the other two men. After they saved the man and woman, they stopped for a moment to mourn the third man. If only there had been another villager here, the doctor thought to himself. As the doctor seemed distressed by his thoughts, the villager eventually broke the silence, asking 'good doctor, didn't you know there is a crazy man on the bridge a few miles upstream who throws people in the river? If you are concerned about these dying people, you should go to the head of the river to stop this killer'.

This story captures what prevention is all about. The practice of public health seeks to identify the underlying causes of health that lie upstream from where doctors work. What good does it do to pull more bodies out of the river, only to return them to the society that made them sick in the first place? It is always better to prevent poor health than to step in when it is already too late (although oddly enough some people do argue for deliberate human sacrifice, a point which we address in earlier sections).

Healthcare is society's last line of defence, picking up the pieces when all other supports have failed. Even the best standards of care in the world would not be able to stop their rising incidence of chronic diseases because, just a few miles upstream, people are throwing more bodies into the river. Big Tobacco is the most well-known serial killer on the bridge, but Big Food also has claimed many lives, and government leaders and health decision-makers are equally guilty for not intervening in a timely manner (see Chapter 2).

Troubled by the growing numbers of bodies they see, doctors have begun calling for help (for example, see Figure 5.1 in Chapter 5 about the growing calls to action). Too bogged down saving patients who come into their offices they rarely can make it all the way upstream. Their voices are being heard by leaders, but still go unanswered. Ministers of health from Uganda, for example, say, 'We know what to do [about chronic diseases]. We have no budget' (242a).

The powerful incentives driving the development of healthcare and public health centre on medical models of care. More patients are pulled out of the river and into the medical system, feeding the interests of the pharmaceutical sector, while preventative approaches tend to be neglected.

In this chapter we discuss what we know and don't know about how to act upstream to prevent people from suffering from avoidable chronic diseases. In the first section, we cover a range of interventions, spanning individual medical treatments to population-wide policies. In considering what works, we must not just look to what is effective from a medical and public health perspective, but also to what can be achieved within limited budgets and existing political structures. Thus, in the second section, we consider how to choose appropriate interventions to reduce the burden of chronic diseases, contrasting prioritization based on cost-effectiveness criteria with community-driven systems of setting priorities. In particular, we focus on how community-led interventions, tackling the upstream killers, staffed with community health workers, responding to the doctors' cries for help, provides a democratic model to empower communities to address their ever-changing health needs. In the third and final section, we draw together the insights of the entire chapter in a case study of how community interventions could work on the ground.

What works to prevent chronic disease?

Before proceeding we need to take a moment to set out a broader definition of the health system than we used in the previous half of this chapter. Often when the public thinks about health, they think about the medical care system. More appropriately, this component of the health system involving health professionals should be called the sick care system, because it deals with people once they are already drowning in the river.

The full health system covers the full range of things that make people healthy, not just those that protect them once they are already ill. This reflects how WHO defines health as 'a state of complete physical, mental, and social well-being and not merely the absence of disease or infirmity' (although it has been argued that this can only be achieved through the help of mind altering drugs). As set out in the embedded hierarchical model of Chapter 2, what makes people healthy includes a broad set of factors, including the agricultural system, providing incentives or disincentives to farmers to grow fruits and vegetables; urban planners who can build healthy cities with cycle lanes and sports fields for play or instead emphasize the dominance of the automobile; owners of restaurants, supermarkets, and other food outlets that can give customers the information they need to make healthier choices; private industry, that could use advanced tactics to market unhealthy or healthy products to kids.

Evidence about the effectiveness of chronic disease interventions

In public health a common assumption is that prevention is better than the cure. But how much do we know about what actually can be done upstream to prevent someone from getting sick?

It might seem logical to categorize our interventions into prevention and treatment, but where does prevention end and treatment begin? Systems that do attempt to classify treatment and prevention into so-called primary, secondary, tertiary, and quaternary components are somewhat arbitrary; in some cases what is classically thought of as treatment, such as treating HIV-positive patients with ART, is in fact one of the most effective strategies at population prevention. When it comes to an infectious agent, there is a clear difference; either you have been exposed to a disease-causing agent, initiating the disease process, or you have not. Of course, chronic diseases do not spread (although there is growing evidence of their social communicability), but the analogy nonetheless holds—it may be more effective to reduce morbidity by giving patients a pill combining drugs to reduce cholesterol and blood pressure (so-called 'polypill') than trying to modify life-styles. Tobacco can be 'treated' using tobacco cessation aides (such as nicotine replacement therapy) or 'prevented' using taxes. To the extent that the chronic disease process is degenerative, as risk accumulates over the life course, all treatment is prevention in the sense that intervention aims to prevent debilitating sequelae of the disease. To some degree, prevention and treatment is a false dichotomy—ultimately the aim is to reduce risks and promote good health by whichever policies can be feasibly implemented.

The gold-standard for evidence about reducing risks, either through prevention or treatment, comes from the randomized controlled trials. This enables researchers to isolate whether a treatment (such as eating more fruits and vegetables) actually improves an outcome (such as reducing the risk of a heart attack). Randomization is important because, if done correctly, it evenly distributes across both groups all possible major differences that could be driving the changes seen other than the treatment itself (i.e. removing confounding by some other factor that is related to both the exposure and outcome). For example, people who use tobacco might also eat too few fruits and vegetables so that the researchers accidentally observe that consuming too few fruits and vegetables has a bigger effect than they actually do because they failed to account for risks caused by tobacco.

Many randomized controlled trials have provided strong evidence that reducing exposure to the key risk factors can decrease risks of chronic diseases. For example, dietary changes that have been shown to lower risk of CVD include decreasing saturated fat intake; increasing consumption of linoleic acid, fish and fish oils, vegetables and fruits, and potassium; and maintaining low to moderate intake of alcohol (34, 243). Moderate levels of physical activity, including brisk walking or 20 minutes of exercise per day, have also been convincingly found to decrease the risk coronary heart disease, stroke, some cancers, type 2 diabetes, osteoporosis, high blood pressure, and high cholesterol (244).

These studies give us a strong evidence base for action, but do these findings apply in the real world? What we learn from a highly selected clinical setting may not easily translate into effective intervention in people's environments and household situations (a so-called settings-bias). The strongest results of randomized controlled trials can literally disappear in real-life settings.

There is convincing evidence that health improves when people are able to reduce their risk behaviours in their environments from studies of smokers. One study, for example, found that smokers who successfully quit experienced drops in risk of developing CVD by up to 36% (245). However, a few studies have found unintended and adverse effects of individual efforts to lose weight. One study found that people who tried to lose weight without medical supervision had higher risks of death, thought to relate to the stress involved in rapidly changing lifestyles or the pressure from peers and family members. These unintended consequences relate to a general problem in epidemiology: the real world is not like the laboratory (see for example the debate about salt reduction in Box 4.4). To overcome these challenges, there is a need to do randomized experiments in more real life, generalizeable settings.

Strategy 1: Conducting randomized experiments in real-life settings, not just laboratories, can improve our confidence in their ability to be effective when scaled up to communities and entire populations.

Nonetheless, apart from a few exceptions, there is a strong evidence base showing that reducing people's exposure to risk factors of chronic disease can achieve major gains in individual health.

Clue 1: Randomized-controlled trials provide strong evidence that when people successfully reduce their exposure to risks of chronic diseases their health improves.

How can these behavioural changes, desirable from a public health perspective, be achieved and extended to entire populations?

Box 4.4 Debates about salt intervention

Since the 1970s there has been debate about whether salt causes hypertension and, as a result, CVD. Many epidemiologists, commenting in the late 1980s, felt that 'I don't accept salt and hypertension . . . If you really look at the data, it's very unclear what the facts are' (28). However, more and more observational studies, such as the Framingham Heart Study, began to provide evidence that salt was strongly correlated with hypertension, which was also found to occur in many patients who had CVD. Extrapolating from these findings, researchers began suggesting that in the US alone between 194,000 and 392,000 quality-adjusted life years and US $10–24 billion in healthcare costs could be saved. Commenting in *The New England Journal of Medicine*, researchers called it 'compelling evidence for public health action to reduce salt intake' (246). Other doctors and epidemiologists disagree (some of whom are funded by the industry-sponsored Salt Institute). They pointed out the randomized controlled trials focused on lowering blood pressure among a small group of the population (247). Other trials that the researchers did not consider had found that the level of salt reduction needed to lower blood pressure would also increase nerve activity, decrease insulin sensitivity (increasing risk of diabetes), and, in fact, could increase blood pressure (by activating the renin–angiotensin system and stimulating aldosterone). They also had shown that in some patients, reduced salt intake resulted in increased risk of being put in the hospital and even dying. They also note that, despite rising population consumption of salt over the past three decades, people's biological levels of salt have stayed about the same. This happens because of homeostatic mechanisms that ensure salt intake equals salt output, like an internal 'salt clock' that maintains an equilibrium. As a result, it is possible that any intervention would be neutralized and a waste of time and money. On social grounds, the researchers question how overall calorie intake might be affected, noting that individuals might compensate by consuming more of what they were eating before (potentially increasing obesity rates) or switch to fattier or more sugary foods (potentially cancelling out the reduced CVD from salt reduction or even increasing diabetes rates). Thus, researchers suggest that, instead of the 'rash route', the public health community should follow the cautious path. Moreover, some public health researchers deplore such a singular focus on salt, viewing it as a diversion from tobacco or unhealthy diet, and caution about an 'over-zealous and non-tested policy actions against salt intake' (248), calling for more 'comprehensive lifestyle and pharmacological approaches for multiple risk factor control for prevention of vascular diseases'.

Individual and population interventions

Consider a few main, although very different, ways to reduce cardiovascular risks. One approach is to deliver mass quantities of preventative medicines. Another approach is to deliver mass quantities of a product like steel-cut oats, rich in fibre, and proven to reduce risks of developing CVD. A third approach is to focus on people's societal and environmental conditions that make unhealthy choices the easiest choices. If we could figure out how to eliminate the avoidable inequalities in chronic diseases by social class or education, the reductions in the levels of chronic diseases would be greater than the first two strategies (1). Each approach plays a role.

In general the public health strategies target two kinds of groups: high-risk individuals and entire populations. We discuss each in turn.

Individual-level interventions

When asked, 'what is the evidence that individual interventions can reduce a population's consumption of salt, sugar, fats and increase physical activity?', one editor of a top epidemiology journal said explicitly, 'I don't know of any'. As a recent systematic review of multiple interventions using counselling or education to reduce risks of CVD concluded, they have 'no effect on mortality . . . [and] limited utility in the general population' (249). Similar evidence has emerged from systematic reviews of education-based interventions on childhood obesity and consumption of fizzy drinks.

This is unsurprising. As described in Chapter 2, the main causes of rising chronic diseases are largely beyond individual control, so even though individuals can change their behaviours, these people are fighting an environment that provides disincentives to do so. However, with this caveat in mind, there is evidence that some interventions—both clinical and education—can help individuals modify their risky behaviours.

Medical interventions

We cannot cover all the drugs and medical solutions being proposed for treating diabetes, heart disease and other chronic diseases, so instead we discuss two: the polypill and tobacco cessation therapy.

Faced with the prospect of rising chronic diseases in resource-deprived settings, researchers have been struggling to find a low-cost way to prevent premature deaths. Unlike malnutrition, no clear magic-bullet like oral rehydration therapy existed for chronic diseases. However, in 2001, researchers proposed one such medical magic-bullet, the 'polypill'. Later patented by two researchers, Wald and Law, the pill would combine a statin to lower cholesterol, three drugs to lower blood pressure, aspirin, and a key vitamin, folic acid. Controversially, the researchers estimated that if everyone over age 55 and who had CVD took the drug it could prevent more than four out of every five heart attacks and strokes (250), increasing the years of disease-free life by over a decade. Such remarkable results led some researchers to call for adding it to the water supply in low-income countries, or even offering it for sale at fast-food outlets. Since all the medications are off-patent, the costs of providing these essential medicines would be very low (but this also means that pharmaceutical companies may not try to encourage their use if it could diminish their profitability). Whether patients will actually heed their doctor's advice and take the medicines is a problem, but this adherence to what doctors suggest improves because patients only need to take one daily pill instead of a complex regimen of five or six at alternating times and days.

To date, the polypill has neither been fully tested nor rolled out in countries. One component of the pill, aspirin, has been found to cause negative health consequences when taken continuously. Other side effects caused by the long-term use of the polypill and its six interacting components are unknown. Many people in public health find the medicalized and magic-bullet approach of the polypill to CVD prevention preposterous. A tongue-in-cheek article in the *British Medical Journal* proposed the 'polymeal', including a daily regimen of wine, fish, dark chocolate, fruits, vegetables, garlic, and almonds (251), as a 'tastier and safer alternative to the polypill'.

A similar pursuit of a medical magic bullet is occurring with smoking. Realizing that it is very difficult for people to quit, especially those who are disadvantaged, pharmaceutical companies developed nicotine-replacement drugs and other quitting aids. These drugs do help, but the vast majority of successful quitters do so without medicine (252). These cessation technologies could be an element of a comprehensive tobacco reduction strategy, but they should not substitute for tackling the tobacco companies that got people hooked in the first place.

Strategy 2: Quick-fix medical solutions can reduce risks of chronic disease, but should not substitute for addressing the upstream causes that place people at risk.

Information and education interventions

Slightly further upstream from medical interventions on people's bodies are approaches that attempt to reach their minds. The classic public health campaign to prevent chronic diseases is to tell people what is good for them: Eat more fruit and vegetables. Brush your teeth. Watch your weight. Wash your hands. (leading some critics, such as the Centre for Consumer Freedom, to believe that public health practitioners are secretly calling for a 'nanny state'). Indeed, these kinds of policies can be quite intrusive and reinforce a divide between the public health experts (who act like they know better) and the populations whom they seek to serve.

These recommendations can make a difference in some cases. One of the most successful examples of education-based prevention is to brush teeth. From early life parents teach children what to do, routine dental checkups take place, and the consequences of failing to brush teeth are immediately apparent when children get cavities or toothaches. To some extent this model works for chronic diseases risk factors. Studies found that when doctors tell their patients they should quit smoking, they sometimes do (245). Similarly, over the past 10 years clinical trials have shown that when doctors recommend weight loss, a healthier diet, and exercise, people are in some cases able to change their behaviours.

When people are successfully able to do so, especially among high-risk groups, the risk of type 2 diabetes significantly drops (253). Table 4.1 summarizes a few studies that have reported successes in getting people at high risk to change their behaviours. Attempts to modify people's lifestyles tend to be most effective when they target both diet and physical activity, mobilize social support, use established behavioural change techniques, and maintain frequent contact (254).

The effects of such interventions can be substantial. Randomized controlled trials from the US, Finland, Japan, China, and India found that high-risk persons (such as those with impaired glucose tolerance) who began exercising moderately, about 20 minutes per day, and eating a healthier had a greater reduction in risk of developing diabetes (more than 50% reduction in several studies) than taking a series of preventative drugs (254).

Clue 2: When public health education interventions successfully lead people to eat healthier diets and be more physically active, their risk of chronic diseases drops significantly, often by as much, if not more, than as occurs through medical interventions.

Information interventions rely on strong assumptions about people's ability to change in the context of an unhealthy environment. Different groups have varying abilities to convert information into positive behavioural change (a notion referred to as 'self-efficacy'). When research revealed that tobacco was a cause of lung cancer, inequalities in tobacco use and tobacco-related deaths began to emerge by socioeconomic status. Subsequently, it was found that while both rich and poor desired to quit smoking in places like the UK, the rich were much more successful at actually doing so.

Whenever interventions rely on people to act based on information and education, underlying differences in their capabilities and resources for converting this knowledge into behaviour change can lead to a net result in widening health inequalities (a point returned to in discussions about the effects of nutrition labelling). Individualized, education- and awareness-oriented approaches, as well as high-risk screening and targeting, may widen socioeconomic inequalities since they are better understood (and thus heeded) by better-educated, higher-income groups (58, 255).

Clue 3: Information interventions can widen inequalities in health because higher socio-economic groups tend to be more capable of modifying their behaviours than lower socio-economic groups.

Consistent with psychological theories of behaviour, however, public health information and education interventions have been found to have a limited effect on people's behaviour when

Table 4.1 Outcomes of selected randomized clinical trials that aimed to prevent diabetes by modifying people's behaviours

Study	Duration of intervention (years)	Behavioural goals	Weight loss achieved at 1 year (kg)	Risk reduction
Chinese Da Qing IGT and Diabetes Study (294)	6	Weight loss + maintenance of a healthy diet + exercise	NR	Diet 31% Exercise 46% Both 42%
Finnish Diabetes Prevention Study (DPS) (295)	4	5% weight loss on low-fat, high-fibre diet + 30 min exercise per day	4.2	58%
Diabetes Prevention Program (USA) (296)	2.8	7% weight loss + 150 min exercise per week	7	58%
Japanese Trial (297)	4	Reduction in BMI to ≤22 kg/m^2 by 30–40 min exercise per day	2.5	67.4%
Indian Diabetes Prevention Program IDPP-1 (298)	3	Weight maintenance by diet low in refined carbohydrates and fat + 30 min exercise per day	0	28.5%
Diabetes Prevention Program (USA) (296)	10	7% weight loss + 150 min exercise per week, with additional lifestyle support as compared to original DPP study	—	Lifestyle group 34% Metformin group 18%

Source: Adapted from (253) Notes: DPP, Diabetes Prevention Program; NR, not reported.

delivered in isolation. For example, one study of Thailand found that knowing more about the risks of smoking had no effect on the decision to smoke. Information campaigns can also be manipulated, as with Philip Morris's campaigns aimed at adolescents, in which children interpreted the 'smoking is only for adults' message as encouragement to act out their grown-up aspirations. Stressing the need to avoid an undesirable behaviour can perversely make people more likely to do it (256). Moreover, as discussed in Chapter 5, these interventions could backfire politically, making it easy to blame sick people by spreading a myth that they could have easily avoided their health problems through a combination of individual will and the right information.

A social reason for limited effectiveness of education interventions relates to the fact that they fail to address the circumstances that lead people to choose unhealthy options. An implicit assumption of the education campaigns is that people smoke or drink because they do not understand the risks to their health. Instead, many people who abuse alcohol do so to self-medicate (257). Substance abuse is most prevalent among those faced with depression and anxiety, making it difficult to decide which came first, the drugs or the mental health problems. No amount of education would solve this kind of excessive drug use without addressing the chronic stressors that cause people to use tobacco and abuse alcohol. Other reasons relate to differences in ways people living pay day-to-pay day in resource-poor settings tend to value the present more than the future as compared with persons who have greater economic security (what has been called a 'dictatorship of the present'). Recently some creative approaches for overcoming these barriers have been devised that tap into insights from behavioural psychology and economics (see Box 4.5).

Box 4.5 Enhancing information interventions with insights from behavioural psychology and economics

A common, mistaken view underpinning educational interventions is that people make decisions based on a careful and dispassionate weighing of the evidence. This is especially untrue in regard to smoking, where addiction plays a key role. Many smokers continually say 'I will quit tomorrow', but tomorrow never comes (the hyperbolic time discount problem, see Chapter 3). One famous anecdote is that of Ulysses in the Iliad. His boat was approaching the Sirens—famed for their beautiful, alluring song that would enchant men, who they would subsequently devour. He longed to hear the Siren's voice, but knew he could not withstand the deadly temptation, so he had his men tie him to the mast of the ship to protect himself against, well, himself.

Recently some creative approaches have been developed to help people do what they say they want to do. In one programme, people make a commitment to a healthy behavioural change (e.g. quitting smoking, weight loss, healthier eating) and wager against themselves in order to stick to the plan. Another innovative programme was set up by a local bank to create savings accounts for people that were trying to quit smoking. Each day, the amount of money that would have been spent on cigarettes was deposited into the account. At the end of the programme, successful quitters received the lump sum saved. Unsuccessful quitters, however, lost all their savings. These strategies create disincentives to reneging on a commitment to change and found been found to increase people's likelihood of exercising or quitting smoking given that they have decided they wish to do so (256, 258, 259).

Other strategies seek to make healthy choices the default choices at restaurants and supermarkets, so that people have consciously to choose to be unhealthy (affecting their availability and effective price). Studies found, for example, that organ donors were much greater in US states where people were organ donors unless they opted out of the programme. Similarly, coffee shops which make lattes using semi-skimmed or skimmed milk, unless people specifically request whole milk, are passively encouraging healthier choices. Another example is in urban design. If the elevator is central, people are unlikely to search for the stairs located to the side. But when stairs are more convenient, people are more likely to use them. These kinds of approaches could be thought of as white glove kinds of policy initiatives to achieving behavioural change (256).

In the context of limited availability of healthy choices, education offers very little help. What good does it do to tell someone to eat fruits and vegetables if there is simply a lack of fresh supplies in their neighbourhood?

Clue 4: Information campaigns cannot address structural barriers to healthy diets, such as the unavailability of healthy foods or their relatively high price.

We must also bear in mind that public health information campaigns are but one small piece of information in an environment where people are bombarded with conflicting messages designed to generate profits. Marketing of food products has been shown to have significant effects on people's behaviour, both in the real world and the experimental setting (see Chapter 2). Whatever degree to which public health interventions seek to influence the behaviour of individuals is likely being counteracted by a much more powerful set of existing interventions that aim to encourage people to make unhealthy choices and consume larger quantities.

Clue 5: Public health information interventions to encourage healthy choices tend to be underfunded compared with marketing campaigns that encourage people to make unhealthy choices.

Population-wide interventions

As the famous epidemiologist Geoffrey Rose noted, 'The efforts of individuals are only likely to be effective when they are working with the societal trends' (1985). When the root causes of rising chronic diseases are at the societal level (as outlined in Chapter 2), it follows that the solutions should also be directed at entire societies. Such approaches can help make it easy for people to be healthy (while doing nothing continues to maintain the unhealthy status quo). This sounds like a great theoretical idea—but can it be delivered to populations as an intervention?

Here we provide a few concrete examples of how magic-bullets in health policy, such as taxes, subsidies, and regulation can powerfully affect the main economic risk factors of unhealthy diet set out in Chapter 2, including price, availability, and marketing. We then cover a series of urban and architectural design intervention identified by WHO as helping people regain control of the way their societies are being built, re-engineering them to be healthier and suited to people's changing lives.

Fiscal interventions—taxes and subsidies

Just as price is one of the most powerful determinants of making a risky decision, so are financial interventions among the most powerful levers of public health change. Two main types of financial policies can be used to influence price: taxation and subsidies.

Tax and price policies applied to tobacco and alcohol products in many countries have provided persuasive evidence that they decrease consumption. Taxes on tobacco are the single most effective intervention to reduce demand for tobacco. One study estimates that a price increase of 10% would reduce smoking by about 4% in high-income countries and by about 8% in low-income and middle-income countries (260). It has been estimated that a 70% increase in the price of tobacco could prevent up to a quarter of all smoking-related deaths worldwide (261), with the added benefit that increasing tobacco taxes by 10% generally leads to increases in government tobacco tax revenues of nearly 7% (262). In the UK, tobacco taxes make up nearly 80% of the price of a packet of cigarettes, but most resource-poor countries have tax rates below 50%, leaving considerable scope for intervention.

Applying these taxes to alcohol or food is more challenging than tobacco because they are not global bads. Food taxes are now being called for in a variety of forms as 'junk food tax', 'calorie tax', 'luxury tax', or 'fat tax', but have yet to be implemented. One exception is Romania, which in 2010 became the first country to implement a junk-food tax on snacks and crisps, cakes and the candy-making industry, soda, and fast-food products. One article reported that fizzy drink consumption decreases by 7.8% for every 10% increase in price (83), estimating that a penny-per-ounce excise tax could raise $1.2 billion in New York State alone.

One important limitation of taxes is that they tend to impact most the incomes of the poor. However, as discussed in Chapter 3, there is surprising evidence that the poor report being happier as a result of these interventions, as the tax helps them achieve their desired goals of breaking addiction that they could not achieve without additional support.

An alternative approach is to use subsidies to promote healthier choices. One US community-based study found that price reductions of low-fat snacks sold in vending machines in secondary schools and worksites in Minnesota resulted in substantially higher sales of these foods compared to usual price conditions (263), even though average vending machine profits were not significantly affected.

It is also possible to target suppliers to discourage production of unhealthy foods, although there are few successful examples. One problem is that the effectiveness of supply-side mechanisms depends on how readily substitutes are available. For example, attempts to curb tobacco supply are frustrated by industry-supported initiatives to smuggle tobacco from neighbouring countries (also used to circumvent taxes) (see Chapter 7.1).

Another instrument is a price floor, especially important for alcohol control, given 'all-you-can-drink' specials in bars at rock-bottom prices. This also prevents supermarkets from using alcohol as a loss leader to attract customers. Maintaining a minimum price can help avoid giving desperate substance abusers an easy means to harm themselves (and others).

Other types of fiscal instruments exist, such as conditional-cash transfers, which are becoming increasingly popular as a mechanism to give people direct incentives to be healthy.

In general, fiscal instruments work extremely well. Its success is indicated by the vigorous response of tobacco and food companies to avoid any interference with the price of their product.

Strategy 3: Fiscal interventions to increase the price of unhealthy foods (using taxes) and decrease the price of healthy foods (using subsidies) are among the most powerful public-health interventions for preventing chronic diseases.

Regulatory interventions

Public health's second main instrument is regulation. Regulation gives a mandate to conduct audits and routine check-ups. In rich countries, this occurs in most food industries (for example, noting Upton Sinclair's descriptions of conditions in the meat-packing industries). To regulate successfully, the state has to be free of influence from those who they are regulating (typically corporations). Unfortunately, this is not always the case. The Food and Drug Administration and Environmental Protection Agency both have revolving doors of industry executives and top federal appointments to positions in these agencies.

The alternative situation is for the industry to regulate itself. Self-regulation is the industry's preferred solution. To crowd out public regulation, many industries implement price floors, nutritional changes, or marketing restrictions (see Chapter 6). These efforts aim to prevent the state from introducing taxes or regulating their practices, prospects viewed as typically being more stringent.

Here we describe bans and providing information as two examples.

Banning risk factors or limiting their use

Bans can limit the harm that products can cause to others, such as second-hand smoke, and reduce people's access to the means of self-harm, such as cheap alcohol. These strategies decrease availability (increasing their effective price), making unhealthy options more difficult to choose.

Do bans work? There is now convincing evidence that banning tobacco in public spaces reduces heart attacks. In 2004, a small study conducted in Helena, Montana, USA found that hospitalizations due to heart attacks decreased during the 6-month long smoking ban, compared to rates before the ban was implemented and after the ban was lifted (264). Rates in a comparative community without a smoking ban (a type of 'control' group) did not decrease during that same time, further supporting the causal role of the smoking ban in reducing heart attacks. Similar results have been observed in diverse settings, including Italy (265) and New York 202); few studies of bans in low-income countries have been done but one can imagine similar effects.

Are they feasible? Restaurant owners initially opposed smoking bans, on grounds that their profits would be diminished. In most settings this has proven to be incorrect—in fact, profits rose as many people who avoided restaurants or bars because of undesirable second-hand smoke were liberated to partake and enjoy public spaces without having their health suffer.

In an effort to reduce tobacco use, WHO used its treaty-making powers for the first time to put in place an international framework that signatory countries would agree to implement and allow independent audits of the outcomes of their activities (the Framework Convention on Tobacco Control) (34). Several countries are now implementing nationwide smoking bans in public and work places (including bars and restaurants). In 2004, Ireland was the first country to enact a workplace smoking ban. Norway, Scotland, and England have since followed. However, the Framework Convention on Tobacco Control is an example of the limits of voluntary, self-regulation and, as such, the WHO has no authority to enforce it. As of 2009, fewer than 6% of signatory countries had implemented the bans on tobacco use in public spaces to which they had agreed.

Regulatory approaches also exist to prevent manipulation of children by advertising. Strategies include removing fizzy drinks from school vending machines, limiting the density of fast food restaurants in neighbourhoods (decreasing availability), and requiring chain restaurants to offer 'healthy' alternatives. Some local authorities are banning trans fats from restaurants and seeking to regulate the sugar and salt content of foods.

One radical example of banning a risk factor was Gorbachev's antialcohol campaign in the Soviet Union between 1985 and 1987. Remarkable improvements in alcohol-related mortality occurred, as age-standardized death rates dropped in half during the ban. Diseases related to alcohol, suicide, CVD, and TB also fell markedly among working-age men, as life expectancy rose by 3 years. One of the most successful initiatives in public health history in the past half-century, it was also one of the most unpopular, in part contributing to Gorbachev's political ouster in the 1990s (266).

Strategy 4: Banning a risk factor or reducing its availability is a powerful intervention to prevent chronic disease.

Providing information and curbing misinformation

When people lack access to information to make decisions that reflect the priority they place on being healthy, competitive markets will fail to price them appropriately (see Chapter 3). To fix this problem, regulations can label foods so that people better understand their calorie content and health implications. Even if only a few people respond, it can potentially drive changes through the marketplace to affect producers and suppliers. Restaurants, for example, might not sell enough of an unhealthy product, taking it off the menu. Or more consumption of the healthier products could lead to prices falling. As noted above, these strategies tend to widen health inequalities, as typically the best educated groups are able to find, understand and change their behaviour in light of new information.

Examples include posting calorie counts on fast-food menu boards or labelling foods with a 'red light' if they contain high levels of fat or sugar. Providing information in restaurants is particularly important because in places like the US people eat about one-third of their food away from home, where they spend close to half of their food budgets.

Consider a common dilemma that you might face when trying to decide between a burger and a pasta dish. Both have the same price, and both are equally tasty. If you knew that the pasta had twice the calories, salt and fat (owing to a sauce used), you would likely choose the burger, or perhaps ask for the sauce on the side. Of course, some people might be indifferent to this information and continue to choose the unhealthy option even if they know it is unhealthy. But the basic idea is that those people who know it is healthy will respond, markets will react, lowering prices and, possibly, driving unhealthy products off the menus. These processes help people make healthy choices easier choices for themselves and others.

Does labelling food lead people to make healthier choices? So far, the results have been mixed. Studies of restaurants indicate that the extent to which people look at nutritional information depends on where it is placed and the size of the font (267). None of the restaurants studied thus far has reported a drop in profits, and some have reported increases (268, 269). The groups who make decisions also matter. Restaurants with wealthier clientele appear to report the greatest reductions in calories consumed (269). In some cases, while parents did not change what they purchased for themselves at fast-food restaurants, their decisions on behalf of their children did reduce their calories consumed by more than 100 calories per meal when labelling was present (270).

Lastly, we point to efforts to curb misinformation by marketers. False advertising happens all the time, to such an extent that we sometimes fail to pay attention. A classic piece of misinformation is called the 'puff', an advertising slogan that is clearly false, such as 'We have the best fish and chips in Britain'. One egregious form of misinformation is marketing products to people who are incapable of making informed decisions, especially children. This has provided scope to ban advertising to children in order to protect them from manipulation. It started with banning cartoon-style images, like Joe Camel, to children, but has extended to advertising fast-food on children's TV programmes. This is spurred by evidence that children who are more greatly exposed to junk food ads on television have higher risks of childhood obesity (271).

Many of the approaches described above seem simple to do. But whenever vested interests, typically tobacco, food, or pharmaceutical companies, stand to lose profits from them, implementation will not be straightforward. As seen with tobacco control, at every juncture, industry attempted to frustrate the expansion of effective public health policies to tax and ban cigarettes. The companies produced fraudulent studies and shifted debates to issues that were peripheral to their core interests of getting people hooked on nicotine. So far, by supporting an elaborate system of smuggling and new, unregulated tobacco products, as well as offering gratuitous financial support and cultivating friendships with finance and agriculture ministers they have been able to stay a step ahead of public health efforts to curb tobacco in resource-deprived settings. We are at the early stages of a much longer process to catch up with food and alcohol industries.

Strategy 5: Regulating food, tobacco, and alcohol marketing practices can curb misinformation and psychological manipulation of dietary choices—especially among children—thereby preventing chronic disease.

Broader social policy interventions: health in all policies

So far we have focused on interventions that affect proximal risks. We can venture further upstream, examining the broader choices about society and welfare that can affect people's risks.

One common slogan in public health is not just 'Health for All' but 'Health in All' policies (272), pointing out that 'every minister is a health minister'. These calls draw on the observation that many of the causes of the risk factors are beyond the control of the formal healthcare system. Commonly they are referred to as intersectoral policies, because they integrate the work of many non-health sectors that provide crucial inputs to health.

There is substantial evidence that social policies outside the healthcare system can have a powerful, albeit indirect, influence on the more proximal drivers of chronic disease risk, such as price, availability, and marketing. This can be clearly seen in urban design practices.

Urban planning and transportation policies

Cities have been engineered in unhealthy ways, so that when people move en masse from the countryside to the city centre their risk of chronic diseases increases. Several tried and tested approaches can steer urban development to encourage healthy behaviour. One recent WHO review found that the most important elements of the urban environment for determining if people would be physically active were whether parks and green spaces were available, attractive, and safe; public buildings and daily amenities (such as post offices, banks, libraries, supermarkets and grocery stores, and restaurants) were nearby, and there existed a functioning and desirable public-transportation system (273).

Many of these factors were determined by how streets were laid out. For example, street design can emphasize bikes over cars or vice versa. One example to make it easier and safer to cycle is an intervention to promote physical activity in Bogota, Columbia (Ciclovia). In 1995 city leaders invested resources in improving public transit and building accessible sidewalks and cycleways (building about 260 km of pathway and 16 bicycle routes by 2009). City planners also closed about 120 km of roadways on Sundays, leaving these streets free for use by pedestrians and bicyclists. Unsurprisingly, travel by car dropped from 17% to 12% during peak travel times in the working week, as people chose to walk or bike to work (274).

A remarkable example of a combination of healthy urban planning and transportation policies comes from Curitiba, the fastest-growing city in Brazil during the 1970s. Prior to its rapid growth, urban planners developed an innovative public transport system starting in 1965. The planners specifically set out to build environments that took account of locations and densities of homes, work, recreation, transport, and public services to optimize the opportunities for being physically active (275). As a result, people travelled less frequently by car: in Curitibas, gasoline usage is approximately 30% lower than in other Latin American countries and air pollution is among the lowest in the country (276).

The preceding examples of how planners decided to close certain areas to provide opportunities for activity or design areas for specific activities are types of zoning regulation. These policies can create or limit the availability of healthy products and activities. Zoning regulations can, for example, prohibit fast-food chains from opening new branches near schools. This is important because the concentration of fast-food restaurants within walking distance of schools correlates with increased risk of childhood obesity (277, 278). Similarly, they can prevent pubs from being located alongside each other, found to prevent binge drinking in hotspots.

Urban designers can also provide resources to encourage physical activity. In addition to building sidewalks or cycle lanes, they can provide the means of physical activity, such as by providing free public bicycles. For example, in summer 2007, the Socialist mayor of Paris, Bertrand Delanoe, implemented the Velib public bicycle rental programme, which provided 10,000 bicycles available for rental at low cost at 750 automated rental stations throughout the city. Since that time the number of bikes has grown to 20,000 bicycles and 1639 stations, with one station approximately every 300 meters throughout the city. The programme has been embraced both by Parisians (who use the bicycles for daily commuting as well as for leisure) and tourists (who use the bicycles to explore Paris) alike. In the first year, there were approximately 27.5 million bike trips made, most of which were daily commutes.[2]

In short, urban planning can harness uncontrolled forces of rapid urbanization, but requires foresight by policymakers as well as public resources and investment. The benefits could be substantial over the long run, redesigning societies to be safer, have a stronger sense of community, and be healthier. Unfortunately, this needed public capacity to wrestle back control of social development and provide public goods like parks has been crucially lacking in resource-deprived countries, precisely where the fastest and most dangerous urbanization of poverty is taking place.

Clue 6: Urban planning can steer urban development so as to prevent chronic diseases or pose additional risks.

Strategy 6: Several strategies are immediately available to urban planners for preventing chronic diseases, such as providing bicycles and cycle-ways as well as zoning development so to limit the availability of unhealthy fast-food and alcohol outlets.

Social protection and the welfare system

The expansion of social welfare tends to coincide with the development of health systems. Starting with financial relief to the unemployed, social welfare systems offer services and protection to people against the risks across the life course (including housing support, unemployment insurance, old-age pensions, disability support). However, they also provide public resources to improve the quality of people's lives, counteracting some of the harmful aspects of society's current engineering.

These social programmes offer substantial protection against chronic disease risks. For example, family-support programmes, a type of social welfare policy, can provide more time to mothers to cook healthy meals for their children and encourage active play. Although people are less active overall, they are in fact choosing to exercise more than ever in their free time to prevent obesity. In the US, for example, people's leisure time has declined as hours worked has risen; overall, Americans work more than 20 additional days out of the year than their European counterparts. Social supports can give people more control of their lives.

Social protections can also help prevent people from initiating risky behaviours in response to psychological stressors. Active labour market programmes can help people who lose jobs get back to work faster as well as prevent them from becoming depressed, harmfully using drugs, and experiencing heart attacks or strokes. A growing body of evidence reveals that social protections can improve many health-related outcomes, both infectious and chronic, in several cases more so than healthcare spending (279, 280).

Clue 7: Social spending on family support, housing subsidies, job reintegration programmes, survivor benefits, and disability support can prevent chronic diseases.

Since the 1970s WHO and a plethora of other organizations have called for intersectoral, whole-of-government approaches to promoting health, including social protections. Why aren't they being implemented?

In practice these approaches are politically difficult to achieve. One problem is that people working in the health system often try to engage other sectors as a mendicant: 'Please education, will you help promote health? Please agriculture, will you realize that your subsidies are worsening health? Please finance ministers, will you invest in the public health system?' Studies show that intersectoral action is most likely to happen when there is clear mutual benefit and clearly defined roles about who should take the lead (281). It sounds obvious, but rarely happens. Perversely, incentives mitigate against it. Organizations are too busy with their own agendas; there can be countervailing arguments and vested interests; and leaders in public health, protecting their own fiefdoms, might be reluctant to give up responsibility to a different part of government.

Clue 8: Activities to prevent chronic diseases across multiple sectors are most likely to occur when there are clearly defined roles for each group, mutual benefits, budgetary support for planning, and an institutional basis for engagement.

How do we choose appropriate interventions? Cost-effectiveness versus community-driven approaches

Thus far we have covered interventions ranging from individual medical therapy to the global legal frameworks. The next logical question is how can we implement the most effective interventions to save the most lives and reduce suffering?

The pursuit of an answer dominates thinking in public health, but it is actually not the question driving public health policy. Instead, the issue most central to people in power tends to be: 'how can we save the most lives at low cost?' and 'how do we decide which few among the range of interventions to implement?'.

Here we return to the debate about Selective Primary Health Care, as its reliance on the technology of cost-effectiveness embodies this policy tradition. Building on its successful drive to help eradicate smallpox in the 1970s, the Rockefeller Foundation launched a project, Good Health At Low Cost, in the 1980s to identify why some countries were doing better with fewer resources (cajoled as 'Good Health In Spite of Poverty' (282)). The project, led by the architects of Selective Primary Health Care (283), concluded that poor countries simply could not afford PHC on the basis of cost-effectiveness considerations:

> The selective approach to controlling endemic disease in the developing countries is potentially the most cost-effective type of medical intervention. On the basis of high morbidity and mortality and of feasibility of control, a circumscribed number of diseases are selected for prevention in a clearly defined population. Since few programmes based on this selective model of prevention and treatment have been attempted. The following approach is proposed. The principal recipients of care would be children up to three years old and women in the childbearing years. The care provided would be measles and diphtheria-pertussis tetanus vaccination for children over six months old, tetanus toxoid to all women of childbearing age, encouragement of long-term breast feeding, provision of chloro-quine for episodes of fever in children under three years old in areas where malaria is prevalent and, finally, oral rehydration packets and instruction.

This emphasis on deciding what to do to promote health based on economic considerations was not new. It could be traced back to the period of resource scarcity during the Great Depression. Policymakers wanted to know how to do more with less money. Methods for answering these questions, to show how much public investment returned to society, were originally developed in departments of defence, but soon extended to all areas of the public sector.

In the WHO's 2000 World Health Report the cost-effectiveness paradigm played a central role in judging the performance of medical care systems. Three main criteria were employed: effectiveness, responsiveness and fairness of financing. Central to the values informing the WHO report's model and vision of healthcare systems were studies of cost-effectiveness. According to this view, the role of healthcare systems was to provide healthcare services that could help the most people at the lowest cost. As the lead author stated, 'our emphasis is not on more money for health but on more health for money' (284).

To assist this process of choosing appropriate interventions, the authors of the WHO World Health Report created a metric to evaluate health systems along multiple indicators of service performance. However, by collapsing numerous difficult-to-assess statistics into one common health system indicator, the WHO report resulted in some difficult results to interpret. Haiti's health system was given the same 'score' as China's, and several systems experiencing significant patient complaints, access deficits, and poor patient outcomes received high scores without it being clear what factored into such a score. Spain, ranking surprisingly high, was at the time experiencing civil riots in response to its poor quality of healthcare (285).

The WHO report came under vigorous critiques from both the left and right, the most significant of which were by Vincent Navarro, focusing on the values expressed in the report's measurements and methods. First, the report's measure of effectiveness was based on health; but the greater health was viewed as an indicator of better healthcare, an assumption which cannot be made (see Chapter 2 and discussion above). Second, the report's measure of responsiveness led to a radical shift of planning from people's needs to market demand. It focused on responsive consumers in the market to drive up quality in healthcare. Thus, the US was deemed the most responsive healthcare system. As the report stated, countries should give more importance to reforms that aim at 'making money follow the patient, shifting away from simply giving providers budgets, which in turn are often determined by supposed needs' (222, 285). Third, the report judged fairness by the percentage spent on healthcare by different income groups. According to such a measure, massive inequalities could persist in a 'fair' system, such as when the poor in Brazil spend 10% of their income (a few US cents) and the rich spend 10% (amounting to several million dollars). While the report acknowledged that regulating the private sector was an important challenge facing health systems, it advocated a weak regulatory model put forward by Enthoven (who inspired the Thatcher-era privatization reforms).

The focus on cost-effectiveness in Selective Primary Health Care is sometimes used to legitimate a focus on infectious diseases. It is often argued that treating chronic diseases are too costly compared with infectious diseases. For example, World Bank authors argue that if chronic disease are seen as consequences of affluence and old age and are expensive to treat given their very chronic nature, we should not bother with them at all. People see how expensive cardiac care is in rich countries, hear about how they are breaking the bank, and wonder how it could possibly be contemplated in poor countries. At the same time, people see countries like Cuba put an emphasis on developing advanced tertiary care, yet at times lack basic equipment, like surgical gloves.

However, even working within a cost-effectiveness paradigm, the common assertions that chronic diseases are too costly to treat are untenable. Two types of economic studies reveal this: cost-effectiveness and cost–benefit analysis. (Others exist, such as broader measures of cost-utility analysis, but we bracket them here.) These typically assess the cost per unit of health benefit, typically in disability- or quality-adjusted life years. One commonly used international threshold says that an intervention is cost-effective if it saves one disability-adjusted life year at the price of $30,000 USD. Another one that is applied regards an intervention to be a good buy if it saves one disability-adjusted life year for less than a country's average income per capita.

Nearly all of the interventions discussed above are as, if not more, cost-effective than many available infectious disease interventions (286). In fact, some of them are among the most affordable and cost-savings strategies available to politicians. Tobacco and alcohol taxes, for example, can be a clear win-win: reduced healthcare costs, increased government tax revenues. (The situation is slightly more complicated in countries which export tobacco as part of the trade specialization model discussed in Chapter 2 and 7.) Several medical interventions are cost-effective, including tobacco-cessation programmes, contextually appropriate mass-media education campaigns to improve diet, community-based physical activity programmes, and secondary prevention through pharmacological interventions (such as the diabetes reduction programmes). Many of these are below US $1000 per disability-adjusted life year saved. Salt reduction to levels recommended by WHO are estimated to cost about US $0.04–0.32 and prevent about 8.5 million deaths over 10 years (287).

Yet, the net costs are sometimes disputed. Some critics argue that reducing a risk factor will extend life, leading to an overall rise in the medical care a person consumes. Countering this argument, it was proposed that by reducing the degree of sickness a person experiences (morbidity), that overall costs would be lower. Firing back, other people question this model, wondering whether it is realistic for people to live healthy lives until they reach to their average lifespan, then go out like light bulbs—the most affordable way to die (28).

Sometimes there is great difficulty in estimating the full costs and benefits, more of an art than a science. How do you count the costs of agricultural policies that subsidize unhealthy foods? They help farmers, but harm public health. How do you quantify people's lost freedom, in terms of changes in market choices, or altered property values when commodity prices change? How do the spin-off benefits, such as better education when children eat healthier foods, get included in the equation? Another challenge is figuring out what is the alternative scenario. Is the drug cost-effective to not treating patients at all or once they have reached an advanced stage of disease? Often these latter scenarios are the case in resource-deprived countries.

As another example, school-based education interventions are often estimated to be ineffective in cost terms because they take decades for the health benefits to accrue. Does it make sense to do nothing to protect children because it is simply cost-ineffective? Cost-effectiveness, with its focus on immediate impacts, has a bias towards downstream, medical interventions and magic-bullet policies or medicines, rather than focusing on structural reforms to the societal risks that increase people's risk in the first place.

Returning to the World Health Report, the emphasis on 'more health for money' over 'more money for health' mistakenly treats these two approaches as a zero-sum game. In fact, choosing a strategy that initially gets less health for money, such as helping children, could yield more money for health in the long run, both by saving money in the future and by creating political space to attract more resources (increasing the amount of money available for intervening, see Chapter 5). Further, squabbling over a small pool of resources, however scientific it might seem to practitioners of cost-effectiveness, could perversely make that pool of resources smaller, as policymakers may come to view public health resources being ineffectively allocated or scientifically imprecise.

Debates continue; what is clear is that for every cost-effectiveness study, counterpoints will be raised and assumptions questioned. It is not as clear-cut a scientific means for selecting policy as its advocates would like decision-makers to believe.

Clue 9: Taxes on tobacco, alcohol, and junk-food are among the most highly cost-effective interventions available and typically are cost-saving because they generate revenue.

Clue 10: Regulations to reduce salts, sugars, and fats are also highly cost-effective.

Clue 11: Defining the costs, effects, and counterfactual in cost-effectiveness studies is a difficult task which involves many assumptions of debatable validity.

Clue 12: An overemphasis on cost-effectiveness as a decision-making criterion can result in the neglect of interventions that can yield significant benefits in the future (such as prioritizing immediate, quick-fix approaches over longer-term early childhood interventions).

Clue 13: Despite clear evidence that chronic disease interventions are highly cost-effective, it cannot be assumed that they will work in resource-poor settings.

Community-based, -participatory, and -driven interventions

The inverse of the cost-effectiveness paradigm, whereby a set of Western scientists define the costs, effects, and set of appropriate interventions in a fixed budget, is the classic PHC mantra—power to patients and their communities. This tradition has been most visibly taken up by a growing body of work on community-driven interventions (288). Rather than focusing on pre-conceived models developed outside of communities by Western experts, community-driven approaches recognize that those most affected by disease also have their own thoughts, opinions, and locally-contextualized perspectives about how to reduce their risk.

We regard community-driven interventions as an illustration of liberatory medicine because it enables communities to define their needs and methods for solving problems, while working closely with experts in public health and medicine. While community participation has become a buzzword in development circles, this generally involves focus groups or a survey incorporated into the planning of an already-developed development programme. In contrast, true participation actually involves giving community members the power to describe the ideas behind programmes, their logistics, and evaluation (i.e. community-driven). Few community driven interventions have been tried. However, community-based interventions, with elements of community participation, have been applied to a range of health issues, spanning individual medical treatment to underlying social determinants of health (289).

Often touted as the first and most effective chronic disease population intervention to date, the Finnish North Karelia project exemplified important features of the community-based participatory model (there is debate about the extent of community participation in the design of the project). Giving voice to communities, the public health community employed mass media, education, community organizing, and environmental change to identify and act on the causes of CVD. From the programme's start in 1972 to long-term follow-up in 1995, the community of North Karelia experienced reduction in mortality rates due to CVD by three-quarters among working-age populations, a remarkable outcome. However, the apparent success of North Karelia has been critiqued. Its community's rates of decline in CVD were similarly experienced in other regions of North Karelia and occurred in periods of economic downturn and stagnation (290) (see Chapter 2).

Shortly after the early effects of the North Karelia Project were reported, several well-known community-based interventions took place in the US including the Stanford Five-City Project, the Minnesota Heart Health Project, and the Pawtucket Heart Health Project, although, unlike North Karelia, they were mainly education interventions applied at the community level. These projects failed to reproduce the apparent success of the North Karelia project. While strategies focused on education, mass media campaigns, community organizing, and social marketing, results encouraged alternative methods for accelerating change. Final reports from Minnesota Heart Health Project and Pawtucket Heart Health Project suggested the potential benefits of partnering the education and social marketing used in their studies with structural strategies focused on macro-oriented policy and environmental changes. Drawing insights from these successes and failures of community programmes, WHO began recommending that community-based approaches integrate policy and environmental changes with education and social marketing. The most recent and important example of this approach is the Shape-Up Somerville project, jointly funded by the US Centers for Disease Control and Prevention, the PepsiCo Foundation (initially through PepsiCo's subsidiary company, Dole), and other funders. Academics teamed up with communities in diverse settings to seek community-defined ways to prevent childhood obesity. The project team reported that the intervention community had less weight gain in children over the 8-month study period (289). Another project in France, translated from French as 'Together, let's prevent obesity in children', applied a community-based approach to communicate the importance of healthy eating and active lifestyles, successfully reducing childhood obesity rates by 9% The programme is now being extended to 200 towns throughout Europe and being applied in Mexico.

Nearly all community-based initiatives for chronic diseases have been in high-income countries, with a few important exceptions we discuss here. Among the most cited examples in middle-income countries are the Isfahan Healthy Heart Program in Iran and the Agita São Paulo programme in Brazil (extended recently to some other Latin American countries). Both followed a community-based approach (but were not led by the community) and emphasized structural interventions, but in practice emphasized education-based modification of lifestyles, mainly through promoting exercise and teaching people about how to make healthier food choices.

The Isfahan Healthy Heart Program, a comprehensive community-based program started in 1999 in Iran, a country known for its historical embrace of PHC principles (291). Strategies included a broad range of interventions from policy changes in food production to television shows promoting physical activity, targeting both high-risk groups and entire populations. After 4 years the Isfahan Healthy Heart Program achieved significant increases in the percentage of individuals with a healthy diet and mean lifestyle score (a composite score combining smoking status, nutrition, and physical activity levels); no significant change was reported individually for daily smoking, daily physical activity energy expenditure, or leisure time physical activity. Isfahan Healthy Heart Program applied a universal, predetermined package of specific interventions, but provided scope for tailoring the appropriate package to the needs, culture, and lifestyle of the community. For example, the community in Isfahan identified that the use of hydrogenated oils in cooking was a large contributor to consumption of trans fatty acids in the regional diet. Responding to these community priorities, Isfahan Healthy Heart Program included an emphasis on switching to healthier cooking oils, focusing on women.

Such small-scale approaches can deliver real change in resource-deprived communities. The second example is Agita São Paolo, meaning 'Move São Paulo', in Brazil's São Paulo state. The programme is a multi-level physical activity initiative aimed at increasing the public's knowledge of benefits of physical activity. Agita has widespread reach, with close to three-fifths of the population reporting having heard about the programme and over one-third knowing its purpose. Physical activity levels have increased because of the programme (292), which was also found to be cost-effective. The World Bank estimated that scaling it up could save one disability-adjusted life year for US $247. The programme, described further in Chapter 7.4, is being extended throughout Latin America.

The programmes in Isfahan and São Paulo have resulted in significant improvements to public health, but aside from being focused on middle-income nations, the benefits within these countries have been seen mainly among the more affluent sectors of society. The Agita programme has mostly benefited those who are employed, who have private insurance, are literate, or have access to schools. The Isfahan programme similarly has had relatively low efficacy among women, those with low educational status, and those who live in rural areas.

Projects are underway to assess whether community-based or community-driven prevention programmes can similarly reduce risks of chronic diseases. One example is Community Interventions for Health, a PepsiCo Foundation funded project to design, implement, and evaluate interventions in China, India, and Mexico. Using a mapping tool, the researchers collect and integrate information about the accessibility, availability, and affordability of dietary products, physical activity, and tobacco to identify 'hot spots' for intervention implementation. Community members and researchers work together to map environmental risks. This can help mobilize communities around shared risks. For example, in conducting the mapping activity, the CIH-China team identified a need for food labelling. This has set the stage for further discussions around a national labelling scheme.

Despite gaps in the evidence base, this process of community-led decisions about what to do and how to do it, in combination with experts who experiment and replicate policies while helping accumulate evidence, is one way how resource-limited communities can address the rising burden of chronic diseases while building a more equitable society.

Clue 14: Innovative projects that begin in low-income communities can spread to high-income settings and vice-versa.

Strategy 7: Community-led decisions about what interventions to do and how to implement them, in combination with experts who experiment and replicate policies while helping build the evidence base, can effectively address the rising burden of chronic diseases at low cost in resource-poor communities.

In the next section, we describe the logistics of how to implement community-driven interventions in a resource-poor setting.

Putting it all together: a global agenda for local programme development

We return to the first chapter, where we described the risk to women of COPD in a small South Asian farming community. This story provides several important lessons about how to manage chronic diseases in resource-poor settings, from identifying the leading causes of avoidable death to intervening using community-driven, cost-effective strategies.

Identifying local causes, priorities and solutions—community epidemiology

It should not be assumed that because the US and Europe have had greater familiarity with chronic diseases, their models of intervention are necessarily the most appropriate in other settings. In most of the world, COPD is a result of tobacco smoking. Yet, in this agricultural community in South Asia, the main cause was indoor air pollution.

Had the doctors simply emphasized a narrow set of interventions, such as smoking bans or tobacco education efforts as in the US and Europe, they would have failed to address the majority of COPD cases. Tapping community-specific knowledge was a crucial step to identifying the local causes of disease. Investigating community-specific risks and potential interventions involves taking a close look at the daily realities of the risks and living experiences of patients.

Community epidemiology overcomes the false dichotomy of 'rich country versus poor country' solutions. This latter approach often limits funding for poor communities under the premise that quick-fix, easy-to-do interventions are 'appropriate technology' for the poor, whereas comprehensive interventions can only be done in rich nations. Rather, such a community-driven approach is needed to support groups ranging from a rural community in South Asia to diabetic patients in the Bronx to slum dwellers with high rates of CVD in Cape Town.

Strategy 8: Community-based approaches offer one possible way to tailor investigations of chronic disease causes and their management to individual communities.

Addressing the structural causes of poor health

The most commonly implemented public health interventions in resource-denied communities do not affect the balance of resources, but merely provide educational messages. If the physicians in the South Asian example solely lectured women on the risk of smoke inhalation, as opposed to building chimneys above their stoves, could we have expected a reduction in COPD rates in their community?

Many of the poorest people affected by chronic diseases are also exposed to risks, such as smoke and stoves that cause respiratory disease, that are inescapable in the context of poverty. Addressing these factors grounded in the daily realities of poverty requires material resources, such as greater access to improved household appliances, power, or agricultural technologies (to avert 'slash and burn' agriculture or incineration of trash, two sources of daily smoke inhalation in poor communities).

Greater reductions in chronic disease rates among poorer households have been observed when actual resource allocations to the poor have increased, permitting greater freedoms to control one's lifestyle. For example, the Community Interventions for Health (CIH) programme targets not only education, but also changes to living and working environments, such as building exercise facilities in public places, providing access to sports equipment and bicycles, cultivating family vegetable gardens, and expanding health services delivery through trained community health workers.

Strategy 9: Re-engineering the development of unhealthy societies can have a much greater impact on health than information and education interventions that ask individuals to adapt to unhealthy circumstances.

Defining the means and ends of community-based programmes

The starting point of intervention is often unrealistic. The health fantasies to reduce the burden of disease by 90%, albeit often cited, provide little help in practice. WHO's broad definition of health has been critiqued as 'utterly unrealistic'. As one former director of Médecins Sans Frontières put it: 'For WHO, health does not consist of the absence of disease or handicaps; it is the state of complete well-being, physical, mental, and social . . . It has nothing to do with the concrete world, with real people, with actual diseases, or with typical expectations about health'.

It is crucial to set out specific policies for achieving specific goals. Even when these ideas are set out, however, they can be the subject of dispute. One concrete perspective was recently elaborated by Dr Giles (a pseudo-name has been used to conceal the identity of the doctor) of the Rockefeller Foundation, arguing that 'Our goal . . . is not to achieve immortality, or to extend our lives beyond normal ranges'. He pointed out that in spite of great advances to living conditions and medical technology people over the age of 65 are not living much longer than they have before. Instead, more people should have an opportunity for a reasonably long life, instead of dying too young from avoidable causes, so that the average lifespan increases. He continued:

> 'Our objective is that we can prevent diseases for the duration of a normal lifetime. That is, we can be born and experience a good childhood, a healthy young adulthood, and be free of disease until a reasonably old age, when our bodies should arrive at a point where they essentially fall apart and we disappear instead of being a burden. And at this achievement of medical research, this prevention of the diseases we now face, we will be saving millions of dollars in averted medical bills along the way'.

This is an extreme version of a goal referred to as the compression of morbidity (see Chapter 1), which aims to reduce the period in which people suffer before dying. According to it, people will live to their natural age, then, as one epidemiologist said it, 'drop like flies' (28).

One fallacy in Dr. Giles' statement is the oft-cited claim that primary prevention will save money. In reality, averting diseases among youth and young adults may avert those immediate costs, but people will become ill of other diseases at older ages, contributing other costs, often more expensive costs. We may prevent measles in infants, and TB in young adults, but then these saved lives will face heart disease after retirement or cancer and strokes when elderly. Unsurprisingly, a series of studies have found that reducing obesity, over the course of a lifetime, noting 'prevention [is] no cure for rising healthcare expenditure' (293).

We could attempt to create massive cost-effectiveness studies to determine exactly what to do, but the metrics of quality-adjusted life years and disability-adjusted life years that we calculate to generate these studies are highly subject to judgement and modelling assumptions, often lacking statistical validity or reproducibility among researchers, particularly when they are manipulated to show that the researchers' own intervention is necessarily cost-effective (as described in preceding sections).

Rather than focusing on cost-effectiveness and lifetimes, one goal is to reduce the avoidable suffering resulting from disease through a community-specific focus. From this perspective, saving money is not its own virtue; rather, we will spend money, but can do so reasonably, with the reduction of human suffering as our goal. Just as with education, public health is 'sunk cost' whose benefit will not be reaped in direct economic results, but only in diffuse community-wide, long-term ones. Some of the money may go to primary prevention, but we must acknowledge the limited efficacy observed among primary prevention initiatives. People will get sick, and our goal must include mitigating the severity of their disease and the suffering that results from it, for both themselves, and their families and communities. Diabetic patients often lose limbs, or die prematurely, adversely impacting upon their ability to act as parents, as employees, and as contributors to community life. Individuals addicted to tobacco regularly spend money on cigarettes that would otherwise go towards education of themselves or their family members, and towards better quality housing, food, or social opportunities (see Chapter 3).

Clue 15: People will get sick no matter what we do.

Strategy 10: One key goal of interventions is to reduce the levels of avoidable and unfair suffering due to chronic diseases (as often indicated by social inequalities in health).

If we adopt this perspective that our goal should be to reduce the avoidable suffering resulting from disease through a community-specific focus, how can we develop chronic disease prevention and management programmes in settings that have been denied healthcare resources?

Building on commonalities in managing non-communicable and infectious diseases among the rural poor

What practical steps should we take to construct and administer chronic disease management programmes? What should be the focus of such programmes, who will administer them, what will be their day-to-day operations, and how will we know if they're effective?

These questions are increasingly being posed to a growing body of 'operations researchers', who make a living by testing projects in many different communities. An abundance of acronyms for new programmes, claims about which projects are 'models', and competing publications and pamphlets have appeared from dozens of agencies, non-profit, and institutional groups. The result has been a complex web of instructions about how we should proceed in a diverse mix of environments and populations. Unfortunately, little of this knowledge provides practical guidance about how to address chronic diseases among the world's most deprived communities.

At the time of this writing, most interventions for chronic diseases have demonstrated limited efficacy and been subject to testing over only short durations. Of these studies, most have been conducted in high-income and middle-income countries; only a few have been done in urban locales of poorer countries, and rarely include the rural poor who constitute the majority of the world's population and the largest population facing chronic disease risks.

The most widely-studied models of disease prevention and care for the rural poor focus on managing infectious diseases. In the cases of TB and HIV treatment, these serve as potential templates for chronic disease, as these conditions are effectively chronic. TB treatment requires at least 6 months of daily therapy, and HIV treatment currently involves a lifetime of therapy. Diabetes and pulmonary disease treatment, and the care of many chronic heart diseases, share these requirements. The most commonly assessed form of therapeutic delivery in the community is DOTS, in which patients are supervised during daily administration of medications. Several DOTS programmes achieve among the highest treatment success rates in impoverished settings for both HIV and TB.

Many successful community-based infectious disease programmes rely on community health workers to deliver care. Rather than a more paternalistic focus on daily supervision in a clinic, these programmes appear oriented towards delivering care near or at patients' homes, reducing the transportation and associated cost barriers to adhere to sometimes complex medication regimens. They also provide a daily nursing supporter who can provide emotional, informational, and psychological support to patients through the course of illness.

Community health worker programmes are commonly used not only for TB and HIV therapy, but also for maternal and child health programmes, the treatment of basic respiratory infections, and malnutrition or diarrhoea treatment programmes. Why not chronic diseases?

The advantage of this approach is that it is already being introduced rapidly and extensively into the poorest rural populations on all continents. As a result of the extensive initiatives to introduce ART and TB therapy into poor communities, community health workers are trained and deployed in hundreds of settings, often with carefully coordinated systems for ongoing training, payment, retention, and evaluation. To create a parallel system for chronic diseases may be a waste, particularly as the same households faced by infectious diseases and maternal and child care problems addressed by community workers are often the same households facing the burden of chronic diseases.

The most effective community health worker programmes in sub-Saharan African countries have revealed that they are most effective when providing preventative services. Health education alone appears to strip community workers of respect in the community and autonomy, whereas permitting them to deliver medical treatments with some visible curative potential, as simple as oral rehydration salts, bolsters their community position and, as a result, long-term sustenance of delivery programmes.

There has long been a mantra that the rich countries get doctors; poor countries get community health workers. An important caveat is that community health workers do not replace qualified medical practitioners, but rather serve as an auxiliary to existing health clinics and hospitals. This frees up time for doctors to focus on specialized tasks, while allowing for community-based follow-up treatments, medication dispensation, earlier diagnosis and triage. This is especially important to dispersed rural populations who would otherwise face barriers to accessing care and pharmaceuticals required for managing chronic disease on a daily basis.

All countries, rich and poor, can take advantage of the potential to mobilize community health workers to respond to the challenge of chronic diseases in unhealthy societies. Their involvement can help transform healthcare systems to a preventative, patient-centred delivery system—a chronic care model—of long-term care.

Strategy 11: Community health workers can be mobilized in both rich and poor settings to deliver chronic care that is tailored to the needs of communities.

Keeping track: creating the metrics for good outcomes

Irrespective of how chronic care is delivered, it is vital that programmes are responsible to the communities they serve. Part of this responsibility is to evaluate their performance and improve critical deficits in service. In the current era of Millennium Development Goals, cost-effectiveness analyses, and complex health system indicators, most metrics of health programme performance are far removed from actual day-to-day logistical concerns of clinical and public health services. While complex metrics may be useful for detailed epidemiologic analysis, they risk being fundamentally undemocratic and excluding communities in shared efforts to improve local programmes and care services.

Simple, easy-to-measure metrics, which can be collected and understood by healthcare workers with potentially limited educational backgrounds, are likely more appropriate. For example, syndromic surveillance by tracking basic symptom complaints, number of vials of drugs used, number of clinic visits attended, number of times visits were missed due to transportation costs or other issues, can serve as replicable indicators of how well a home-based diabetes or COPD programme is working. The key to such simple indicators is that they provide a constructive criticism of programme logistics, so that their presentation at community meetings or to community health staff provides a clear indication of where programmes must improve from year to year.

For those regions with more extensive infrastructure, laboratory-based programme indicators can be used to track individual patient outcomes, such as the change in the haemoglobin A1c of diabetic patients or spirometry ratings among COPD patients (clinical indicators of disease control).

But there are rarely indicators of programme performance at a population level for chronic diseases; usually full prevalence studies, requiring extensive resources and are rarely if ever performed, are used to track population disease status. Household surveys of laboratory indicators not only monitor individual patient performance, but also provide a sense of the population-level changes in risks of time. For example, cross-sectional surveys of the haemoglobin A1c levels among randomly chosen households over time can provide a population-level indication of diabetes control. Community spirometry clinics, similarly, can track lung disease outcomes, just as blood pressure clinics at markets can obtain random comparable samples to evaluate prevalence of hypertension in a community.

Strategy 12: Community-based epidemiologic approaches can keep track of successes and failures using simple metrics so to create awareness of chronic diseases, identify emerging needs, and ensure responsibility to communities.

Summary

All scientific work is incomplete . . . That does not confer upon us a freedom to ignore the knowledge we already have, or to postpone the action that it appears to command at a given time.

Austin Bradford Hill, 1965

In public health, debates have long occurred about the merits of upstream and downstream approaches. What good is it to heal an ill person but send them back to the environment that made them sick in the first place? Approaches that focus on unhealthy environments can help make it easy for people to be healthy (while doing nothing continues to make it more difficult for people to be healthy).

It seems sensible that any comprehensive control strategy must focus on prevention. There is, unfortunately, little evidence that individual interventions can be scaled up to improve the health of populations. This is because the real world is often not like clinical settings. Here the lack of a biological model, as discussed in Chapter 1, and the lack of a theoretical model of human behaviour, can mean that even the most efficacious interventions may be ineffective or lead to unintended consequences when applied to an entire population.

Part of the problem is that we often falsely leap to the conclusion that the prevention of NCDs is a matter of education. This assumes a great deal of agency and choice among the affected population. When designing interventions for poorer members of a community, such as the women affected by indoor air pollution, we must recognize the constraints to human behaviour. Structural interventions that have directly targeted the burdens of living in poverty and stresses associated with it have been observed to have the greatest effectiveness at mitigating tobacco and alcohol (and other drug) use among the poor.

Instead, some of the most promising (and low-cost) interventions require reverse-engineering some of the changes in society that have led more people to become ill. Taxes and regulations are the two most powerful levers of public health interventions, helping make healthy choices the easy choices.

Urban planning can also harness uncontrolled forces of rapid urbanization, but requires foresight by policymakers as well as public resources and investment. The benefits could be substantial over the long run, redesigning societies to be safer, have a stronger sense of community, and resources for being healthy. Unfortunately, this needed public capacity to wrestle back control of social development and provide public goods like parks has been crucially lacking in resource-deprived countries, precisely where the fastest and most dangerous urbanization of poverty is taking place (a point returned in the country case studies of Chapter 7).

Many of the approaches described above seem clearly beneficial and easy to do. However effective and cost-effective they appear, they face opposing vested interests and formidable political barriers. It cannot be assumed that interventions are simple to do when vested interests stand to lose profits from them. Even the most basic interventions, such as tobacco control, have proven to be extremely challenging. At every juncture, industry attempted to frustrate the expansion of effective public health policies to tax and ban cigarettes. So far, by supporting an elaborate system of smuggling and new, unregulated tobacco products, they have been able to stay a step ahead of public health. In cases where there has been political support, it is unclear that actual action on the ground occurs. When health information campaigns were implemented to raise awareness among youth about risks of tobacco, the industry attempted to frustrate efforts at all turns, making it seem 'cool' to engage in an unhealthy behaviour. With regard to food and alcohol we are at the early stages of a much longer process to catch up.

How do we choose among the range of possible interventions?

One option is for scientists to define the costs, effects, and set of appropriate interventions in a fixed budget. Usually the criterion is cost-effectiveness. It is not so clear-cut as a scientific criterion for choosing policy as its advocates would like decision-makers to believe. For example, choosing a strategy that initially gets less health for money, such as helping children, could yield more money for health in the long run, both by saving money in the future and by creating political space to attract more resources (increasing the amount of money available for intervening, as discussed in Chapter 5 in summaries of strategies used to prevent HIV).

An alternative strategy, embodying the principles of PHC, is to let communities decide. Only by undergoing a process of self-determination, jointly with experts, can lasting change be achieved, breaking the cycle of dependency and illness. Analogous to the chronic care model as applied to doctor–patient relationships, participatory, community-based approaches aim to achieve a balance of power among experts and patients and their communities in sharing values and setting priorities.

Nonetheless, to our knowledge, no existing studies have compared actual chronic disease management programmes among the rural poor. Testing alternative models of programme delivery for chronic diseases in poor rural communities could help ascertain which logistical models of care delivery can have the greatest impact. These types of metrics are only now being evaluated in a few pilot projects—their results are still pending at the time of this writing. The sphere of testing and operations research remains largely empty and available for public health and medical researchers to engage with rural poor communities as they encounter NCDs.

Despite these remaining gaps in the evidence base, there is robust evidence that something can be done at reasonably low cost through community-led interventions. Experts will continue to squabble over the relative merits and cost-effectiveness of programmes. This is wasting time. The price of inaction on tobacco numbers billions of deaths. We can begin working with communities now. Treatment can lead to prevention; prevention can lead to treatment; there are many sequences to action. The key is to start.

Weak health systems add to the challenge of getting these programmes off the ground. Where there is little or no surveillance, interventions are like driving without a dashboard. With surveillance we can adjust our speed and fine-tune action. But this should not stop us from starting the process of joining with communities to decide key priorities, identify risks, and strategies for intervention, as experts help set up experiments, replicate them, and learn from their successes and failures while building the evidence.

The next chapter about the political economy of NCDs considers these substantial challenges to increasing the priority and action on NCDs, reviewing how past social movements have overcome these barriers to achieve remarkable improvements in public health.

Endnotes

1 This is not to be confused with liberation medicine, a different movement building on traditional healers and religious practices of medicine combined with faith-based intervention approaches.

2 The programme is financed by JCDecaux Advertising, which invested nearly $142 million in start-up costs, in exchange for free advertising throughout the city of Paris (this is why rental costs can be kept so low). However, costly problems that have been encountered include vandalism and theft.

Chapter 5

Politics of chronic disease

- What action is currently happening globally?
- Where is the money coming from, where is it going, and is it enough?
- Why are chronic diseases neglected?
- How can the priority of chronic diseases be increased?

David Stuckler, Sanjay Basu, Lawrence King, Sarah Steele, and Martin McKee

Part 1

Political economy of chronic disease

Key policy points

1 Despite repeated calls to action on chronic diseases over the past decade, there is a critical lack of funds and resources available for chronic disease control.

2 Less than 3% of $22 billion in global health funds went to chronic diseases in 2007. The top global health funders, Gates Foundation, Global Fund to Fight HIV, TB and Malaria, and World Bank commit less than 2% of their budgets to NCDs. The top funder of chronic diseases, WHO, allocates about 9% of its budget to NCDs (and about 38% of its core budget), totalling close to $200 million.

3 About half of all global health money comes from private foundations or companies. This money is channelled through budgeting systems that are inconsistent and difficult to track. Close to one-third of the money earmarked for health is spent on unidentifiable activities.

4 Overall, there is little or no correlation between global health funding and the disease burden, suggesting factors other than need are driving the global health agenda. This inconsistency occurs in spite of donors' commitments to align aid flows with national health needs.

5 The misalignment between health needs and health allocations is the greatest for private donors, who assign the least priority to chronic diseases. Many of these private donors have potential conflicts of interests, as they are in close contact with, sit on the boards of, or own substantial shares in food and pharmaceutical companies.

6 Ultimately, the failure to prioritize and act on chronic diseases is a political, rather than a technical issue.

Key practice points

1 The most important questions to ask about global health interventions are: who wins and who loses?

2 Global health is ruled by a few private donors who make decisions in secret. The capacity to decide what is relevant and how it will be addressed is in the hands of very few, who ultimately are accountable to their own interests. A challenge for global health is to identify these interests and bring them to the light of day, holding them to standards of transparency and public accountability.

3 Studying who rules global health is difficult, because power cannot be directly observed and involves complex relationships. Three questions to ask are: Where does the money come from and how much? Who sits on the executive board (and what are their histories and whose interests do they serve)? Who wins conflicts (in this case, deliberately choosing to exclude NCDs from their priorities)?

Key practice points *(continued)*

4 There are five major ways people view global health: as foreign policy, security, charity, investment, and public health. The last listed tends give the highest priority to chronic disease, but also tends to be the weakest in driving global health policy. While there are signs of change, the agendas of top global health funders generally focus on narrow, vertical, and technical interventions for infectious diseases ('smallpox paradigm'). Development agencies tend to view global health as an instrument for achieving foreign policy and security goals.

Political economy of chronic disease

In view of the health and social consequences of rising chronic diseases (set out in Chapters 1 and 3) and the potential for low-cost prevention (set out in Chapter 4), one might expect that leading health organizations, such as WHO and national health ministries, and development institutions that focus on poverty, such as the World Bank and UN Development Programme, would be scaling up efforts to combat chronic diseases. Yet, several academics have recently argued that this is not the case, instead claiming that global chronic diseases are 'neglected', 'silent', 'a hidden epidemic', and that the failure to act is 'scandalous' (see *The Lancet* special issue about 'the neglected epidemic of chronic disease').

A stock take of progress against chronic diseases over the past decade appears to support this view. Despite repeated calls to action, which pointed to the urgent need to address the avoidable and unfair burden of chronic diseases (see Figure 5.1), little seems to have changed. Five years have passed since *The Lancet* and the WHO began calling for a 2% reduction in NCDs each year. Thus far, the trends in disease burden appear to have continued along the same path as predicted in the 'no change' case described in 2005 *Lancet* chronic disease series.

One possible reason for neglect is a feeling that little can be done to tackle chronic diseases. Of course, everyone must die from something, but these chronic disease deaths are highly preventable, as described in Chapters 1 and 4. Certainly, many interventions for chronic diseases are more complex than, say, immunizations or distribution of insecticide treated bed nets (although in reality nothing is simple, given evidence that, in some places, bed nets are used

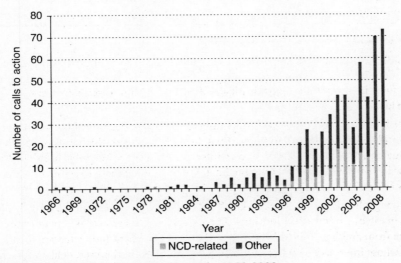

Fig. 5.1 Calls to action published in medical journals: 1966–2009.
Source: Medline, adapted from 298a.

instead for fishing). However, there are some straightforward measures that could be taken now that would impact markedly on the burden of chronic diseases in low- and middle-income countries, such as scaling-up treatment of hypertension and implementing tobacco control measures (although questions remain about whether countries have the capacity to implement them if resources were provided).

It is also possible that chronic disease control is a victim of inadequate overall resources for global health. This argument is less tenable in view of the sharp increase in funding for health since the 1990s. Between 2000 and 2007 the main source of global health funding, development aid for health (DAH), rose from $5.6 billion in 1990 billion to $22.0 billion in 2007. Health was the second fastest growing sector of development aid, receiving the largest share of aid commitments earmarked to a specific sector.

A third possibility is that the burden of chronic diseases is unrecognized or invisible, so that its low priority simply reflects a lack of awareness. This argument could have been sustained until about a decade ago, reflecting what has been described as a 'scandal of ignorance' whereby deaths of adults in much of the developing world (unless it was in childbirth) were invisible beyond those immediately involved (54). However, the intervening period has seen enormous efforts to expand vital registration and, where that has yet to be achieved, to implement sentinel surveillance systems and refined modelling techniques. Evidence from many countries has established that chronic diseases will continue to dominate the overall burden of disease (55) (see Chapter 1).

Why do chronic diseases continue to have low political priority in spite of a growing number of doctors, advocates, and patients who are deeply concerned about them? What lessons can be learned over the past decade that can benefit the movement for global health improvement in general?

In this chapter we seek to understand the potential reasons for this failure to act. The first part of this chapter evaluates the political economy of chronic disease by mapping the programmes and budgets of eight key institutions involved (or not) in the prevention and control of chronic diseases (private donors, national development agencies, academic institutions, nation-states and health ministries, international financial institutions, the UN, and WHO). It provides a preliminary analysis of 'who rules' global health: How are priorities set? Who controls the agenda? And who wins and who loses? Building on this understanding of the global health political system, the second part of the chapter identifies a series of tactics that could be combined to create a social movement to increase the political priority given to chronic diseases.

Who rules global health? Mapping the budgets and priorities of key global health institutions . . .

Based on previous reviews of literature, we have identified eight institutions and groups that are currently or potentially active in chronic disease prevention and control: private donors (including for-profit and non-profit organizations), national development agencies, academic institutions, nation-states/national health ministries, International Financial Institutions, UN development agencies and WHO. Figure 5.2 depicts a simplified web of interrelationships among these groups. In the course of the discussion, we also include the group of health leaders referred to as the H8 (Gates Foundation, WHO, World Bank, GAVI Alliance, the Global Fund, UNICEF, the UN Population Fund, and UNAIDS) (299).

How do we assess power and influence of these institutions in global health? Power is difficult to measure, because it cannot be directly observed and involves complex relationships. Typically, political economy studies rely on three indicators:

1 Where does the money come from, how much is it, and where does it go?

2 Who sits on the board of directors (and what are their histories) and whose interests do they serve (sometimes visible in the mission statements)?

3 Who wins conflicts (in this case, why have they chosen to prioritize chronic diseases or not)?

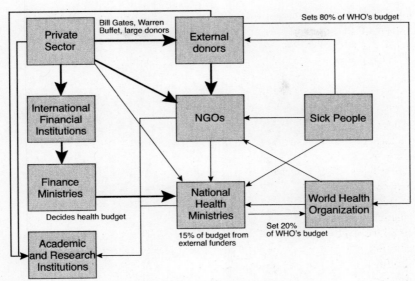

Fig. 5.2 Who sets the agenda: power structure of global health.
Notes: Shade of arrow denotes strength of effect based on authors' judgements of the weighting of financial flows, as described in the main text. External donors broadly include private foundations and national development agencies. For a more comprehensive framework see 298b.

Related to decision-making and control of the agenda, notions of "soft power" (299a) and Lukes' third dimension of power (299b) emphasize the importance of power expressed not only through concrete, observable decisions and financial flows but also in hidden and more subtle, yet powerful, influences such as through shaping perceptions, cognition, and preferences, and influencing what is "kept out" of agendas. This dimension of power is arguably the most powerful; it is ideological in nature and addresses how decisions are made by the foundation about what issues are funded and how (e.g., the foundation will fund child health but not HIV, or will fund programs in Africa but not in Asia), and the cultural influence of funders on the overall field to which the philanthropy is being directed (e.g., emphasizing individual rather than collective responsibility, or focusing on technological interventions rather than indigenous capacity building). However, this dimension of power is also more difficult to observe, as it is indirect, informal, and may not be made explicit (299c). The first of these measures, financial data, are the most widely available and relevant indicator. True commitment can only be judged by the decision to spend money. However, the financial data are of very poor quality. As one scholar notes, the 'data are terrible' (300). Figuring out where the money comes from and where it goes—or whether if ever reaches the poor—is a terribly difficult job. A recent analysis of these data concluded that 'the fragmented, complicated, messy and inadequately tracked state of global health finance requires immediate attention' (301).

Despite these limitations, these financial data reveal the priorities of these global health agencies which, in many cases, are set behind closed doors, hidden from the public's eye. We first describe the overall allocations of global health funds to chronic diseases.

Where is the money going?

Out of the $22.0 billion of development assistance for health in 2007 it was only possible to ascertain where about two-thirds of it went. A small portion of these unidentifiable funds went to 'health systems', supporting health infrastructure, multiple disease projects, and multisectoral health projects. The rest did not have any defined purpose other than 'health' (302).

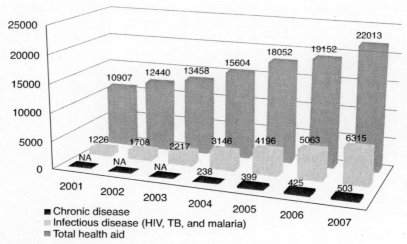

Fig. 5.3 Trends in Official Development Assistance for Health, 2001–2007.
Adapted from: Nugent, RA, Feigl, AB. 2010. Where have all the donors gone? Scarce donor funding for non-communicable diseases. Center for Global Development. Working Paper 228. Washington D.C.: USA.

Of the two-thirds of DAH for which project-level information could be ascertained (about $14.5 billion), $6.2 billion was for HIV/AIDS, TB, and malaria, and $0.9 billion for health-sector support (see Figure 5.3). About $668 million went to chronic diseases in 2008 (<3% of the total). This marks a slight improvement over the situation observed in a study of ODA in 2001 which found less than 0.1% of assistance provided by OECD (Organisation for Economic Co-operation and Development) countries went to chronic disease (303).

Since these data are based on commitments, not actual disbursements or spending, they overestimate the fraction of funds that actually reach the poor. Considerable money leaks from the health system. Recent studies have found that for every $1 of DAH only about $0.40 more is being spent on health (304). The remaining $0.60 ends up in reserves, military spending, or other areas where it was not intended, or displaces existing government health spending. A recent analysis found that when countries were exposed to lending programmes from the IMF, typically setting targets for governments to maintain low levels of government spending, there was complete displacement of resources (i.e. $1 additional donated added nothing to the health system's resources) (305).

Clue 1: More than half of global health aid money leaks into unintended areas, such as military spending, education, or reserves, and displaces government health spending.

Where is the money coming from?

The bulk of development assistance for health now comes from private foundations and NGOS (about 40% in 2007) (301, 302). In 1990, only about one-third of these funds came from publicly accountable UN agencies. By 2007, this fraction dropped to 14%. The World Bank contributed about one-fifth of development assistance for health in 2000, at the time when it was the leading financier of global health, a proportion which since has dropped to 7.2% in 2007.

These health aid resources are increasingly concentrated in low-income countries, (20, 304), where they make up a significant fraction of their system's overall health spending. In the lowest income countries in 2005, an average of 14.5% of health funding consisted of donor contributions, an increase from 11.1% in 2001. In some countries, as much as half of the health budget comes from external sources (including private donors, development agencies, and NGOs, mostly in the form of ODA) (20).

Critics of this high level of external financing have suggested it creates dependency on donors. These critics point out that the global health aid system potentially skews budgetary priorities by privileging the interests of private Western financiers over the need of populations (306). Indeed, these data reveal that private donors have come to dominate much of the global health agenda in terms of their sheer financial power (a passive 'privatization of global health'). The net effect of these billions of dollars in additional financing from donors has been to transfer power to from publicly accountable systems to private donors, who increasingly set the global health agenda.

Clue 2: Current systems of global health aid transfer the power to set priorities from publicly accountable systems to private Western donors.

Clue 3: The rising reliance on private donor financing of health is a passive privatization of global health.

Is it enough?

On the surface, it appears that money for chronic diseases has risen substantially, from less than $5 million to more than $500 million per year. Yet, in view of the scale of the problem, and the availability of cost-effective interventions, they appear to be underfunded relative to the burden of disease they cause. In 2008, about $0.78 was given per disability-adjusted life year caused by chronic diseases in low- and middle-income countries, compared with about $23.9 per year of suffering due to infectious diseases (HIV, TB, and malaria) (see Table 5.1).

A series of analyses have revealed that donor funding misaligns with the burden of disease, measured at global, regional or country levels (302, 303, 307, 308). Figure 5.4 depicts this misalignment in the budgets of WHO, World Bank, Gates Foundation, and Global Alliance for AIDS, Malaria and Tuberculosis. This situation occurs in spite of commitments by private donors to 'align aid flows with national priorities' and 'adapt and apply aid to differing country situations', as set out in the Paris Declaration of 2005 and Accra Agenda of 2008. (Some donors refer to these two documents as their 'Bible'.)

Clue 4: Donor funding misaligns with the burden of disease; factors other than need appear to be driving the agenda.

Why is there so little funding of chronic diseases and such a weak correlation of health resources with health needs? Why do donors appear not to be heeding the commitments set out in the Paris Declaration and Accra Agenda? To help answer this question, we now investigate the activities and priorities of the major global health institutions, starting with the most powerful group— private donors.

Table 5.1 Development Assistance for Health for chronic disease, infectious diseases, and all causes of death per disability-adjusted life year (DALY) and per deaths in low- and middle-income countries (LMICs)

	2008 DALYs, LMICs (million)	Health Development Assistance (US$)	Funding per death	Funding per DALY
Infectious diseases (HIV, TB, and malaria)	264	6.32 billion	$422	$23.9
Chronic disease	646	0.50 billion	$18	$0.78
All health conditions	1,338	22.09 billion	$16.4	$16.4

Source for 'Infectious disease' and 'All conditions' funding: (302);
Source for 'NCD' Funding: CGD Funding Analysis;
Source for DALYs: (18)

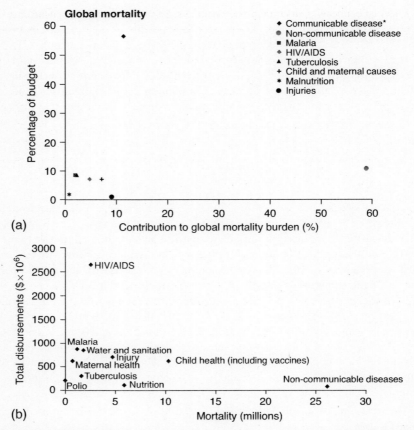

Fig. 5.4 Relation between global health budgets and burden of disease. a) WHO budget allocations and the global burden of disease, 2004–05. b) World Bank, US Government, Bill & Melinda Gates Foundation, Global Fund to fight HIV/AIDS, Tuberculosis and Malaria budget allocations and global burden of disease, 2005.

Sources: a) Stuckler D, Robinson HR, McKee M, King L. WHO budget and burden of disease: a comparative analysis. *Lancet* 2008; **372**:1563–9; b) Sridhar D, Batniji R. Misfinancing global health: a case for transparency in disbursements and decision making. *Lancet* 2009; **372**:1185–91.

Private donors (for-profit and non-for-profit organizations)

Private donor funding (for profit and not-for profit combined) made up a little over half of chronic disease funding in 2007. As shown in Table 5.2, six of the top ten financiers of chronic diseases are private philanthropic foundations and non-profit organizations—Wellcome Trust (a UK-based public charity), Bloomberg and Gates Foundation, Novo Nordisk (diabetes pharmaceutical company), General Electric Foundation, International Diabetes Federation, and Hilton Foundation.

Relative to the extent of funding for work on global health, very few of the private philanthropic organizations provide significant funds to address chronic diseases. Of this funding for chronic diseases, little has been for diet-related chronic diseases. Bloomberg Foundation and Gates Foundation support cervical cancer vaccines and tobacco control. There is also modest support for tobacco control from the UN Foundation, the Open Society Institute, and Rockefeller

Table 5.2 Top global health and chronic disease donors, 5-year totals, latest available data

Chronic disease	Purpose	5-year total (2004–2008)
1 WHO (including PAHO)	General NCDs	$873 million
2 Wellcome Trust	General NCDs	$458 million
3 Bloomberg and Gates Foundation	Tobacco and cervical cancer	$250 million (combined)
4 World Bank	General NCDs	$183 million
5 Novo Nordisk	Diabetes	$58 million
6 General Electric Foundation	General NCDs	$41 million
7 InterAmerican Development Bank (Latin America)	General NCDs	$21 million
8 National Institute of Health	Tobacco	$27 million
9 International Diabetes Federation	Diabetes	$18 million
10 Hilton Foundation	Sense organ diseases	$12 million
All global health	**5-year total (2003–2007)**	
1 US	$20,655 million	
2 Corporate Donations	$10,646	
3 Other (incl. private donors)	$8639	
4 UK	$6910	
5 Unallocable	$4035	
6 Japan	$3994	
7 Bill & Melinda Gates Foundation (BMGF)	$3683	
8 France	$3394	
9 Germany	$3237	
10 Debt repayments (IBRD)	$3099	

Adapted from: Nugent, RA, Feigl, AB. 2010. Where have all the donors gone? Scarce donor funding for non-communicable diseases. Center for Global Development. Working Paper 228. Washington D.C.: USA.

Foundation. Hilton Foundation provides funding related to sense organ diseases. General Electric Foundation provides money to general chronic disease programmes. The largest funder, the UK Wellcome Trust, supports considerable research for chronic diseases (except cancer, which in the UK is supported by other large charities), totalling $458 million over the past 5 years.

Private foundations and non-profit organizations mainly receive their money from private companies or philanthropists in the form of investments and endowments which provide income. These organizations are defined negatively as 'not public charities', and their primary purpose is usually to make grants to other organizations. These foundations provide some tax-exemptions to parent companies and separate their liability from the foundation's activities.

Public charities, on the other hand, such as the American Cancer Society, are set up with a legal mandate to promote the public interest (although this meaning is in practice somewhat ambiguous),[1] often receive government funding, and directly conduct charitable activities and services as well as make grants. In the British usage of the term 'charity', the Wellcome Trust is considered a charity. Its aim is 'to foster and promote research with the aim of improving human and animal health'.

Non-profit organizations' grant-making decisions are usually made by a board of directors or trustees. In the case of corporate foundations linked to corporate entities, such as PepsiCo or Coca-Cola Foundation, these priorities are usually set by the chief executive officer of the corporation or by a committee appointed by the foundation's board of directors (which can and often includes corporate officers). These grant-making decisions can influence the global health agenda by promoting a particular philosophy or viewpoint.

Many private foundations working in health have promulgated views that chronic diseases are individual problems. In the 1970s the Rockefeller Foundation espoused the view that 'The solution to the problems of ill health in modern American society involves individual responsibility'. As described in Chapter 4, the Rockefeller Foundation also played a key role in the push for Selective Primary Health Care and an emphasis on cost-effectiveness as part of its Good Health at Low Cost project. In general, these Foundations emphasize market-based, technical solutions to global health problems. They tend to support vertical, disease-specific programmes (the 'smallpox paradigm', see Chapter 4 for a discussion). This is but one example of how Foundations tend to promote particular global health agendas.

Whose interests do these private foundations serve? The answer is not always clear. These non-profit foundations mainly serve the interests of their donors and their causes. Typically these foundations will support (or at least not conflict with) the interests of their parent companies. Although these foundations argue that they are legally independent from their parent companies (which is true from a liability perspective), it is important to note that there are revolving doors and personal linkages between them. As Milton Friedman famously put it, 'the principal objective of a company is to maximize the wealth of its shareholders'. These private companies are legally bound to increase profits. Many of these officers working both in parent companies and setting priorities of private foundations are supposed to separate their roles, but in practice the distinction is blurred, and there are ethical quandaries about the scope of conflicts of interest.

Many of the directors of parent companies of corporation foundations have close ties to food, beverage, agriculture, and pharmaceutical companies, who have vested interests in global health. For example, two of the largest foundations donating to work on chronic diseases have members of their parent companies' boards who also sit on the board of food companies. From Coca-Cola's board of directors, Peter Ueberroth, is on the board of Hilton Hotels (Hilton Foundation, tenth largest donor), and Samuel Nunn Jr is on the board of General Electric (General Electric Foundation, sixth largest donor). Similar ties to the biggest chronic disease donors can be seen with PepsiCo (owner of General Mills), ConAgra, and Kellogg, among others.

It would be surprising if these linkages did not have an influence on these private foundation's priorities. They do not necessarily manifest as neglect of chronic diseases, but, as we return to in the second part of this chapter, these interventions can actually result in increased financial flows to chronic diseases in order to shape the agenda in a direction that protects their companies' interests ('co-opting the social movement'). Some notable examples include how food companies have promoted physical inactivity as the main explanation and point of intervention in relation to diet-related chronic diseases.

Do these mutual roles create potential conflicts of interest? According to the WHO guidelines for its Roll Back Malaria programme (308a):

> A conflict of interest can occur when a Partner's ability to exercise judgment in one role is impaired by his or her obligations in another role or by the existence of competing interests. Such situations create a risk of a tendency towards bias in favor of one interest over another or that the individual would not fulfill his or her duties impartially and in the best interest of the RBM Partnership.
>
> A conflict of interest may exist even if no unethical or improper act results from it. It can create an appearance of impropriety that can undermine confidence in the individual, his/her constituency or

organization. Both actual and perceived conflicts of interest can undermine the reputation and work of the Partnership.

Because of the particular importance of the Gates Foundation in global health, with a larger budget than the WHO, we discuss its influence in greater detail before discussing the roles of other private non-profit organizations:

Clue 5: Private donors tend to give very low priority to chronic diseases as part of their overall global health portfolios and priorities.

Clue 6: Of resources allocated to chronic diseases by private foundations, there has been little focus on diet-related chronic diseases and, to the extent there has been, most has focused on physical inactivity or a skew away from activities related their parent companies' products.

Bill & Melinda Gates Foundation[2]

The Gates Foundation is the largest private financial contributor to global health and the leading funder of research (309). It has a profound influence on health policy and the design of global health programmes (299). Its representatives sit on the boards of many global health partnerships. Gates donates to the World Bank, contributes to 4% of WHO's budget, and finances think tanks (including the Center for Global Development, the International Food Policy Research Institute, and the National Academy of Sciences).[3] As one scholar put it, Gates Foundation is 'creating its own World Health Organization' (310).

There is little doubt that the US$3 billion that the Gates Foundation provides to global health has helped improve the health of millions of the poor. Questions remain, however, as to whether more lives could be saved without this money because of criticisms that its grants potentially distort and monopolize research and create misalignments between global health priorities and the global burden of disease.

As with many private foundations, the Gates Foundation sets its priorities in private. It has no mission statement (although there are 15 guiding principles, such as 'we leave room for growth and change' and 'we treat our grantees as valued partners' and 'driven by the interests and passions of the Gates family'). In describing how its priorities are set, spokespersons from the Gates Foundation state, 'we use our best judgment to determine where our funding can achieve the greatest reductions in health inequity around the world'. According to the Foundation's website, the first guiding principle is that it is 'driven by the interests and passions of the Gates family'. At the time of this writing, none of the members of the Gates Foundation's board was from a low-income country.

Bill Gates writes an annual letter setting out his priorities. The most recent emphasizes how 'technical innovation can save the world'. His most recent letter states, 'overall we have about 30 innovations we are backing. Although the list includes only one new vaccine and one new seed, we are funding vaccines for several diseases (malaria, AIDS, TB, etc.) and new seeds for many crops (corn, rice, wheat, sorghum, etc.) . . . a few things we do, like disaster relief and scholarships do not fit this model, but over 90% of our work does'.

Financial support to the Gates Foundation mainly comes from the private fortunes of Bill Gates and Warren Buffett (who donated over $30 billion). Although the Gates Foundation has severed commercial ties with its parent companies Microsoft and Berkshire Hathaway, both Gates and Buffett have informal social networks to food and pharmaceutical companies, and about half of the Gates Foundation's endowment is invested in Berkshire Hathaway. As shown in the structure of each of the boards of Microsoft and Berkshire Hathaway (see Figure 5.5a), board members of these firms also are on the boards of General Mills (since acquired by PepsiCo, see Chapter 6),

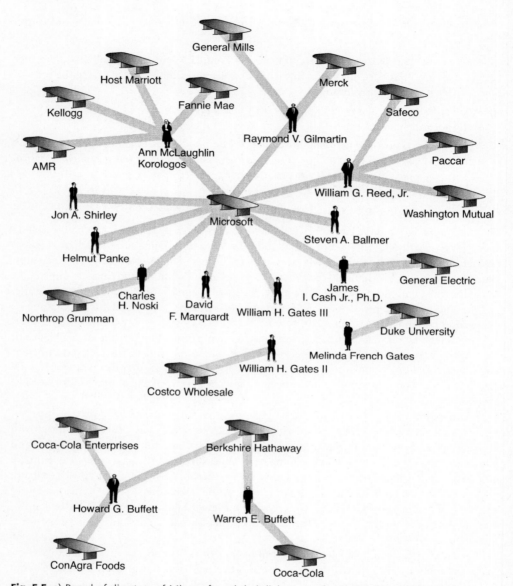

Fig. 5.5 a) Board of directors of Microsoft and their linkages to food, pharmaceutical, cosmetic, supermarket industries and companies with large donations to global health.
Source: Data accessed 30 April, 2010, based on 2004 data from the Securities and Exchange Commission (336).

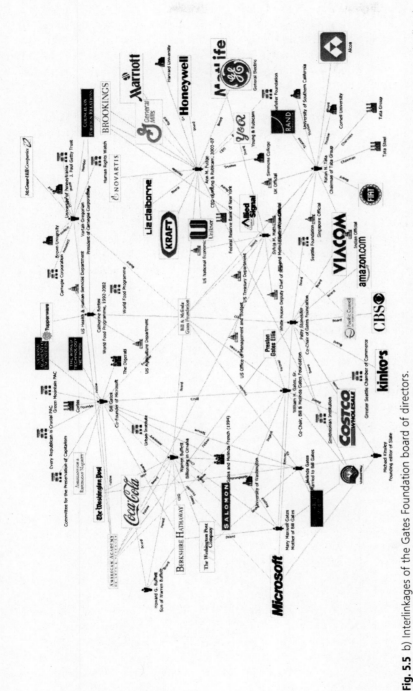

Fig. 5.5 b) Interlinkages of the Gates Foundation board of directors.
Source: Latest available data from NNDB mapper (accessed 10 July, 2010) (337) A Google search of 'Gates Foundation' and the companies listed reveals a series of partnerships.

Kellogg (a major food company, see Chapter 4), and General Electric (the sixth largest donor for work on chronic diseases). There are also close ties between Microsoft and Merck, as a member of Microsoft's board sits on Merck's board. In April 2010 a former Merck executive, Richard Henriques, became the chief financial officer of the Gates Foundation (two other members of the Gates Foundation leadership have held senior positions or been on the board of directors of GlaxoSmithKline). Buffett runs Berkshire Hathaway and and sat on the board of Coca-Cola for two decades (Figure 5.5a), and his son, Howard Buffett, is currently on the board of Coca-Cola Enterprises and ConAgra Foods (which emphasizes modern seed technology). Berkshire Hathaway also holds another 8.3% of Coca-Cola.

These interlocking directorates of food companies and the parent companies of the Gates foundation may indicate a strong relationship of mutual interest, a weak one, or none at all. At a minimum, they imply that the same people are making decisions over huge organizations and reveal the informal social networks that are involved in the command centres of the Gates Foundation.

As shown in Table 5.3, it is also clear that the fortunes of the Gates Foundation and Buffett are highly intertwined and heavily invested in food companies. About half of Gates Foundation is invested in Warren Buffett's company, Berkshire Hathaway (and Bill Gates is a director on its board). Warren Buffett's gift of $31 billion in 2006 to the Gates Foundation came in the form of shares of Berkshire Hathaway most recently with 24.7 million shares in July 2010. Currently, the Bill & Melinda Gates Foundation is listed with the SEC as a 10% owner of the Berkshire company. Coca-Cola is Buffett's largest stock holding, making up 20% of his portfolio. Buffett also owns 9.3% of Kraft (although at the time of writing there are talks of selling this holding) as well as a significant portion of GlaxoSmithKline. These purchases in 2008 led to headlines asking why Buffett purchased these two companies: e.g. 'Buffett buys into GlaxoSmithKline turnaround' Gates does not directly own healthcare companies, but does own significant shares in McDonald's (7.4 million shares) and Coca-Cola (6.7 million shares). Taken together, Berkshire Hathaway, Gates and Buffett's fortunes come close to a controlling interest in Coca-Cola of about 20% (not counting the contribution of Howard Buffett). In 2009 the Bill & Melinda Gates Foundation sold extensive pharmaceutical holdings in Johnson & Johnson (2.5 million shares), Schering-Plough Corporation (14.9 million shares), Eli Lilly and Company (about 1 million shares), Merck & Co. (8.1 million shares), and Wyeth (3.7 million shares). Gates also owns significant shares in the world's high-tech recycling company, Waste Management; a company with close ties to R.J. Reynolds tobacco and a partner of PepsiCo (311).

Overall, the Gates Foundation provides very little funding to work on chronic diseases. In 2008, the Bloomberg Foundation and Gates Foundation partnered to donate $250 million over 5 years to tobacco control and develop cervical cancer vaccines. The rest of the Gates Foundation's health and development programmes (totalling more than $3 billion) relate to infectious diseases. Its 2008 annual report does not mention any chronic disease risk factors, and mentions 'chronic' only once in relation to chronic hunger. In 1999, the Gates Foundation gave $750 million grant to start the Global Alliance for Vaccines and Immunization.

Nearly all of Gates Foundation's core health projects relate to drugs produced by Merck and GlaxoSmithKline (Box 5.1). For example, with regard to Merck, these include partnerships to test pneumonia and rotavirus vaccines (through the ROTATEQ partnership as well as Merck Vaccines network partnership with the Global Alliance for Vaccines and Immunizations network), experimental malaria vaccines (through an NGO, Medicines for Malaria Venture), cervical cancer vaccines (through an NGO, PATH, and Merck's vaccine Gardasil) and HIV interventions (through the Africa Comprehensive HIV/AIDS partnership). Typically Merck donates

Table 5.3 Summary of Bill & Melinda Gates Foundation stock portfolios, 2010. (299c)

Entity	Holding	Portfolio Rank	US Dollars Billion	Portfolio Share	Company Share
Bill & Melinda Gates Foundation Trust	Berkshire Hathaway	1	5.89	49.75%	3.19%
	McDonald's	2	0.62	5.21%	0.88%
	Coca-Cola	4	0.51	4.31%	0.44%
	Waste Management	5	0.49	4.15%	3.25%
	Walmart	7	0.44	3.75%	0.13%
	Coca-Cola FEMSA	9	0.35	2.97%	2.47%
	Costco	10	0.34	2.83%	1.39%
	Monsanto	>20	0.02	0.19%	0.20%
	Total	–	11.85	–	–
Berkshire Hathaway	Coca Cola	1	10.0	21.58%	8.68%
	Procter & Gamble	4	4.7	10.08%	2.75%
	Kraft Foods	5	2.9	6.34%	6.03%
	Johnson & Johnson	6	2.4	5.25%	1.50%
	Walmart	7	1.9	4.04%	1.07%
	Nestle	23	0.16	0.35%	0.09%
	Sanofi-Aventis	29	0.12	0.26%	0.15%
	GlaxoSmithKline	34	0.05	0.11%	0.06%
	Total	–	46.44	–	–

Notes: (1) Because one-half of Gates endowment is held in Berkshire Hathaway, a figure which will rise in the future, we also report the holdings of Berkshire Hathaway. Data retrieved from http://www.sec.gov/edgar.shtml (accessed 30 June 2010). Company share calculated based on dividing number of shares held by the total company shares outstanding.

Doic10.1371/journal.pmed.1001020.t003

Source: Stuckler, D, Basu, S, McKee, M. (2011) Global health philanthropy and institutional relationships: How should conflicts of interest be addressed? *PLoS Medicine* v8(4): e1001020.

experimental drugs to NGOs to test in the field but retains the possibility of partnering the drug. In other words, Gates funds programmes that accelerate R&D for private pharmaceutical companies, which the Gates Foundation's donors and endowments are in turn invested in (312).

These large grants from the Gates Foundation have come under criticism for monopolizing the field and distorting global health priorities (299, 315). One study of Gates' Foundations' $9 billion for 1094 global health grants between 1998 and 2007 found that 82% went to recipients based in the US; one-third was allocated to research and development (mainly for vaccines and microbicides). According to a chief malaria officer at the WHO, this has created a situation where

Box 5.1 Example of Gates' influence on research: Malaria, Merck, and the Gates Foundation

In the 1990s about $84 million a year was spent on malaria research, mainly by US military and health institute. The situation changed with the influx of Gates funding, now the largest driver of malaria research. It invests so heavily that, in 2009, the chief of malaria operations for the WHO complained that Gates funding was monopolizing the field. As he put it, Gates had malaria scientists 'locked up in a cartel' so that independent reviews were increasingly difficult.

In 2009, Merck donated an experimental antimalarial drug to an NGO, Medicines for Malaria Venture, heavily funded by the Gates Foundation ($137 million in 2005) with the aim to 'to further develop and accelerate antimalarial discovery and development projects'. As Reuters reported, 'by donating the new drug to the Medicines for Malaria Venture, the U.S. company hopes its clinical development will be accelerated . . . Merck will have the option to partner the drug after completion of mid-stage tests' (313), as press releases heralded how 'Wellcome Trust and Merck launch first of its kind joint venture to develop low-cost vaccines'.

In other words, non-profit groups, funded by Gates, do clinical trials; if it works, Merck still gets the profits. Merck and the Gates Foundation also have close ties through partnerships to donate antiretroviral medicines, such as the African Comprehensive HIV/AIDS partnership (314).

Gates also gave $1 billion to PATH-International, an NGO focusing on vaccines and collaborating heavily with Merck to conduct vaccine trials (previously PATH had about $15 million). In 2010, Merck teamed up with PATH to conduct a 'demonstration project' of Gardasil, a cervical cancer vaccine. It is not part of the India's universal immunization programme. According to local news reports, villagers were told that Garadasil was an expensive vaccine that they would not be able to afford once the company's project was over. Indian government suspended Merck's vaccine following the recent report of the deaths of four girls and several cases of complications (although there is now dispute about the causes of the deaths). The drug has generated $1.4 billion for Merck.

it is difficult to find independent peer-review, and researchers are afraid to criticize each other, out of fear that they may not get grants from the Gates Foundation.

The Gates Foundation has also come to dominate health surveillance systems and the monitoring of the disease burden. It invested $105 million to set up the Institute for Health Metrics and Evaluation at the University of Washington. It hired WHO's chief scientist who led the Global Burden of Disease Study (see Chapter 1), the source of the most widely used data in global health, and the lead author of the WHO's health system report (see Chapter 4).

Commentators have interpreted these patterns as evidence that the Gates Foundation is constraining research, making undemocratic funding decisions, and forcing people to engage in one man's agenda based on his self-created statistics about what is important, defining the framework for 'what matters' before those most affected can say anything. As the authors of an investigation about the Foundation's priorities and decision-making processes concluded: 'What we have is a private actor with a huge degree of influence, but not really a mechanism by which that influence is held to public account' (299). As the editors of *The Lancet* point out, 'although Gates is driven by the belief that "all lives have equal value", it seems that the Foundation does not believe that every voice has equal value, especially voices from those it seeks most to assist' (315).

Some people will respond that the Gates Foundation, as a private philanthropic organization, should be allowed to do whatever it wants with its money within the remit of the law. Potential conflicts of interest exist everywhere, they argue, and as long as it is declared it should not be an impediment to action. Others suggest that, in view of potential conflicts of interests and adverse effects on global health, there is a need to create greater transparency and public accountability of these private philanthropic institutions, as well as divestment and financial separation from corporations which may benefit from the philanthropic work (for more details see 299c).

Clue 5: Many global health donors set their priorities in secret and have strong ties to food, beverage, and pharmaceutical companies that may benefit from their activities.

Strategy 1: In view of potential conflicts of interest and unintended adverse effects on global health, there is a need to critically assess the effects of global health funding on health and hold private donors to standards of public accountability.

Other private non-governmental and non-profit organizations

Few private, non-profit organizations provide a substantial share of their funds to work on chronic diseases. Most relate to diabetes, heart disease, or cancer, such as the International Diabetes Federation (the ninth largest chronic disease donor), the World Diabetes Federation (funded by Novo Nordisk), the World Heart Federation, and the International Union against Cancer. Most of these groups receive funding from pharmaceutical companies.

One of the few private non-profit organizations seeking to make chronic diseases a development priority is the Oxford Health Alliance. Its mission is 'preventing and reducing the global impact of chronic disease'. Its funding mainly comes from Novo Nordisk and PepsiCo. Oxford Health Alliance's research and action programme, Community Interventions for Health project, described in Chapter 4, is funded by the PepsiCo Foundation (US$5.3 million in 2007–2010).

Historically, there have been concerns about NGOs set up as pseudoscientific front groups for industry. One example is the International Life Sciences Institute (ILSI), funded by PepsiCo, H.J. Heinz, Coca-Cola, and a consortium of industry partners. Maintaining a special consultative status with WHO, the ILSI produced evidence and attempted to lobby WHO that the sugar targets set out in its chronic disease strategies were scientifically inaccurate.

A Swiss non-profit foundation, the World Economic Forum, which brings together business leaders, finance ministers, and non-governmental organizations, consistently ranks chronic diseases as one of the top three global risks to the economy and one of the top five most likely risks to occur (192, 316). Their insights draw on the observations of US companies, such as General Motors, which faced major costs of paying healthcare insurance of its workforce (in 2009 jokingly referred to as a 'healthcare company that sells cars'). As described in Chapter 3, US managers report healthcare costs as their top concern about the sustainability of their business.

Several NGOs receive support from global UN institutions. For example, WHO has helped support the development of coordinating mechanisms for NGOs, such as the Framework Convention Alliance. This alliance was established to support the ratification and implementation of the Framework Convention on Tobacco Control, now includes more than 180 NGOs from over 70 countries and has established itself as an important lobbying alliance. In 2009 WHO launched NCDNet, a voluntary collaborative arrangement involving WHO member states, UN agencies, NGOs, WHO collaborating centres, the World Economic Forum, and other international partners. An NGO-chronic disease alliance was established to support NCDnet, representing more than 700 organizations including the International Diabetes Federation, the International Union Against Cancer, and the World Heart Federation, responded to a call from the Latin American countries (CARICOM) to lobby the UN to create a special envoy of the Secretary General for chronic diseases (as exists for HIV/AIDS) and dedicate a summit of the UN General Assembly to chronic diseases (317).

More than 25 public–private partnerships address diseases of poverty, but few focus on chronic diseases broadly. As highlighted by the debates in Chapter 6, there is disagreement about whether and under what circumstances food companies can interact effectively with public sector health groups. Standards for engagement remain unclear. Specific chronic disease advocacy groups, such as World Heart Forum and Oxford Health Alliance, have begun partnering with the private sector.

Clue 6: Many non-governmental organizations and their activities involved in chronic disease control are funded by food, beverage, or pharmaceutical companies with potential conflicts of interest.

National development agencies

National development agencies provide very little money for chronic disease control compared with their other objectives (including aid agencies such as the Canadian International Development Agency and Swedish International Development Agency). The UK Department for International Development donated a modest amount of funding in the past to chronic diseases, but in 2010, partially as response to the financial crisis, eliminated all funding for work on chronic disease.

The US is the largest global health donors (about $21 billion in 2003–2007), but did not spend any money directly on chronic diseases until recently. In 2009, the Millennium Challenge Corporation, an independent US foreign aid agency, awarded US$17 million to Mongolia as part of a 5-year $285 million compact to reduce poverty and promote economic growth. The Obama Administration's US Global Health Initiative is set to provide $63 billion of development aid for health over the next 6 years. The US is also largest donor to the WHO's budget. Its goals, set out in the Institute of Medicine's report *The U.S. Commitment to Global Health: Recommendations to the New Administration,* treat 'global health as a pillar of U.S. foreign policy' (318). None of the current US global health strategies specifically mentions chronic diseases. Even though the Institute of Medicine report included chronic diseases, its recommendations did not make it into the US global health strategy. Although the Obama administration has set up innovative chronic disease programmes to address childhood obesity, US development authorities have raised concerns that implementing them on a global scale could harm US exports (313a).

At present, the only national development agency considering chronic diseases as a focal development priority is the Danish agency, DANIDA. Recently it held a conference about the importance of tackling chronic diseases to promote development in Copenhagen, sponsored by the Danish pharmaceutical company, NovoNordisk. Many representatives from national development agencies, including the US and UK, were invited; very turned up other than representatives from DANIDA.

In general, it appears that development aid agencies have expressed little interest in supporting work on chronic diseases, although there are glimmers of change at the UN High Level meeting scheduled for September 2011.

Clue 7: There is little concern or participation in global chronic disease prevention and control among national development agencies.

Academics and research institutions

Grant-making and research institutions

There is often a mistaken view that because rich countries invest heavily in research on chronic diseases, that there is little need for research on global chronic diseases. As described in Chapter 4, few of the advanced, expensive and technologically- and medically-based solutions being developed in Western universities are applicable or can be easily transposed to resource-poor settings.

Research funds come from a variety of sources, both public and private. As previously mentioned, the Gates Foundation is the largest funder of global health research. The US and UK are the two largest funders of medical research (hence in this book many examples have been drawn from studies of these countries), although China and other emerging economies are beginning to invest heavily as well. In the US, most funding comes from publicly funded bodies, such as the NIH. As shown in Table 5.2, the NIH is the ninth largest funder of chronic disease support to low- and middle-income countries. Medical funding is largely driven by commercial interests. There are also alliances between pharmaceutical companies and food companies. As one of many examples, Bristol-Myers Squibb has members on the board of both PepsiCo and Coca-Cola.

How are these grants awarded? Mostly they are awarded through a system of peer-review. However, it is well known that some of them are conferred through patron-client linkages. In academic medicine, an up-and-coming student might need to find a 'sugar daddy', an established academic who is willing to support his/her research agenda. These patrons typically have links to the grant-making institutions. Especially when reviewers are not blinded, there can be an exchange of favourable reviews among researchers, making them reluctant to criticize each other and making it difficult for outsiders to dominant research groups face to obtain funding.

The importance of these networks is indicated by studies that demonstrate the existence of strong relationships between academics and pharmaceutical companies.[4] A paper published in 2007 in *The Journal of the American Medical Association* found strong ties between individual faculty members and companies. The study surveyed 459 department chairs of 125 medical schools and 15 teaching hospitals. It found that two-thirds had a personal relationship with industry, about one-quarter having worked as a paid consultant or served on a scientific advisory board. Seven per cent had been a chief officer or executive of a company, and 9% were founders. The authors concluded 'failure to address the existence and influence of industry relationships with academic institutions could endanger the trust of the public in US medical schools and teaching hospitals' (319). To quote the former editor of the prestigious *New England Journal of Medicine*, 'Medical centers increasingly act as though meeting industry's needs is a legitimate purpose of an academic institution'.

In relation to chronic disease funding, given the stated priorities of the main funders of global health research, it is unsurprising to find that the major growth of international research funding in recent decades has not been proportionally allocated to chronic diseases. Most international funders of research focus on infectious disease.

There are some important exceptions, such as the Wellcome Trust in the UK, which is now the second largest donor for chronic disease-related global health activities. Responding to a set of grand challenges, published in *Nature* (as further described below), a Global Alliance for Chronic Disease was created in 2009, bringing together leading health research agencies collectively managing 80% of public health research spending worldwide (including Australia's National Health Medical Research Council, UK Medical Research Council, Canadian Institutes of Health Research, Indian Council of Medical Research, Chinese Medical Research Council, and US NIH).

Another important funder of chronic disease research is the Fogarty International Center at the US National Institutes of Health. The Fogarty Center allocates one-third of its resources to chronic disease research and training in resource-poor countries. Recently it has launched a $1.5 million-per-year recurring grant programme to build research capacity on stroke, lung disease and cancer in resource-poor countries (2008). The US National Heart, Lung and Blood Institute, also part of the NIH, has partnered with UnitedHealth Group, one of the largest US healthcare suppliers, to fund 11 centres of excellence across the globe for CVD and lung disease control (320).

Academics and universities

The lack of research funding makes it difficult for academics to build a career in areas related to global chronic diseases. In medicine and public health most academics have to chase after grant funding, because, as one academic put it, 'they have to eat'. Promotions and performance is heavily tied to the successful ability to bring in grants. In many schools as over 80% of a professor's salary may come from grant money.

Despite limited resources, academics have made substantial contributions to global chronic diseases. For example, they have achieved scientific consensus about what should be done: *Nature*, one of the world's leading science journals, has published a set of 'Grand Challenges for Chronic Diseases', listing the top 20 policy and research priorities in preventing and controlling chronic diseases emerging from an international Delphi exercise organized by the Oxford Health Allliance (321). There is also high awareness among academics of the importance of global chronic diseases. As shown in Figure 5.1, there has been a growing number of 'calls to action' identified from a search of Medline over the past four decades (as of March 2010, 575 could be identified in medical journals), showing that chronic diseases have attracted no greater share of this type of attention over the past decade.

Yet, in spite of efforts by academics to increase the priority given to chronic diseases, the attention it has received relative to other conditions appears to have remained about the same. Many other health issues are felt to be neglected, all invoking 'calls to action' (largely reflecting the distribution of global health funding). Promoting slogans in *The Lancet* such as 'Fight for a fairer trading system', 'Climate change is the biggest global health threat of the 21st century', and 'No health without mental health', researchers compete with the chronic disease community for priority and resources for 'their disease' or issue. So far chronic diseases have featured twice among over twenty special issues of *The Lancet*. Furthermore, the academic market for 'neglect' is already crowded. 'Neglected Tropical Diseases' (NTD) lay claim to special consideration, having established a special category of illness, since recognized by the WHO (322), while searching for the phrase 'neglected infectious disease' turns up many more hits than for 'neglected chronic disease'.

Most international public health training occurs in the US, where global chronic diseases attract little attention (as indicated by core requirements of members of the Association of Schools of Public Health). Emphasis remains on primary healthcare and infectious disease, although selected institutions, such as Johns Hopkins, Yale, and the University of North Carolina at Chapel Hill, address obesity in nutrition courses and have international tobacco seminars. The University of Copenhagen in Denmark has started a master's course on global chronic diseases and the Metropolitan University, also in Copenhagen, has launched a global nutrition course with a focus on chronic diseases. Courses in global nutrition and chronic diseases are also offered at institutions across Australia.

Clue 8: There is scientific consensus about key priorities for addressing global chronic diseases.

Clue 9: Over the past 5 years, academics have published more than 100 calls-to-action on chronic diseases, but meanwhile over 300 have been published about other areas of global health that are similarly felt to be neglected.

Clue 10: Few international training courses about global chronic diseases exist in universities.

National health ministries

Like many public health academics, health ministers are well aware of the health risks of chronic diseases, but have few budgetary resources. A 2001 WHO survey of 167 countries' health ministers found that virtually all health ministers recognize chronic diseases as a key priority, yet nearly two-thirds of those ministers surveyed did not have a budget line for chronic diseases.

Another survey of 20 chronic disease managers working low- and middle-income countries found that political influence and few resources were key barriers to increasing action on chronic diseases. Responses included a lack of 'political will'; 'political pressure from some lobbies (especially private and welfare organizations)'; 'lack of finances in this field'; 'lack of professionals'; 'lack of experienced staff'; 'lack of a national plan on chronic disease'; and 'non-existence of chronic disease strategy'. Several managers stressed a need to create formal chronic disease bodies to provide political representation, reflected in responses such as 'Establishment of the department of chronic diseases at the ministry of health', and 'national centres of excellence for prevention and management of chronic diseases.'

Within the health system, several managers responded that there were 'No political opportunities' and 'there are no leaders'. As one manager put it, 'We have people with orientation in some areas of chronic diseases like diabetes or cancer, but we haven't leaders in the prevention and control of chronic diseases in general'. Another responded, 'There are people who could be leaders in chronic disease control but to display leadership they have to do only that kind of job, not to do at the same time some other very serious job'.

Why are there so few resources available for tackling chronic diseases, in spite of high levels of awareness and concern? It reflects a combination of the level of the health budget and how the priorities within the health budget are set.

First, in most countries, the level of resources available to health ministers is mainly determined by finance ministers. Especially in resource-poor countries, decades of structural adjustment policies have resulted in stagnation of the development of the public health sector (see Chapter 2). Finance ministers in these countries, seeking to attract foreign investors and forced to comply with IMF lending conditionalities (although they often fail to in practice), aim to keep inflation low and implement strict fiscal austerity programmes. These austerity policies deprive health systems of money, forcing them to rely on donors, private sector growth, and external resources for health.

Second, the authority of health ministers to set priorities has also been weakened, because of decentralization and a reliance on private donor financing. Decentralization has sought to increase responsiveness to local concerns but implicitly weakened the influence of the public sector, undermining efforts to mount effective population-wide responses to rising chronic diseases. Since private donor money is mostly earmarked to a narrow set of infectious diseases (vertical programmes), there is little democratic process for allocating these resources to population needs.

Even if health ministers received a larger budget that they could allocate themselves, they would have little authority or influence over the global economic forces that drive increasing risks of chronic diseases from tobacco, alcohol and unhealthy diets (see Chapter 2). Taking action on the societal determinants of chronic diseases, such as trade liberalization, export-oriented agriculture and unhealthy food subsidies, pits health ministers against trade, agricultural and finance ministries. Health ministers usually lose these debates and need to seek areas of mutual benefit to increase their effectiveness.

Clue 11: Health ministers in low-income countries have high awareness of the threat of chronic diseases, but lack budgetary resources with which to respond.

Clue 12: Health ministers and managers have their hands tied by global economic forces largely beyond their control.

International financial institutions: World Bank and International Monetary Fund

Two of the most powerful global health institutions are the World Bank and IMF (see Chapter 2). Each institution has a differing mandate and vision for global health policy:

World Bank

The World Bank comprises the International Bank for Reconstruction and Development (IBRD) and the International Development Association (IDA). The World Bank's specific focus, as set out on their website, is 'to reduce global poverty', focusing on the Millennium Development Goals, to achieve 'a world without poverty'. The agenda is split between the IBRD, which aims to reduce poverty in middle-income and creditworthy poorer countries', while the IDA 'focuses on the world's poorest countries'. They do this by focusing on six themes: the poorest countries, post-conflict and fragile states, middle-income countries, global public goods, the Arab world, and knowledge and learning. In theory, chronic diseases fit within global public goods (see Chapter 3 regarding market failures), which includes 'climate change, infectious diseases, and trade'.

In the late-1990s, the World Bank set up a policy that every country receiving 'highly indebted poor country' relief aid would author a Poverty Reduction Strategy Programme (PRSP), setting out how the countries would seek to address poverty. These contained many good ideas, such as greater country ownership and including voices of the poor. Yet, NGOs such as Oxfam have raised concerns that, despite successes, the PRSPs do not fully permeate the work of the Bank, transparency is lacking, and these institutions do not release key documents so that their potential impact on health can be assessed (and if they are ever released for public scrutiny, it is often after the processes of privatization or liberalization has been completed).

The World Bank's work is complemented by the International Finance Corporation, Multilateral Investment Guarantee Agency, and the International Centre for the Settlement of Investment Disputes. The International Finance Corporation, for example, 'provides investments and advisory services to build the private sector in developing countries', created in 1956 as 'the first step . . . to foster private sector investment in developing nations'. It lends to private sector companies in high-risk environments, and benefits from the World Bank's bond rating (in turn depending on limiting debt defaults and forgiveness).

Between the mid-1990s and about the year 2000, the World Bank was the leading financier of global health, contributing about one-third of all development assistance for health. In 1993 the World Bank published a seminal report, *Investing in Health*, that reinforced its model of Selective Primary Health Care as part of its Health Sector Reform model emphasizing private sector development (see Chapter 4). About the same time, the World Bank's advisors published major reports emphasizing the health of adults (323). Together with Harvard economists, they worked to develop new methods, such as the disability-adjusted life year, which better captured the suffering of adults.

Attention to chronic diseases at the World Bank has begun to rise through a series of policy reports. In 2000, advisors at the World Bank advocated the position that 'any shift in attention from communicable diseases to non-communicable ailments . . . would work to the detriment of the poor . . . [and] the shift's primary beneficiaries would be the rich, who would therefore gain at the expense of the poor' (324). Nonetheless, the World Bank commissioned two recent important papers that could help embed chronic diseases into their programming. The first is a paper, summarized in Chapter 3, which spells out that the risks of poverty caused by chronic diseases. The second is a public policy report, *Public Policy and the Response to the Challenge of Non-Communicable Chronic Diseases*, concluding 'the case for the World Bank and its clients to respond . . . is compelling' (48), identifying chronic diseases as a key barrier to economic growth.

During the 1990s the World Bank provided chronic disease-related loans to Eastern European countries (63, 303). In 2005 the World Bank allocated about 2% of its health budget to chronic diseases, amounting to $3.2 per chronic disease death versus $160 for infectious diseases (excluding HIV and TB).

International Monetary Fund

The IMF, similar to the World Bank's PSRPs, has a Poverty Reduction Growth Facility. The name basically sets out what it aims to do: reduce poverty through economic growth. As the IMF's former director, Michael Camdessus put it, 'Our primary objective is growth. In my view there is no longer any ambiguity about this. It is toward growth that our programs and their conditionality are aimed' (325). The Fund's history is reviewed in greater detail in Chapter 2. The IMF provides no resources to chronic diseases. However, since about 2000 the IMF has begun to provide support for HIV/AIDS, conditional on countries agreeing to implement their economic policies (often which de-fund the public health sector or undermine chronic disease control) (121) (see Chapter 2).

Lastly, there are rising Global South banks that place a higher priority on chronic diseases. Since 2007, the Inter-American Development Bank (IADB) started funding two chronic disease projects totalling $21 million, becoming the seventh largest chronic disease donor (320a).

Clue 13: *The World Bank and IMF's stated agendas focus on poverty alleviation and economic growth.*

Clue 14: *Some of the most effective public health intervention policies involving taxes, subsidies, and regulations conflict with the dominant free-market ideologies of the World Bank and IMF, except when these measures can be proven to correct market failures.*

Strategy 2: *Arguments about impacts of chronic diseases on the economy and the market failures which cause chronic diseases will help create opportunities for integrating chronic diseases into the agendas of the World Bank and IMF.*

Strategy 3: *Arguments about unhealthy market-distorting, agricultural subsidies will resonate with the stated agendas of the World Bank and IMF.*

United Nations Development Agencies

Many UN development agencies play major roles in setting out principles and goals to guide action. The UN's social development agenda, the Millennium Development Goals, designed for 'reducing poverty and improving lives', does not include chronic diseases. Millennium Development Goal number 6, 'Combat HIV/AIDS, malaria, and other diseases', theoretically refers to chronic diseases which fit in the 'other' category, in practice they receive little or no attention.

This policy to exclude chronic diseases was deliberate. As Jeffrey Sachs, the economist who led the WHO's Macroeconomic and Health Report, and a well-known advocate of free-market policies, argued: 'the reason that the MDGs do not explicitly address noncommunicable diseases such as cardiovascular or psychiatric is because the MDGs focus on the gap in health status of rich and poor countries, a gap mainly accounted for by infectious diseases, malnutrition, and unsafe childbirth. The goals were crafted to address these large gaps rather than to solve all pressing health problems' (326). This echoed the argument put forward by the World Bank that chronic diseases were second-order concerns. Reflecting this focus, a Global Fund for AIDS, TB, and Malaria was set up in 2002 with $19.3 billion of approved funds after a 2001 UN General Assembly Special Session committed to create such a fund.

The lack of funding has led to exclusion of chronic diseases from the operations of UN institutions. For example, the UN Children's Fund's (UNICEF) goal-setting programme, *A World Fit for Children* (2003), does not include chronic diseases or risk factors among its 25 action points to 'promote healthy lives'. The International Labor Organization's (ILO) major reports do not refer to chronic diseases. The UN Population Fund (UNFPA) does not incorporate chronic diseases in its strategy on population and development (2007).

Conflicts arise between WHO and UN agencies about trade and agricultural interests. Reports are written, but policy does not change. For example, WHO co-authored a report with the World Trade Organisation, entitled *WTO Agreements and Public Health*, indicating how trade agreements, such as General-Agreement on Tariffs and Trade (GATT) can reduce national policy capacity to control chronic diseases. Nonetheless, the WTO GATT has concluded that import restrictions on tobacco do not qualify as a 'necessary' exception to circumvent treatment as a 'non-tariff trade barrier' on the basis of health impacts. Similarly, the Food and Agriculture Organization has jointly with the WHO published the report *Diet, Nutrition and the Prevention of Chronic Disease* (2003) setting out the need to re-assess unhealthy agricultural subsidies, although the Committee on Agriculture of the FAO disapproved of the WHO Strategy on Diet, Physical Activity and Health because of perceived threats to the sugar industry.

In 2010, a series of UN meetings, sponsored by Pfizer and promoted by fifteen Caribbean countries (CARICOM) has resulted in a dedicated UN session to chronic diseases, to be held in September 2011. The outcome of those efforts at the time of this writing is uncertain. There appears to be a low possibility of incorporating chronic diseases into the existing Millennium Development Goals, a rallying point for many NGOs like the World Diabetes Federation.

> Clue 15: *Conflicts arise between WHO's objectives to prevent chronic diseases and the policies of other UN development agencies which can unintentionally spread chronic diseases and undermine their control.*

> Clue 16: *The deliberate exclusion of chronic diseases from the UN's symbolic agenda, the Millennium Development Goals, has perpetuated a situation where many private donors and development agencies focus squarely on HIV, malaria, and child health, to the neglect of many other conditions, including chronic disease.*

> Strategy 4: *Two main strategies to influence the UN's agenda are to argue that chronic diseases should be a core Millennium Development Goal in their own right in view of their effects on poverty and development and to argue that chronic diseases are crucial to meeting existing goals.*

World Health Organization

Established in 1949 as a specialized agency of the UN, WHO was set up in a period when infectious diseases were dominant threats to health. Historic focus, operations and capacity on infectious diseases, along with difficulties changing WHO's structures, has left organizational changes lagging the disease burden (so-called institutional inertia). WHO's two main roles are setting health norms and providing country support. In this latter capacity, WHO gives advice on policies, evaluates treatments, especially for poor countries, maintains a network of laboratories and sends international teams to fight outbreaks of diseases.

WHO's power has waned over the past three decades. Until about the mid-1990s, it was the leading financier of global health until it was overtaken by the World Bank, but today it mainly has advisory and technical assistance roles. Leaders of the organization are concerned that, with the rising influence of Gates, the World Bank, Global Funds, and other international health partnerships (like the IHP), the WHO is becoming redundant. A bit tongue in cheek, one analyst asked 'Who needs WHO?' Nevertheless, when it comes to NCDs, the WHO is the single greatest funder, spending over US$812 million dollars on NCDs between 2004 and 2008 (see Table 5.2).

Where does WHO's money come from? There are two main pools. One is assessed from member states as a portion of their ability to contribute and allocated at the World Health Assembly. The other is given by private donors, and allocated according to their wishes. In the early 1970s, about three-quarters of WHO's money came from member states. However, since the US ambassadors began calling for holding the WHO regular budget at zero nominal growth in the 1980s, the fraction of WHO's budget allocated by private donors has risen from less than one-quarter of its budget in the early 1970s to more than 80% in 2008/2009. In the 2008/2009 period, the WHO's yearly budget for 2006/2007 from private donor contributions was US$3.3 billion and from member states assessed contributions about $0.96 billion. By comparison, the Gates Foundation's operating budget in 2008 was US$3.8 billion (327).

As shown in Table 5.4, the largest country donors to the WHO were the US and the UK (about US$600 million), while the largest institutional donors were other UN agencies (about US$230 million) and the Gates Foundation (about $150 million). In terms of finances, these four groups control the finances behind about 30% of WHO's agenda.

Within WHO there has long been awareness of the health importance of chronic diseases. Since 1956, when the Indian health minister put forward a resolution on cardiovascular diseases to at the World Health Assembly (WHA), there have been more than 50 resolutions to increase the priority of NCDs. In 1998 WHO established a cluster dedicated to chronic diseases at its headquarters. In 2004, a Global Strategy on Diet, Physical Activity and Health was approved at the WHA. A 2005 WHO report, *Preventing chronic diseases: a vital investment* has the potential to

Table 5.4 Sources of WHO private donor contributions (extra-budget), 2006–07

Top 10 Member States	US dollars	Percentage of total
US	305,668,404	21.5
UK	303,593,823	21.3
Canada	150,849,285	10.6
Norway	102,395,274	7.2
Sweden	87,274,166	6.1
Netherlands	65,053,198	4.6
Italy	58,924,491	4.1
Japan	46,223,718	3.2
Spain	36,720,013	2.6
Australia	34,979,931	2.5
Total Top 10	1,191,682,303	83.4
Total Member States	1,422,331,985	—
Top 10 other sources		
UN*	232,070,782	21.6
Gates Foundation	148,174,632	13.8
European Commission	128,127,194	11.9
Rotary International	27,038,394	2.5
World Bank**	24,204,713	2.3
Novartis, Switzerland	11,933,675	1.1
Asian Development Bank	10,871,000	1.0
World Lung Foundation	10,395,059	1.0
Sanofi-Aventis, France	9,909,802	0.9
Kobe Group, Japan	9,000,000	0.8
Total top 10	611,725,251	56.9
Total other sources	1,075,731,946	—

Notes: See WHO A61/20, p. 3–16 for more details. Other sources include only those organizations that contributed more than US$10 million out of a total of 400 contributors during this period. Data do not sum to 100% because of rounding errors. *Excludes funds for UNAIDs and the Global Fund, which WHO administers. The amount drops to $106,198,595 if funds for emergencies are excluded. **Excludes funds for Global Alliance Vaccine Initiative but includes funds for Tropical Disease Research and Reproductive Health.

stimulate global action. Significant capacity for tobacco control has built around the development and passage of the Framework Convention on Tobacco Control, when WHO used its treaty-making powers for the first time.

In the past, vested interests have sought to influence WHO's agenda. Tobacco industry documents reveal that they felt a need to 'attack WHO . . . the leading enemy'. Their strategies were multi-faceted, aiming to 'discredit key individuals' and 'contain, neutralize, [and] reorient WHO'.

Nonetheless, there have been efforts at the highest level to raise priority of chronic diseases. The President of the 61st World Health Assembly, Dr Leslie Ramsammy of Guyana pointed to the 'glaring omission [in the] MDGs [which] failed to identify the NCDs, in spite of the fact that these diseases account for fully 60% of the global mortalities . . . most of the morbidity and mortality caused by the chronic diseases are preventable [This is] a serious omission [and] I propose we seriously consider an MDG +, which would set goals for the chronic diseases, as we have done for other . . . challenges'.

On the whole, these resolutions and calls to action have yet to be responded to with significant financial support. In 2007, the WHO's budgetary allocations for chronic diseases were about 12% of its budget. One study estimated that the WHO spends only $1 on each chronic disease death in the developing world, compared with $15 for every death from infectious disease (WHO 2003). Across regions, the WHO's budget also misaligns with needs, as shown in Figure 5.6 comparing the budgetary allocations and health burdens of Western Pacific and Africa regions. Africa has about one-quarter of its disease burden caused by chronic diseases and three-quarters by infectious diseases, whereas in Western Pacific the reverse situation occurs. Yet, both groups of countries have more than three-quarters of the budget allocated to infectious diseases (328).

This misalignment in priorities results from the WHO's agenda being captured by private donors. As shown in Figure 5.7, the budget allocated by private donors gives less than 10% to chronic diseases, but the budget set by the health ministers through the democratic World Health gives significantly more resources to chronic diseases, about 38% of the overall budget in 2006/2007 (307).

This critical lack of funds has meant that, although regional and country offices have mandates to address chronic diseases, the capacity to implement programmes on the ground is weak.

WHO has begun to recognize the potential conflicts from private sector funding. Its 2010 World Health Assembly is the first to include a special section on the role of the private sector in global health financing. WHO's board has called meetings to assess how the organization can address the potential impact of its extra-budget on its global health agenda.

Clue 17: *Four-fifths of WHO's budget is set by private donors (mainly including foundations and development agencies), which has resulted in a continued focus on infectious diseases.*

Clue 18: *The remaining one-fifth of WHO's budget is set by health ministers, which assigns more than four times as much priority to chronic diseases as do the private donors.*

Clue 19: *In global health, food and pharmaceutical companies are virtually omnipresent, affecting almost every philanthropic and non-profit effort to reduce chronic diseases.*

Sick populations

Finally, we come to those who the global health system is intended to serve: sick populations. People can leverage an influence on global health. Those people who have loudest voices live in the global North. It is therefore important to ask, what does the average 40-year-old American person think about when he/she thinks about global health?

To shed light on this question, we created a synthesis of key words, a so-called word cloud, based on collecting text from an Internet search about global health (Figure 5.8). We drew this

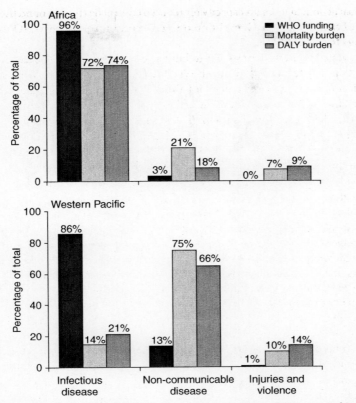

Fig. 5.6 Relation between WHO budget allocations and the burden of disease in Africa and Western Pacific regions.

Notes: WHO allocations are from 2004–05 budget cycle. Data for global mortality and disability-adjusted life year (DALY) are from the WHO Global Burden of Disease, 2002 edition. DALYs are the sum of years of life lost because of premature mortality and years of life lost because of disability. Data do not equal 100% because of rounding errors.

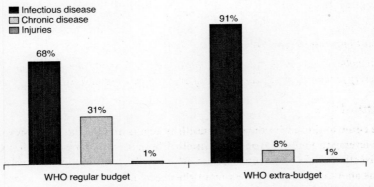

Fig. 5.7 WHO's budgetary allocations, private donors (extrabudget) versus health ministers (regular budget), 2006/2007 fiscal year.

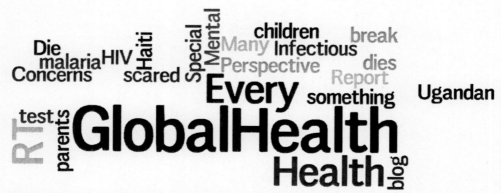

Fig. 5.8 What do people talk about when they talk about global health? What is an ordinary person in the West exposed to when thinking about global health? We created a word-cloud from messages on Twitter (a social networking site catering to all-ages, albeit mostly youth). As shown in the cloud, key words 'scared', 'children', 'concerns', 'infectious' were among the most prominent. At the time of our search, messages were being communicated about Haiti's post-earthquake mental health situation (analogous to what occurred after the Sri Lanka tsunami). This resulted in mental health being the only clear NCD-related phrase appearing in internet media. *Source:* Search on Twitter, 6 April, 2010. Word cloud created using wordle.com.

material from Twitter, a live feed of global health stories from public users. Albeit not perfectly representative, it does give a sense of what people talk about when they talk about global health. As shown, the key themes were 'children', 'die', 'malaria', 'HIV', and 'scared'. Many of these themes are inconsistent with the discourse about chronic diseases.

Unsurprisingly, the views of the public about what is killing people in poor countries are grossly out of sync with the actual situation (Figure 5.9). As one example, we draw on a survey of Americans which asked what people believed were the leading global causes of death. In response, the majority of the Americans believed that HIV and starvation were leading killers. Actually, heart disease and stroke are, as shown in Chapter 1.

Clue 20: The average person living in rich countries holds views about what is killing people in poor countries that grossly misalign with the actual situation.

In our next chapter and book's conclusion, we discuss strategies for helping build a social movement to raise priority of chronic diseases.

Public health and politics

It is within this context of power and politics that the public health community operates. As described above, the grant-making system creates significant constraints on the capabilities of academics. Nonetheless, it is also clear that calls-to-action (see Figure 5.1), awareness, and scientific consensus about what to do have been spurred by the academic community.

How have public health leaders sought to translate this awareness into priority and action on chronic diseases? Mostly by focusing on the scientific evidence. Their approach is often underpinned by an ideal, evidence-based view: rational policymakers should align global health investments to the areas where they could maximally reduce the burden of disease at the lowest cost.

Reflecting this narrow perspective, experts working in global health often build cases for action based on public health (and more recently economic) evidence, appearing to assume that

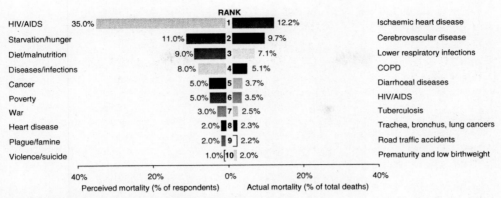

Fig. 5.9 Perceived versus actual burden of disease.
Notes: Perceived mortality data is from Research!America's in response to question, 'What do you think are the two leading causes of death in [*poor or developing countries/countries other than the US*]?' Data represents only 'first mentions'—i.e. the percentage of respondents choosing each health issue as the leading cause of death. Actual mortality data is from the Global Burden of Disease (GBD) Study 2004 Update. COPD = chronic obstructive pulmonary disease.
Siegel KR, Feigl AB, Kishore SP, Stuckler D. "Misalignment between perceptions and actual global burden of disease: Evidence from the U.S. population" *Global Health Action* 2011, **4**: 6339.
DOI: 10.3402/gha.v4i0.6339.

policymakers will make rational decisions on the basis of their evidence. Thus, the case for action usually begins by describing how large the burden of disease is, and how much could be reduced at low cost:

'An impressive body of evidence supports the case for urgent action in response to the growing burden of chronic disease in developing countries' (329). 'It is clear from the high death rates projected for lower-income and upper middle-income countries for 2015 that these countries also need urgent interventions to control and prevent chronic diseases' (3). 'The NCD epidemic is growing faster in poor countries . . . This makes it imperative to take urgent action to address the double burden of disease, dealing effectively with both infections and NCDs' (19). 'Alcohol consumption is one of the major avoidable risk factors, and actions to reduce burden and costs associated with alcohol should be urgently increased' (330). 'A serious scaling up of the response to stroke and other chronic diseases is urgently required in all low-income and middle-income countries' (331). 'Urgent action is needed by WHO, the World Bank, regional banks and development agencies, foundations, national governments, civil society, non-governmental organizations, the private sector including the pharmaceutical industry, and academics' (332). 'We call for urgent and intensified action from all stakeholders to respond to the chronic disease epidemics on the basis of all the available evidence, including that presented in this Series. The evidence is unequivocal: major and rapid health and economic gains are possible with only modest investments in prevention and control of chronic diseases' (332).

Unfortunately, these epidemiological considerations are only one, often minor, factor for most of the people who make important decisions. It could be thought of as a 'scientific' or 'rational' component to decision-making. Yet as a large body of work has made clear, 'policy change is not simply a technocratic process based on rational analysis, and that knowledge alone is not sufficient for policy change. Policy change is a profoundly political process' (282).

Nevertheless, the next sequence in the case made by public health experts typically involves explaining how policymakers should respond urgently to 'the emergency of chronic diseases'. Making the case that health and the economy could be improved, advocates next point out 'something should be done', spreading awareness, raising calls to action, typically in the form of calls to 'political will':

> 'A prerequisite [for action] . . . is strong political will to confront chronic diseases . . . local political will is therefore essential' (332); Other scholars explain differences in the extent to which countries have implemented the Framework Convention on Tobacco Control as reflecting the fact that 'countries vary greatly in their political willingness and capacity to implement these policy measures' (333). The most recent major report on cardiovascular disease calls repeatedly for 'the political will to support action' (318). 'Real political will is necessary to muster cooperation adapted to today's reality and challenges' (316); 'The WHO, as the lead technical agency in health, must garner necessary resources and cross-sector political will to implement the Global Action Plan for Non Communicable Diseases, 2008–2015' (192).

In other words, to these public health authors the case for action is so clear that it should naturally and voluntarily spring forth. If it does not, it is believed the problem must be that decision-makers are not sufficiently aware about the scope for effective interventions and their economic benefits. People need more information; then they can make better decisions. More calls to action are needed. And so on. 'Political will' will eventually follow, as policymakers, recognizing the error of their ways, will voluntarily decide to make action on chronic diseases a priority.

Such notions do not shed light on how and why policy decisions are actually made. Where does political will come from? How does it emerge? Why is it currently so weak? As one scholar notes, such 'moral exhortation—calling for political commitment and political will—is . . . unlikely to produce positive results in policy formulation or implementation' (282).

Thought about differently, would anyone working in public health suggest that people can solve obesity through individual will? Or put another way, how does one respond to the advice of economists at the World Economic Forum, who point out that WHO needs to get resources and people across diverse sectors to have 'real political will' to support its chronic disease Action Plan—something it has been trying to do for decades through call after call for intersectoral action. In the same way that individuals trying to lose weight are constrained by an unhealthy environment, so too are individual politicians seeking to raise desirable goals like reducing chronic diseases higher on the agenda limited by their political environments and agendas that emphasize more emotional and immediate problems.

Clue 21: Scientific information is one very small component of political decision-making.

Clue 22: Many public health experts seem to believe that priorities will be set based on information and awareness about cost-effective interventions, raising calls to action for political will.

Clue 23: The failure to achieve a higher priority of chronic diseases is ultimately a political, rather than technical, problem.

Strategy 5: It is necessary to account for the incentives of people who have power to make decisions about how to influence the burden of disease.

That is, these calls to action are 'just words'. What makes them come to life politically?

Types of political incentives

It is necessary to take into account the incentives driving the decisions made by people who wield influence over the burden of disease. Five types of incentives have been identified; these are scientific, political, economic, organizational, and symbolic (282) (see Box 5.2).

Which of these incentives prevail depends on the political and institutional arrangements that expand or constrain policy options. For example, consider the implications of six different ways a development agency could set its budget (reflecting its balance of global health priorities):

◆ If the development agency applied a mathematical formula involving the burden of disease, the scientific/technocratic incentives would predominate (although there would be a vociferous discussion to choose how to weight different measures along with hidden struggles by disease groups to inflate their statistics of the disease burden).

◆ If heads of government choose what to do, the political incentives would predominate, as ministers contemplate what they could achieve for their country that would serve their domestic constituents.

◆ If private donors decide, the economic and symbolic incentives would likely predominate, with the outcome depending on which private donor gave more money and the nature of each donor's independent interests (implicitly, this is what organizations like WHO have passively been allowing to happen over the past three decades).

◆ If the health ministers were allowed to decide, there would be a mix of political, economic, and scientific incentives (assuming health ministers motives are to some extent driven by their domestic political prospects, economic forces, and, to some extent, their population's health needs).

◆ If the NGOs decide, there would be a dominance of symbolic and economic incentives, as NGOs rely on donors for funding, where members of the public react to emotive symbols (like dying children) and businesses use NGOs to achieve their economic goals (like opening markets and getting preferential access).

◆ If the development agency let its executive director and board decide (whose tenure covers longer-term political cycles), it would choose diseases that maximized the agency's global reputation as a leading global health authority (tapping into an unresolved debate within organizations such as WHO as it seeks to find its way in a changing global health environment where international financial institutions and private donors have displaced the organization's authority). In this scenario the organizational incentives would predominate.

It is also helpful to examine the key principles and incentives that guide policy choices. In general, groups outside public health view global health interventions as a means to achieve goals as

---

Box 5.2 Five types of political incentives

1 Political: politicians may prefer focusing on a disease with a very low burden, because a small group of advocates in his/her constituency are making a lot of noise about it or lobbyists are threatening to throw resources behind a politician's opponent if that politician does not support their policies.

2 Economic: private companies will seek to skew the balance of priorities towards what best impacts their bottom line of maximizing profits.

3 Organizational: organizations may also act in pursuit of their own survival—to maintain their functions, even if those functions are no longer needed; to increase its own resources and power.

4 Symbolic: symbols and signals can play a powerful role in creating or quelling issues, like the Millennium Development Goals.

5 Scientific: the rational or technocratic perspective of most practitioners of public health tends to be the weakest of all.

See Reich (282) for more details.

diverse as charity, investment, security, or foreign policy (307, 334). These principles inform the global health agendas of different organizations to varying degrees, depending on their core objectives (see Table 5.5). For example, a focus on investment and economic growth is more central to the agenda of the World Bank, whereas foreign policy and security have tended to dominate the discussion about global health in the US (318).

Summary

Despite more than 100 calls to action over the past 5 years, there is a critical lack of resources available for chronic diseases. Less than 3% of official development assistance for health, the main source of global health funding, was dedicated to chronic diseases in 2007. Together, the Gates Foundation, Global Fund to fight HIV, TB and Malaria, and World Bank allocated less than 2% of their budgets to chronic disease in 2005 (308, 328). The bulk of funding to address chronic diseases comes from WHO, which allocates less than 10% of its budget.

Ultimately, this failure to achieve a higher priority for chronic diseases is a political, not a technical, problem, since cost-effective interventions are available. It is not even a problem specific to chronic diseases, but, relates to the overall functioning of global health as a political system and, within it, the effectiveness of the movement to increase the priority of chronic diseases.

Returning to the question posed at the beginning of this chapter: who rules global health? The answer is resoundingly the private donors and the sometimes hidden interests whom they serve. As the director of the WHO's leading tobacco-free programme described the tobacco companies. 'They are cockroaches', he explained, 'they are everywhere'. This chapter has shown that food and pharmaceutical companies are virtually omnipresent. They lie behind almost every philanthropic or non-profit effort to reduce chronic diseases. Their influence is subtle, but can be profound. A challenge for global health is to identify these interests and bring them to the light of day, holding them to standards of transparency and public accountability.

Table 5.5 Five leading global-health metaphors

Principle	Selected goals	Priority diseases	Key institutions
Global health as foreign policy	Trade, alliances, democracy, economic growth, reputation, stabilize or destabilize countries	Infectious diseases, HIV/AIDS	US State Department, USAID, President's Emergency Plan for AIDS Relief
Global health as security	Combat bioterror, infectious diseases, and drug resistance	Avian influenza, severe acute respiratory syndrome, multidrug-resistant TB, AIDS	US Centers for Disease Control and Prevention
Global health as charity	Fight absolute poverty	Famine or malnutrition, HIV/AIDS, TB, malaria, rare diseases	Bill & Melinda Gates Foundation, other philanthropic bodies
Global health as investment	Maximize economic development	HIV/AIDS, malaria	World Bank and IMF, International Labour Organization, private sector
Global health as public health	Maximize health effect	Worldwide burden of disease	WHO, vertical disease-specific non-governmental organizations

Stuckler, D. and M. McKee. "Five metaphors about global-health policy." *The Lancet*. July 2008, **372**(9633): 95–7.

Private donors have begun to dominate the global health agenda, in what has been referred to as the privatization of global health. About half of all global health money now comes from private foundations or companies. Figuring out where their money comes from and where it goes and whether it actually reaches the poor is a terribly difficult job. This money tends to be channelled through budgeting systems that are inconsistent and difficult to track. Close to one-third of the money earmarked for health goes to unidentifiable purposes.

In general, these donors give the lowest priority to chronic diseases. The reasons for this are not clear. Their mission statements, decision-making processes, and the vested interests whom they serve are often hidden from the public. Thus, the capacity to decide what is relevant and how it will be addressed is in the hands of very few, who ultimately are accountable to their own interests. A challenge for global health is to identify these interests and bring them to the light of day, holding them to standards of transparency and public accountability.

Many of the parent companies of private philanthropic foundations have vested interests in food and pharmaceutical industries. This can be seen in the interlocking directorates of leading global health institutions, such as the Gates Foundation and Microsoft Corporation, with Coca-Cola, PepsiCo, Kellogg, and Merck. It also can be seen in the personal fortunes of private donors and the investments of the Gates Foundation Trust in these companies. Whether this potential conflict of interest impedes greater priority of chronic diseases is not known, but it would be surprising if it did not have an influence, even if subconsciously on the people who work in both the world of private philanthropy and leading private food and pharmaceutical companies.

What is clear is that the failure of private donors and development agencies to commit resources is not a result of a lack of awareness or the availability of effective interventions. Chronic diseases were deliberately omitted when the Millennium Development Goals, the UN's agenda for social development, were being set.

This exclusion of chronic diseases from the UN Millennium Development Goals has perpetuated a situation where many private donors and development agencies focus squarely on HIV, malaria, and child health, to the neglect of many other conditions, including chronic diseases. Rich countries and donor agencies are less likely to donate resources for action on chronic diseases on the grounds, they argue, that poorer nations do not identify chronic diseases as a priority. At the same time, resource-poor nations do not ask for funding because they think they have a better chance of securing money for research and treatment of infectious diseases. This creates a low priority gridlock—at least for those diseases 'not on the agenda'.

The resulting inequities are easy to see in practice. Advocates from Ghana ask, 'How is it that HIV, with a national prevalence of 3.2% in Ghana gets multi-million dollar funding from Ghana's development partners, while hypertension, with a national prevalence of 28.7% is ignored?' (335). Why is it that an HIV-positive person can get access to antiretrovirals but, if also diabetic, is left to suffer a prolonged wasting death from lack of insulin?

The next part of the chapter evaluates how to rectify this inequitable situation, influencing and challenging vested interests. It draws on a body of literature about the success and failure of women's suffrage and civil rights movements, identifying tactics to create a social movement for raising the priority of chronic diseases.

Part 2

Creating a social movement to raise the priority of global chronic disease

Key policy points

1 Social movements seek to raise priority of an issue; examples of social movements in global health in recent decades include HIV, child survival, and climate change.

2 Three steps in building a social movement are reframing the debate, creating political opportunities, and mobilizing resources.

3 Reframing the debate will involve putting an emphasis on social injustice and the causes of rising chronic diseases are beyond people's control, their societal, causes.

4 Creating political opportunities will require strengthening the positions of those who support chronic diseases. Strategies include establishing more democratic systems of global health policy and aligning global health budgets with the avoidable burden of disease.

5 Mobilizing resources will involve focusing on common causes of poor health and failed development. This can be done by forging broader alliances by showing how action on chronic disease can achieve other desirable social goals (such as improving education, economic, environmental, and women's outcomes) and by putting an emphasis on the shared risks of poor health in resource-deprived communities (including tobacco, poverty, and poor nutrition).

Key practice points

1 The practice of medicine cannot be apolitical; nor can politics be separated from its impacts on health.

2 In every study we do and every intervention we propose, we should think about how our results will affect the political context in which we operate.

3 Pervasive myths about chronic diseases are being perpetuated by vested interests and, to a lesser degree, the chronic disease community. Overcoming these falsehoods about chronic diseases requires not just rebutting them, but generating a new narrative that evokes a more compelling, symbolic and emotive images of the disease's causes and victims.

4 People's beliefs about the causes of disease have a significant influence on the potential for implementing public health policy. When people recognize that chronic diseases are rising because of causes beyond an individual's control, they are more likely to support effective public health policies to tax risks and subsidize protective factors.

Social movements in global health

In the 19th century consumption was a leading killer of the poor. Medicines were ineffective, but the rich were, through a combination of social measures, able to keep death rates from TB relatively low. Deeply concerned about the inequitable situation, Rudolf Virchow, a public health doctor, came up with a surprising solution—to get rid of the church.

Virchow's argument was that people's outrage at the root social causes of TB, such as poverty and inequality, was being misdirected by fatalistic religious beliefs. Instead of the poorest and sickest members of society seeking social change, they came to believe they would reap rewards for their suffering and sickness in the afterlife. If their beliefs could be changed, to direct their ire at political leaders, Virchow believed there would be groundswell of activity that would command a response to the burden of TB by people in power.

Clearly, we are not suggesting that the church is the reason why chronic diseases have a low priority, but the case of TB and the church illustrates a central challenge: for a social movement to arise people must believe they can make a difference, losing their sense of fatalism. People must believe that the issue is beyond their individual control, requiring broader societal action, and they must believe that, given solutions exist, failing to act would perpetuate a situation that is grossly unfair and unsustainable (338). In short, people must be motivated to reform existing social relationships and structures that are adversely affecting their community or entire society.

As we explored in the first part of this chapter, in the case of chronic diseases the equivalent to the 'church' is a series of social institutions that have agendas and vested interests that deliberately seek to prevent chronic disease from becoming a top global health priority. As the director of WHO's NCD department put it, 'Vested interests are a major constraint. The clearest example is the tobacco industry. Their marketing campaigns are impeding preventive efforts . . . and they have huge lobbying power'. It is a challenge that affects rich and poor countries alike. Writing in the early 1990s about chronic diseases in the UK, one public health expert said, 'We are now in a position where the public health priorities are clear, but where the food policies of the government and of the farming and food industries are geared to completely different goals'.

Addressing the influence of these groups requires an understanding of how the global-health political system works. As one leading chronic disease expert, put it, 'the battle to fight chronic disease has moved from a technical to a political phase.' Accordingly, the top objective of the WHO's chronic disease Action Plan is 'to raise the priority accorded to chronic diseases in development work at global and national levels, and to integrate prevention and control of such diseases into policies across all government departments'.

Several researchers, recognizing this need, have attempted to understand why chronic diseases have a low priority. They point to specific characteristics of chronic diseases—such as how the long-term nature of chronic diseases is misaligned with short-term political cycles, or how chronic disease interventions seem complex and difficult to implement and monitor compared with 'magic-bullet' approaches to infectious diseases. These explanations provide a partial picture, but they lack a theoretical model of the power and politics of the groups that rule global health.

Part of the problem is that these approaches draw on a tradition of understanding politics referred to as 'pluralist', so named because its proponents claim power is distributed broadly in groups who compete with each other for priority. Pluralist theories view politics as a market, where the ultimate political outcomes are determined by a collision of forces involving people, interest groups, and ideas. One leading pluralist framework contains four determinants of political outcomes: leaders, issue characteristics, actor power, and ideas (339).

Clearly, this framework can identify that there are few leaders and weak actors actively engaged in chronic disease control or prevention. But does it help to tell people working in the area of chronic diseases that they lack leaders and therefore need to go find some? (At almost every conference we hear 'We need leaders like those in HIV or climate change'.) Or does it help to tell someone that their ideas about how to control chronic diseases have not been influential, so they should come up with better ones? In other words, even though these frameworks can identify some barriers to making chronic diseases a priority, they tell us little about the powerful interests who sustain this situation or what we can do to overcome them.

In this chapter, we draw on an alternative tradition found in the sociological literature that studies the success and failure of social movements in influencing political processes. Ours is an approach that responds to Geoffrey Rose's challenge: there are 'sick individuals and sick populations'–requiring different approaches for study and intervention (see Chapter 2). Those problems which cannot be overcome by the actions of individuals—such as sick societies—require societal action; our combined efforts to achieve this action can be viewed as a social movement.

Here, we invoke social movements to explore the pathways available to concerned people for strengthening global health interventions on chronic diseases. These movements can be understood as informal groups of concerned people, leaders, and institutions unified by mutual values and a focus on shared goals about societal or political issues (224, 340, 341). They are a valuable mechanism by which ordinary people can participate in political processes and challenge the status quo in society (340). In an effort to bring about social change, these groups mobilize resources which they use to launch sustained, organized campaigns to raise awareness, set the agenda, and increase action on collective issues.

Even though the deprived conditions of the poor can create conditions that give rise to social movements, they rarely arise, chiefly because, as detailed in Chapter 3, these people are often impoverished, ill, and/or disabled in ways that make it extremely difficult for them to organize, mobilize, and act politically. Participating in a social movement demands time, resources, and money that many persons who are afflicted with chronic diseases simply do not have, and may also involve risks and a backlash from authorities that many persons are unwilling to take. Yet, in the face of unequal growth and inequalities in access to healthy diets, physical activity, and medical care, engaging a process of collective action may offer the best promise to change elements of the political, economic, and social systems that are creating our sick societies.

Social movements develop through a series of phases, from an initiating event and circumstances that lead, sometimes slowly, to organized protests, before culminating in their ultimate decline (338, 342). These phases can be broadly characterized as going through initial stages of emergence to coalescing around shared interests, followed by a phase where the movement becomes institutionalized through autonomous structures or social networks. At this juncture, the movement has typically begun to challenge authorities about the injustice of the status quo using a repertoire of strategies, ranging from peaceful protest such as hunger strikes to extreme forms of violence against public officials. These campaigns can lead to outright success or failure, as well as a series of alternative outcomes, such as being repressed by authorities (as in the violent reactions to civil rights protests in the US) or co-opted by authorities (who realize that change is inevitable and better to be a part of) or becoming mainstream (such as the antiglobalization movement) (see Figure 5.10).

To date, groups concerned about chronic diseases have yet to develop into an organized social movement, but there is hope. Many social movements have aimed to change societies so as to improve people's lives: human rights, HIV, child survival, women's rights, gay rights, civil rights, antinuclear, antiglobalization, and climate change movements are but a few illustrations. While there are currently no large-scale protests about the scandal of allowing many thousands of young Africans to die needlessly from diabetes almost a century after the discovery of insulin, civil society has not ignored chronic diseases; as described in the preceding sections, there are passionate and concerned people who have formed numerous special interest groups and NGOs, each advocating greater priority for their disease.

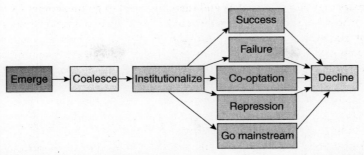

Fig. 5.10 Stages of social movements. Adapted from: Blumer, Herbert G. Collective Behavior. In Alfred McClung Lee (ed). *Principles of Sociology*. Third Edition , pp. 65–121. New York: Barnes and Noble Books, 1969; Mauss, Armand L. *Social Problems as Social Movements*. Philadelphia: Lippincott, 1975; and Tilly, Charles. *From Mobilization to Revolution*. Reading, Massachusetts: Addison-Wesley, 1978.

Why is the current chronic disease movement so weak? How could it be more effective? What strategies can we learn from the successes and failures of other social movements?

To strengthen a social movement on chronic diseases, in this chapter we use an adapted version of a 'Political Process' model that has been used to evaluate a range of social movements, including women's and civil rights (341). In our adapted version, we integrate several leading theories about social movements (such as culture theory, mass society theory, elite theory, and resource mobilization theory). At its core are three strategies: re-framing the debate, creating and identifying political opportunities, and mobilizing resources. In the first section we cover each of these in turn. In so doing, we draw lessons from the successes and failures of other global social movements, such as HIV/AIDS, child survival, civil rights, climate change, and tobacco control. Based on this analysis, each section concludes with a series of tactics that can be used to strengthen a global social movement to put chronic diseases on the global health agenda.

Modelling the political process

Before we begin, pause to consider how to stop a social movement, as though you were a 'maniacal dictator of death', set out to kill people from chronic diseases. What would you do?

First, you might scatter those people who would otherwise form a cohesive movement, and create conditions in which they are distracted and fight amongst themselves. You might generate a vague or contradictory base of information about what key factors were of importance to global morbidity and mortality, leading to endless arguments about what should be done and by whom. By setting priorities that reward individuals for generating high-profile programmes that produce little impact, you could slowly starve the movement of critical resources. You might exclude victims of diseases who are supposed to be the subject of the movement's plans, in so doing establishing these inappropriate models as best practices. To be most effective, these models would not have clearly-observed or defined public health outcomes, but would garner publicity, operating to fragment individuals competing over the wrong issues.

Together, these steps would become self-defeating, creating a political process that rewards individuality or elitism, publicity over substance, and oligarchy over democracy. As this system fails to produce results, you would help spread a feeling of ineffectiveness, dispassionate acceptance, and complacency. You would create a rigid bureaucracy, with few opportunities for advancement, so that everyone would come to be stuck in middle-management positions on large ineffective projects, working on programmes that seem to be far from the passionate roots of the original call for change. Without a clear vision or rewards in place, few of the young and interested could be recruited and become involved in a meaningful way to push forward an exciting agenda for change.

Such a plan is diabolical. But it is precisely what happened to those who might have formed a movement to tackle chronic diseases. The question is how this happened, who facilitated it, and what we can do to stop it.

We start by discussing the tactics for overcoming common myths about chronic diseases.

Strategy 1—reframing the debate about chronic diseases

As we see from the maniacal dictator of death, one major concern that prevents a successful social movement emerging is the dissemination of information that is inaccurate, distracting, or de-moralizing (creating what is referred to in sociology as 'false consciousness'). Information can act not only to limit what we know about a problem, but also how we react.

How an issue is framed crucially affects the scope of intervention. In sociological theory, framing refers to the process by which words, texts, and events derive meaning from an individual's selected understanding of them. These frames can be thought of as cerebral filters that make sense of incoming messages and can powerfully affect how people interpret and respond to them. As one set of scholars put it, 'Like a picture frame, an issue frame marks off some part of the world. Like a building frame, it holds things together . . . We do not see the frame directly, but infer its presence by its characteristic expressions and language. Each frame gives the advantage to certain ways of talking and thinking, while it places others out of the picture' (342a). In other words, the way we talk about chronic diseases influences the potential for political priority and action.

In the next section, we provide an initial analysis of the current discourse in global health and how it relates to the potential for action on chronic diseases.

The main problem: blaming the victim

In the case of chronic diseases, a series of pervasive myths 'blame the victim' or suggest 'nothing can be done'. These frame chronic diseases as:

- ◆ 'Diseases of individual choice', implying that people knowingly accept risks of chronic disease, choosing to drink and smoke, and should be left to their own devices.

- ◆ 'Diseases of ageing', inevitable consequences of progress in healthcare, and that public resources would be wasted on those who have achieved a normal span of life (sometimes called 'a fair innings').

- ◆ 'Diseases of affluence', afflicting mainly rich people in rich countries, with their growth possibly even serving as a marker of social progress.

These myths negate the potential for political action by framing chronic diseases in one of two ways: as an individual problem, requiring no collective policy action, or as a population problem, which is so deeply instilled that policy cannot make a difference—so legitimating the status quo of little or no action.

If chronic diseases are an individual rather than a societal problem, then there is no need for a social movement, only the 'education' of individuals. In liberal societies, social interventions against individual problems are viewed as impinging on people's freedoms; this renders strong public health measures, such as taxation or regulation, illegitimate. Taxes on soft drinks, bans on smoking in public places, and other potentially-effective public health interventions are considered intrusions into personal freedom rather than life-protecting measures, analogous to the automobile safety belt.

As described in Box 5.3, the discourse in global health is dominated by a focus on victims, uncertainty, and fear of disease outbreaks. As shown in Figure 5.10, when people talk about global health, they focus on 'children', 'scared', and 'infectious', framing which spurs a social movement. On the other hand, when people talk about chronic diseases, they focus on 'long', 'normal', and 'ago'—hardly a sense of urgency, illegitimacy, or public concern, as invoked by UNICEF in raising the priority of child health in the 1980s (see Box 5.4).

Several experts from WHO, recognizing these pervasive myths about chronic diseases, set out to debunk them using rigorous scientific evidence. Their data were compelling, at least to the scientists who understood them, ultimately being published as part of the first *Lancet* special series about the neglected epidemic of chronic diseases. Yet, 5 years later, the lead author of the series remarked, 'I thought we got rid of these myths. But they keep coming back'.

This leaves us asking, how can the debate be successfully re-framed to strengthen the potential for a social movement to arise?

Box 5.3 The current debate about global health: infections, victims, and uncertainty

In viewing the current discourse about global health, we immediately see that those afflicted by communicable diseases are commonly, and appropriately, portrayed as victims, either of the circumstances that rendered them vulnerable to infection or of the infectious agent itself.

In contrast, those afflicted by chronic diseases are commonly represented as the agents of their own misfortune, typically because they have freely chosen certain health-damaging lifestyles, such as smoking, hazardous drinking, or overeating (343). Indeed, it is often the exceptions to this general view where there have been the greatest successes in implementing effective action to tackle chronic diseases. Examples include creation of smoke-free public places to protect non-smokers from the dangers of second-hand smoke and restrictions on drinking and driving as a means of reducing road traffic injuries. Yet this 'victim-blaming' approach ignores how, while people do make individual choices about their lifestyles, they rarely do so in circumstances of their own choosing (344).

A second aspect of the discourse on NCD is that of uncertainty. The promulgation by Koch of his postulates paved the way for associating specific micro-organisms causally with diseases (345). Yet for chronic diseases the situation is much more complex, involving the interpretation of relative risks derived from observational epidemiology which, almost inevitably, is subject to caveats related to issues such as measurement of exposure and confounding. Here too, powerful vested interest have played a role, as in the 'confounder' studies undertaken at the behest of the tobacco industry to create scepticism about the effects of second hand smoke (158) or even seeking to redefine 'good epidemiology' practice so as to exclude all but the most prominent risk factors (159).

A third important consideration is the perception of threats associated with rapid spread of a disease. Even in cases where the effective disease burden is zero, such as Avian flu, concerns about danger and threats to security lead to it receiving a higher priority; a disease is framed as a potential 'crisis', 'pandemic' or 'epidemic'. It is difficult to blame victims when there is potential that you could become one of them.[7]

Box 5.4 UNICEF's child health revolution and the World Bank backlash in the 1980s

One example of a successful effort to overcome the challenges in framing the debate can be seen in the explicit movement to 'create a new global consensus' on putting the health of children first. In the 1980s UNICEF produced explicit messages to define infant mortality as a societal problem (part of the debate about Primary Health Care versus Selective Primary Health Care, see Chapter 4). Unabashed, they blamed policymakers for killing babies (obviously babies were not to blame), pointed to simple solutions that could save lives at low cost (such as oral rehydration therapy), and called explicitly for a 'revolution' toward child survival. UNICEF sought to make child health the top global social development priority—and by the 1990s it was largely successful (346).

Of course, the unspoken corollary was that adult health, dominated by chronic diseases (and in due course HIV), would come second. This growing emphasis on children was not pleasing to many other groups, who had a different vision for global health. To many observers, it led to an unfair situation where a child would be cared for, but his/her mother would not. Other analysts deplored the 'short-sightedness of technological fix thinking with respect to the complexities of child survival', calling for a 'larger social, economic, and demographic revolution' (347).

In the 1990s the World Bank sought to reframe the debate by publishing reports that began with stark sentences: 'This book seeks to place adult health firmly on the agenda' (323) and 'Surviving childhood is not the only health hurdle in developing countries' (348). Naturally, the World Bank reports claimed that the debate was not about one disease versus another (seeking to avoid 'an unproductive debate about the equity of investment in adult versus child health'), but implicitly it was.

Case study: histories of HIV and tobacco control

Blatant lies about a disease have been a persistent problem facing groups concerned about HIV, food safety, climate change, child health, and many other issues (349, 350). For example, in the 1980s, people spread hateful, stigmatizing myths about HIV, claiming it was 'God's punishment' for sexual promiscuity (especially among homosexual men); a disease of 'individual choice' because infected people could have chosen to use protection instead; and a disease of 'affluence' because richer people had more sexual partners, to name a few (349). These myths were perpetuated, not just by corporate vested interests, but also government campaigns and coalitions of HIV-sceptics working in global health, concerned about their disease losing money.

The importance of how the debate is framed is most apparent in the history of tobacco control. Tobacco companies, acting like the maniacal dictator of death described above, first argued that the evidence that smoking caused disease was contradictory and flimsy (351). Litigation pursued between the 1950s and 1990s by individuals that tobacco companies were negligent and fraudulently misrepresenting the risks overwhelmingly failed, but as the scientific evidence base grew stronger that tobacco was causing disease, the case was made that there was a need to intervene. Tobacco companies swiftly responded that it was illegitimate to intervene, arguing that tobacco use was an individual choice. The field of public health became fragmented, as some economists opposed tobacco regulation on the grounds that tobacco deaths were saving governments millions of dollars (see Chapter 3). Similarly, tobacco companies attempted to have WHO focus on other lung diseases, as a diversion from tobacco, creating internal fighting within the Union of TB and Lung Disease culminating in a greater focus on TB than COPD and a failure to identify tobacco as a major risk factor for both (352).

One major turning point in the US came when the Surgeon General, David Kessler, began to argue that tobacco was a paediatric disease, which overcame the individual choice argument by focusing on adolescent adoption of smoking. His argument was strengthened by new research making a strong economic case for intervention, and, crucially, the disclosure of tobacco documents showing how choices of individuals were being manipulated through industry lies and efforts to cultivate addiction (increasing awareness of the political determinants of information). This process only came to fruition over four decades after tobacco's effects on health had been demonstrated.

Not only did the damning research result in widespread legislative reform during the late 1990s that regulated tobacco advertisements and required tobacco companies to pay for public health costs caused by smoking-related diseases, but also remarkably across 2000–2010 produced a number of successful personal litigations in which the court awarded substantial damages. In 2009, the US Court of Appeals for the District of Columbia issued groundbreaking judgment that defendant cigarette companies knew nicotine was addictive yet continued to deny and deceive the public of this fact, ruling: 'knew of their falsity at the time and made statements with the intent to deceive' and that their 'liability rests on their knowledge of their falsity'.

Despite these large awards, as noted in Chapter 1, tobacco use continues to rise in resource-poor countries, although there are signs of decline in middle-income countries (see country chapters of Brazil and South Africa), and remains above 20% among youth, groups which tobacco companies view as their main growth markets (29). The cost of political inaction is devastating.

Key solution: emphasizing the societal causes of chronic disease

Similar debates to those about tobacco use are developing about the causes of obesity. Many industry front groups, such as The Center for Consumer Freedom, argue against 'nanny state' interventions to tackle obesity, a label used with remarkable frequency by certain newspapers, such as the *Daily Mail* in the UK. One recent study in the US found that people's beliefs about the causes of obesity strongly influenced their support for different policy interventions (353). Those who believed individual responsibility was an important cause of obesity were much less likely to support taxation, subsidies or other fiscal interventions—some of the most effective measures available to public health.[5] Another study of how diabetes is framed found that people exposed to a social determinants message were more supportive of public policy interventions than those exposed to genetic or individualized frames (354). The city authorities in New York have framed obesity as primarily a social problem (in part as a result of threats of litigation, see Chapter 8), resulting in a requirement that restaurants label menus with calories. Similarly, California has banned trans fats; on the other hand, southern states in which state governments view obesity, and many other health problems, as an individual responsibility have refused such interventions, and they continue to face the highest rates of obesity and obesity-related diseases in the country.

We should also point the finger at ourselves: the chronic disease community, too, unintentionally perpetuates myths about chronic diseases, framing them as individual problems or inevitable. Almost every paper about chronic disease explains their causes as due to some combination of population ageing, nutrition transition, urbanization, economic growth, globalization, and epidemiological or lifestyle transition (see Chapter 2). Yet to most people, these descriptions sound like progress—a process to be encouraged, not a powerful critique of modern society (see Box 5.5).

Overcoming these pervasive myths requires not just rebutting them, but generating a new narrative that evokes a more compelling, symbolic, and emotive images of the disease's causes and victims. Evidence about the addictive nature of many products that cause chronic diseases, especially among children, will need to be acquired either through scientific research or discovery of existing corporate strategy documents, so as to dispel dominant myths.

Box 5.5 Examples of how the chronic disease field perpetuates myths

The phrase 'lifestyle', the most commonly used term by epidemiologists to describe the risks of chronic diseases, sounds like a fashionable development, possibly promoted by designers like Versace or Gucci. It makes it all too easy to blame the victim. To economists, suggesting that chronic diseases are being caused by economic growth, globalization, or urbanization not only sounds inevitable, but like a sign of success, as these are precisely the development strategies they recommend. (Indeed whilst dining with an author of the World Bank's World Development Report, the authors were asked, 'isn't obesity a sign of progress?') To policymakers, saying that 'chronic diseases are the result of population ageing' makes the epidemic sound inevitable. As researchers at the World Bank note, 'an overemphasis on ageing can give rise to a mistaken view that policy cannot make a difference'. Finally, chronic disease epidemiologists often present the wrong disease-metric to describe the distribution of the risks of chronic diseases (see Appendix). When we present data about crude, rather than age-standardized burdens of chronic diseases, we artificially make chronic diseases appear to be diseases of affluence, when the reality is that their greatest risks are, like most causes of poor health, disproportionately concentrated among the poor (see Chapter 1 for more details).

Central to motivating groups to act is to develop an 'injustice frame', that inform individuals, societies, and advocacy groups of misinformation about chronic diseases that they are being fed, and to reshape the assumption that the individual is to blame. Thus, we refer to two kinds of framing: social-generating or social-degenerating. In every study we do and every intervention we propose, we should think about how our results will affect the political context in which we operate.

Thus we have derived our first set of tactics to help re-frame the debate:

Tactic 1: Emphasize the causes of chronic diseases beyond an individual's control—their societal causes.

Tactic 2: Focus epidemiological inquiry on victims of an unhealthy society—especially children and their rates of obesity, tobacco use, high blood pressure and diabetes.

Tactic 3: Find emotive symbols of victims of chronic diseases.

Tactic 4: Conduct research that exposes the vested interests that interfere with effective disease control measures and preventative strategies (mainly food and pharmaceutical companies).

Tactic 5: Build evidence to support a legal case for disclosure of food and alcohol industry documents by showing products are addictive and have health impacts.

Even if these tactics could be successfully implemented to reframe the debate about chronic diseases, they are no guarantee for action and risk being neutralized by competing groups who have incentives to keep things the way they are. Further, it is likely that many food and beverage companies will realize the challenges they face and elect to become part of the movement rather than oppose, in the process attempting to 'co-opt' the movement to limit the potential for taxes and regulation and structural change (a discussion returned to in Chapter 6). Hence, in search for ways to weaken the power of vested interests and their continued neglect as well as potentially adverse influence on chronic diseases, we now look to the powerful forces who rule the global health political system and their histories.

Strategy 2—creating political opportunities

Analogous to the maniacal dictator, there are several groups that are acting, either consciously or subconsciously, to create apathy or a sense of fatalism in ways that limit people's ability to identify political opportunities as well as their motivation to create them. To be motivated as activists, individuals must have a sense of empowerment that they can challenge existing political systems and create real change. There is also a sense of urgency, especially in the case of chronic diseases, where any further diversion or delay in taking effective action results in more avoidable deaths.

The problem: slow pace of institutional change and vested interests

As described in Chapter 4, global health was borne out of 'tropical medicine' and 'imperial medicine' heritage, emphasizing 'magic-bullet' interventions (for example, smallpox paradigm). This culminated in a focus on infectious diseases through vertical, disease-specific programmes, emphasizing simple interventions with high biological efficacy, such as vaccines. Appropriate targets for interventions were represented as 'natives' who have a particular set of archetypal diseases (not Western conditions like heart disease, diabetes or cancer); limited understandings of the people and health systems of poor countries led the director of US Agency for International Development to claim to the US Congress that Africans 'can't tell time' and that health systems around the continent are incapable of refrigeration, in spite of having some of the most modernized cities in the world (355).

As in all political systems, the global health system has a tendency towards no or slow change, a conservative bias referred to as 'institutional inertia'. Without external shocks (such as HIV in the 1980s), institutions typically continue to set priorities in global health along the paths already established, slowly adapting to changes in the disease burden.

The tendency towards little or no change is also driven by vested interests that seek to maintain the current situation. This includes people in powerful positions in global health, who have organizational incentives to keep funding for their laboratories and teams of researcher. It also includes vested interests, such as pharmaceutical companies which attempt to influence the agenda to create a greater market for their drugs.

The current global health political system could be described not as a participatory democracy but as an institutional oligarchy, involving a few powerful institutions and groups which wield excessive power. These include the World Bank, the Global Fund for AIDS, TB, and, Malaria, WHO, and, increasingly, private donors like the Gates Foundation.

This situation has historical parallels. In the US during the late 19th and early 20th century (a period of massive inequality and free trade), 'robber barons' generated unprecedented wealth, giving rise to private philanthropic foundations including the Rockefeller Foundation and Ford Foundation. Much of their efforts to redistribute wealth privately were a subtle way of maintaining control and alleviating social discontent that would call for governments to redistribute wealth through taxation.

Why are rich white men suddenly interested in the health of the poor? Again, one answer is because charity in the private sector is preferable to developing systems of public taxation. It also helps create positive public relations, helping to legitimate massive extremes of wealth. In fact the analogy runs further. Massive global health redistribution by private donors can similarly be viewed as impeding efforts to create a global social health safety net (between-country redistribution, just as taxation and welfare systems have generated within-country redistribution).

It seems unlikely that private philanthropy will support the most effective public health measures to protect populations from chronic diseases, especially when they involve fiscal interventions like taxation, subsidies and regulation of the markets for products in which these philanthropists have invested heavily. One example is the 'Keep America Beautiful' campaign funded by, among others, Philip Morris, which focused on every kind of trash except tobacco waste (even though it makes up 25–50% of all litter on US streets) and subsequently on individual responsibility for waste (356, 357).

In sum, those who would form a chronic disease movement are 'challengers' to the dominant forces in global health. Without a significant change to the status quo, there will likely be a continuation of the current situation whereby a few private groups (including private NGOs and non-profit foundations) focusing on a narrow set of infectious diseases will dominate the global health agenda. It can also not simply be assumed that, eventually, as the burden of disease comes to be overwhelmingly chronic in nature, that priority will be given to chronic diseases. There is a risk that, once infectious disease are controlled (a prospect that has remained elusive for decades), the global health system, rather than extend into chronic diseases, would simply be dismantled—the ultimate vision of several leading development economists who oppose state intervention (306).

How can we create political opportunities for chronic diseases? Again, we can look to how the civil rights movement in the US benefited from identifying and provoking changes in the structure of political opportunities.

Case study: African American civil rights movement

Despite the success of the US abolitionist movement in ending slavery in 1865, black minorities remained geographically and institutionally segregated. A series of laws were passed during the late 19th and early 20th centuries, including the so-called 'Black codes', and the 'separate but equal' doctrine in 'Jim Crow' laws, that created a legal framework that explicitly discriminated against blacks. These laws exposed African Americans to strict penal labour and bondage regimes and deprived them of access to education and financial opportunity. Blacks were also denied the right to vote or have political representation, while also exposing them to state-sanctioned violence.

It took nearly a century for the situation to begin to significantly change when, in 1954, an important legal case, *Brown v. Board of Education*, overturned the separate but equal doctrine, and in 1964, the democratic party passed the Civil Rights Act[6] that banned discrimination based on 'race, color, religion, or national origin' in employment and public services. Nonetheless, the unequal situation persisted for years to come—leaving enduring inequalities that can still be observed in the US (for example, rates of chronic diseases nearly twice as high and wealth five times lower in blacks than whites).

Nevertheless, significant gains were achieved for African Americans through a powerful social movement and a series of concentrated campaigns. Thus, we must ask, what created the political opportunity for the civil rights movement that made it possible realize these goals in the 1960s?

While efforts to launch a social movement at end of the 19th and the beginning of the 20th century were marred by discrimination and violence against African Americans, in numerous ways throughout this period blacks were slowly mobilizing around the hope of gaining better social and economic opportunities, largely through lawsuits and the development of autonomous political and social organizations. For example, the National Association for the Advancement of Colored People (NAACP) was founded in the North in 1909, the African Blood Brotherhood was established in the 1920s, and the International Labor Defense forged a link with the black communists after the 1920s: all three shared the aim of ceasing race discrimination through a strategy of lobbying, litigation, and education.

After the success of the Brown case, which established that separate provision was inherently unequal, created a legal basis for action, the civil rights movement's tactics shifted to 'direct action'—boycotts, freedom rides, sit-ins, and marches—that were directed at gaining mass mobilization, as well as violent and non-violent action. This marked a departure from the traditional approach of seeking incremental, often limited gains, to seeking rapid and systematic changes in the ways in which society was organized.

The potential for these mass mobilization and protest campaigns were largely enabled by the incremental growth of the resources available to the civil rights movement had experienced over the past half-century. This growth of resources was in part caused by industrialization, migration to cities, and the development of autonomous black organizations in urban churches (such as the Southern Christian Leadership Coalition). These resources made it possible for the civil rights movement to reach out to more people and escalate protests, often creating violent reactions from white individuals and, in several outrageous cases, the police.

These protests and violent reactions forced the federal government to step in to protect blacks, but as a result alienated many white voters. While initially hesitant and poorly informed about civil rights, President Kennedy, acting on advice from his brother (a passionate civil rights advocate), decided to try to pick up black votes in the North to offset the loss of white support in the South, sending in troops to enforce the law. This most famously occurred in response to an uprising at University of Mississippi which refused entry to James Meredith, as the governor proclaimed 'no school will be integrated in Mississippi while I am your Governor'. In the process of quelling these revolts by whites, the federal government supported large voting registration drives, helping create new Southern black voters for the Democratic Party from Southern blacks and encouraging further political participation and social organization.

After Kennedy's assassination in 1964, President Johnson continued these efforts, ultimately with the passage, under his leadership, of the Voting Rights Act of 1965 that restored and protected voting rights of 1965 and the Fair Housing Act of 1968 that banned discrimination in housing markets. Realizing the political implications of these decisions, he famously said, 'we [the Democratic Party] have lost the South for a generation.' Nevertheless, African Americans re-engaged in politics across the South, and across the country, youth were motivated to continue to fight for the betterment of the Black community and social equality.

Key solution: strengthening the position of those who support chronic diseases by making global health more democratic

Albeit not nearly so bleak as the situation facing blacks in the US during the periods described, chronic diseases start from a position of institutional stigma and disadvantage, with little or no clear political opportunity. Like African Americans during the late 19th century, those at greater risk from chronic diseases, which as we saw in Chapters 1 and 2 are largely the poor in the developing world, are often politically isolated and voiceless at a governmental level.

Thus, political opportunities need to be identified as they arise, and steps can be taken to create them. The key approaches involve strengthening the position of those who support chronic diseases, either by undermining the power of dominant forces or by changing the incentives that govern the system in which those forces operate. A second major approach is to seek to identify new groups of emerging vested interests.

Thus, we have derived a set of tactics for creating political opportunities:

Tactic 1: Establish democratic systems of priority-setting that include the voices of the poor.

Tactic 2: Seek to align global health budgets with the burden of avoidable disease.

Tactic 3: Make donor priorities, funding, and vested interests transparent and accountable to the public.

Tactic 4: Design new measures of the disease burden that focus on overarching global health priorities, such as unfair and avoidable mortality.

Tactic 5: Help develop National Action Plans focusing on chronic diseases and their socioeconomic risk factors.

Tactic 6: Embed health protections and impact assessments into Free-Trade Agreements so that emerging superpowers such as Brazil, China, India, and Mexico can protect their economies from unhealthy and unfair US and European agricultural subsidies.

Identifying political opportunities that arise from changing balances in power is a crucial step in building a social movement, but it only matters if these opportunities can be converted into real social change. Turning opportunities into action requires assembling resources and creating organizations that can agitate for action, the object of our next strategy to mobilize resources.

Strategy 3—mobilizing resources

Referring back to our maniacal dictator, we see how one key strategy was to starve the movement of resources, creating a self-defeating process of in-fighting and rewards for individuals whose actions were actually being counter-productive. Without the ability to attract money, capture media attention, and forge alliances, many social movements can be rendered impotent. Social movements cannot be effective without people, power, and money; dissent in isolation is rarely sufficient to bring about social change (as a series of tragic stories of lone hunger strikers who starved themselves to no effect can attest).

It is tempting to emphasize the role of money, but if it were the only factor many successful social movements (including peasant movements) over the past century would have never occurred. While previous chapters have noted how deprived groups may lack toilets, they are increasingly gaining access to new technologies and resources, such as cell-phones and the Internet, which create new possibilities and capacities to mobilize, organize, disseminate information, and instigate action. One example is the backlash of the Iranian government to the 2009–2010 election protests that were organized through web media sites like Facebook and Twitter. The government, recognizing this stratagem of mass mobilization, acted swiftly to censor information in an attempt to crush the growing social movement.

This brief discussion reveals that the principal goal of mobilizing around chronic diseases is linked to a need to create alliances and action, potentially drawing upon innovative mechanisms for integrating dispersed groups with shared interests and goals.

Current state: fragmented groups—fighting over irrelevant issues and how to divide a small pool of resources

Few visible, charismatic leaders are actively engaged in the struggle against chronic diseases. In most countries, there is a handful of well-trained, professional staff and, thus, for the most part those specialized and passionate about the cause are lacking. Many countries lack a chronic disease strategy or anyone with explicit responsibility for tackling them within the ministry of health. Outside a few schools of public health, there is little training in global chronic disease control, so that the field tends to lose its best and brightest to infectious diseases; resources are scant, as a very small fraction of the money in global health aid is going to chronic disease prevention and control, depriving the movement of resources for seeking political change.

There have been numerous calls to action, indicating that academics are starting to mobilize around chronic diseases. Shifting the tide of intellectual opinion helps, but it needs to lead to clamour of patient and advocate voices, thunder in the media, and enthusiastic advocates willing to fight to address the unfair and avoidable burden of chronic diseases. Yet, as shown in Figure 5.1, for each the 'calls to action' by chronic disease groups, there are three times as many being made by other disease constituencies. In the context of a small pool of resources, unless the chronic disease community's advocacy efforts are more effective than others, there will be little or no change to the current situation.

The task of mobilizing resources to fight chronic diseases has much in common with climate change. Carbon emissions rise slowly and variably, and there is a long latency period between pollution and depletion of the ozone layer. Powerful corporations oppose the most successful and low-cost interventions, especially taxation and regulation. Climate change pits people against power. It is an issue that remains unsolved, bogged down in political, rather than, technical difficulties.

How can resources be raised if there are so few resources (and so many countervailing resources) in the first place? We can again look to the strategies used by previous global health movements.

Case study: successes and failures of the HIV movement

In the late 1990s members of HIV movement were frustrated. It was clear that low-cost, preventive strategies, such as distributing condoms or advocating abstinence, weren't working. The alternative—treating people with antiretrovirals—compared poorly on international criteria for cost-effectiveness such as cost per disability-adjusted life year.

The HIV movement played the gambit, and importantly, it worked. When donors and advocates observed how patients literally appeared to come back from the dead (the so-called 'Lazarus' effect), it compelled them to even greater action, generating a positive spiral of more funding and more resources. The approach ranks among the most effective interventions in public health history. It has also had a number of important spillover benefits, such as establishing a right-to-care that has formed the beginnings of a global social safety net.

One important lesson from the HIV movement's success is that it is not enough to work within the funding available, but that strategies are needed to increase the overall pool of funds. Most cost-effectiveness evaluations fail to account for the political environment in which they operate—choices about which interventions to pursue create or quell opportunities for additional funding in the future.

We can also learn lessons from the HIV movement's failures and its criticisms. HIV activism was born out of a group of outraged, relatively affluent homosexual groups (358). This activism failed to extend fully to more fragmented poor black communities and among injecting-drug users, where the epidemic remains concentrated in the US. A similar situation characterizes the spread of HIV in prisons in Eastern Europe and mining communities in sub-Saharan Africa.

A key point is that resources mobilize less easily in circumstances where the costs of the status quo are widely dispersed in a population but the beneficiaries are concentrated than in a situation where the costs are concentrated but the benefits are diffuse (as in the case of homosexual men). It is also more difficult to mobilize resources when the baseline of resources is low (such as the case of marginalized and sick populations); and when groups are fragmented (like the injecting drug-users). What we can learn from the HIV/AIDS movement is that strong social movements can dominate public debate, strengthen a civil society response, and improve national policies, but it does not guarantee that an effective response will extend to the most vulnerable and marginalized populations being affected.

Nevertheless, today, the HIV movement has been so successful that it faces a major backlash from within the development community. Being branded as 'exceptional', and critiqued for distorting global health priorities, the HIV strategy of the past decade is being regarded as a failure or misappropriation (306) rather than as a model of mobilization that needs to be extended to other public health realms (353a).

Key solution: forge alliances by focusing on shared risks of daily living in resource-poor settings

Since chronic diseases have to compete against a broad set of other, better organized disease groups for resources, and because attention in development to the challenge of chronic diseases has thus far been limited in comparison to other existing threats, several tactics are needed. A first set of tactics is to increase the flow of resources to global health overall. The second major strategy is to strengthen advocacy for chronic disease resources to be allocated from within global health.

Tactic 1: Forge global health alliances that focus on interconnected risks of daily living in resource-deprived settings (such as tobacco, poverty, low education, poor nutrition, and social instability).

Tactic 2: Forge broader alliances by showing how action on chronic disease can achieve other desirable social goals such as improving education, economic growth, women's equality, and reducing poverty.

Tactic 3: Forge alliances with movements against climate change, sweatshops, and alternatives to globalization by focusing on common causes (such as unfair trade agreements, unhealthy environmental and agricultural policies, and fair labour policies).

Tactic 4: Prioritize chronic disease interventions that provide change that people can see and believe in (such as medicines that deliver visible physical benefits).

Tactic 5: Include community partners in efforts to assess the disease burden and conduct epidemiologic investigations (participatory surveillance and community-led epidemiology).

Tactic 6: Focus advocacy efforts on unfair diseases like tobacco and childhood diseases that could increase potential for greater subsequent action and priority (as entry points).

Tactic 7: Invest in the energy of youth, launching a social movement through innovative social media, such as Twitter, Facebook, and other social network sites.

Tactic 8: Create rewards for leaders, youth advocates, and identify success stories so that people see ways they can contribute and come to feel empowered.

Tactic 9: Adapt existing infectious disease clinics that provide long-term care, such as HIV and tuberculosis clinics to deliver chronic disease care.

Summary

> Medicine is a social science, and politics nothing but medicine at a larger scale.
>
> (Rudolph Virchow, 1848).

Today, Virchow's statement might also read in reverse: 'Social science is medicine, and medicine is nothing but politics at a larger scale'. The practice of medicine cannot be apolitical; nor can politics be separated from its impacts on health.

This chapter has set out a series of reinforcing strategies to create a social movement for influencing this political context. In the first part of this chapter, we showed how power and politics are key determinants of the failure to achieve a higher priority of chronic diseases. As we showed in Chapter 4, most of the key chronic disease challenges are solvable with existing knowledge. The failure to act lies in the economic and political context in which public health decisions are made and in which new threats to health arise.

As public health reaches this crossroads, it must decide which path to take. It has reached the end of the road travelled thus far. The report of the Commission on the Social Determinants of Health acknowledges the tension between the status quo of economic policy and maximizing the best possible public health. Yet one road ahead, putting politics and power back in analysis, is not new at all. In the late 19th and early 20th century, before we had discovered effective medicines, we learned how to control deadly diseases such as TB. The techniques were simple and cheap: providing basic toilets and sewage systems, adequate nutrition, and help to the poor. Today, we stand at the opposite end of the spectrum. We have pushed medicine close to its limits but are achieving diminishing returns from the dominant economic development model, as well as medicine itself. We have medical knowledge but lack the imagination that, in the past, had achieved remarkable progress when technology had little to offer (353b).

Public health is, intrinsically, about making the invisible visible (353b). It can do much by drawing attention to the complex paths from political and economic decisions and the health of nations; studying the immediate causes of disease alone is insufficient and, arguably, counter-productive from a political economy perspective. Members of public health community have long recognized the need to address social determinants of health, but public health practitioners rarely engage with those who drive these determinants. These include the IMF, the World Bank (beyond its Health, Nutrition and Population division), the World Trade Organisation, and

---

Box 5.6 Example of the Political Process Model: WHO's defeat to the World Bank in the Primary Health Care versus Selective Primary Health Care debate

All three elements of the Political Process Model played a role in the struggle of WHO to set the global health agenda:

First, the Primary Health Care model appeared to resemble too closely the principles of the Soviet model, risking Western institutions losing ideological ground in the battle between capitalism and communism for legitimacy. As the debate grew heated, Mahler was blamed for transforming WHO from a technical into a political organization (359) (reframing the debate).

Second, and in part as a result, WHO began to lose its role in global health as the main financier, as its budget was held frozen, by the US, at zero nominal growth, forcing it to rely on donations from private agencies and institutions. As a result, WHO began to lose its resources, autonomy, and agenda-setting power (change the structure of political opportunities).

Third, WHO lost its most powerful allies, UNICEF and the medical profession (mobilizing resources). When James Grant, a Harvard-trained economist and lawyer, son of a Rockefeller Foundation doctor, was appointed head of UNICEF, serving between 1980 and 1995, UNICEF backed away from Primary Health Care. Throughout the 1980s UNICEF began launching a counter-revolution to Mahler's vision—a 'children's revolution' in global health which centred on pushing for the 4 GOBI (Growth Monitoring, Oral Rehydration, Breast Feeding, and Immunization) interventions (360). Deeply ingrained conservatism among the medical profession also came to the fore. Doctors in resource-poor countries were often trained in rich hospitals, resembling the US, and were relatively affluent. They snubbed their noses at Primary Health Care as seeming non-scientific. Their view was seemingly reinforced by the observation that many international consultants became rich off system-wide approaches that were tried under the auspices of Primary Health Care, breeding corruption.

Supported by private foundations and UNICEF, the World Bank's model, won the day. Selective Primary Health Care became the dominant approach. (There is some irony in the observation that the World Bank was a key driver behind the Education for All approach, emphasizing universal access to primary education, launched about the same time as the Health for All debate occurred, in 1990.)

Losing the Primary Health Care and Health for All debate had long-term implications for the future of WHO. When Nakajima was elected successor of Mahler, becoming director of WHO, it marked the end of a political era for WHO and, at least temporarily, prospects for Primary Health Care and Health for All (213).

representatives of finance and trade ministries, but it must do so within a clear set of rules of engagement, based on explicit principles, including transparency.

In the second part of the chapter, we outlined three major strategies—reframing the debate, creating political opportunities, and mobilizing resources—and a series of tactical approaches within them that could help increase the effectiveness of the chronic disease as a social movement. This model of the political process, drawn from sociology, can identify some reasons for the relative success and failure of social movements and who wins and who loses key conflicts involving power and politics (see Box 5.6). It provides a powerful theoretical model that can help guide action and the development of a social movement against chronic diseases. The approaches discussed integrate a series of strategies, spanning top-down agenda-setting interventions to bottom-up grassroots mobilization campaigns.

One school of health policy analysis is simple: ask who benefits? And who loses? Follow the money, and we will find the root cause of many of our most intractable problems. Public health must engage with powerful international financial institutions as the key means of interaction with the powerful corporate and political interests who they represent, but it must do so within a clear set of rules of engagement, based on explicit principles, including transparency.

In the next chapter we step into the realities of current debates with vested interests, presenting two extremes of the existing views about the appropriate roles of food companies in the battle to prevent and control chronic diseases.

Endnotes

1 In US law it is defined as religious, charitable, scientific, testing for public safety, literary, educational purposes, to foster national or international amateur sports competition, promote the arts, or for the prevention of cruelty to children or animals. See IRS Publication 557 'Tax-exempt status for your organization'.

2 This section draws on a comparative analysis of five philanthropic foundations: Stuckler D, Basu S, McKee M (2011) Global Health Philanthropy and Institutional Relationships: How Should Conflicts of Interest Be Addressed? *PLoS Med* **8**(4): e1001020. doi:10.1371/journal.pmed.1001020

3 Indeed, the study of financial aid data that this chapter draws on was conducted largely by Andrea Feigl during her time at the Centre for Global Development, which Gates Foundation gave $26 million over 5 years. Her specific study with Rachel Nugent was funded by PepsiCo.

4 For more details see 355a and 355b.

5 In general, the more individualistic the society (like the US), the more likely that individuals are to misattribute a societal cause to an individual issue (the inverse of ecologic fallacy, an individualistic fallacy).

6 It is also worth noting that in arguing the famous 1954 case of *Brown v Board of Education of Topeka*, Kansas, black lawyers from the NAACP had to argue that segregating whites and black children in public schools had a detrimental effect on black children. Their case focused on how the public system denied black children exposure to other cultures, which adversely affected their functioning as adults, making them victims of the legalization of school segregation.

7 Medicalizing a disease, such as by pointing to the genetic underpinnings of obesity in some individuals, can help overcome 'victim-blaming'. This strategy risks stigma as well as making it more difficult to achieve classic preventative approaches targeting entire populations.

Chapter 6

Activities of the private sector

Part 1

The current and future role of the food industry in the prevention and control of chronic diseases: The case of PepsiCo

Tara Acharya, Amy C. Fuller, George A. Mensah, and Derek Yach

Introduction

Over the past 30 years, quality of life and lifespan have markedly improved. The decrease in child mortality rates between 1978 and 2006 was equivalent to 18,329 children's lives being saved every day. Adjusted for inflation, the world's expenditure on health increased by 35% between 2000 and 2005. Information and communication technologies have positively affected health literacy while other technical improvements have improved infrastructure for health, water, and sanitation systems. Improved nutrition has contributed significantly to the unprecedented global gains in human health (361).

However, there has also been significant regression in some parts of the world. In sub-Saharan Africa, life expectancy has declined for over a decade due to a combination of the HIV/AIDS epidemic and continued food insecurity. With estimates that the world's population will grow by over 70% between 1995 and 2050, agricultural resources and food supplies will need to be tailored to meet regional needs. Latin America and Asia will each require a twofold increase in food supply while Africa's needs top out at five- and sevenfold increases depending on the type of regional staple crop (362). The industrialized world's demand for food may remain flat or even decline, though the nutritional quality of food products in these countries deserves more attention and research. Even in developing countries there are nutritional issues beyond basic supply. Globally, nearly 4 million women and children under 5 years of age die each year because of factors related to undernutrition while millions of adults die prematurely due to unhealthy diets (363, 364). Life expectancy among men in Russia has declined as consumption of unhealthy foods, alcohol, and tobacco has increased (365). Links between stunting in early childhood and obesity in late childhood are also creating risks for chronic disease.

In most countries, particularly in the developing world where the impact of a nutrition transition is most prominently seen, substantial changes in the types and quantities of foods currently consumed will be required for sustained improvement in dietary outcomes and reduction in chronic disease risk. The food industry is a crucial member of the spectrum of stakeholders needed for successful development and implementation of nutrition and public health programmes. Among the many actions the food industry can take, the most important include provision of safe and nutritious food to people at an affordable cost and produced in a sustainable manner.

Nutrition and health overview

There is a rising global burden of nutrition-related chronic diseases (366). In 2005, chronic diseases in adults accounted for 60% of the estimated 58 million deaths worldwide (367). The leading chronic diseases that contributed to these deaths were CVDs such as heart attack, stroke, rheumatic heart disease, and other disorders of the heart and blood vessels; cancers, chronic diseases of the lungs, diabetes, and mental and psychiatric conditions (see Chapter 1). Nutrition transitions in developing countries are among the most worrisome, with resulting chronic illness causing increased prevalence of and mortality from ischaemic heart disease, stroke, and diabetes.

Dietary changes in both industrialized and developing countries play a role in the increasing prevalence of chronic disease. For example, several epidemiological studies have shown that a diet low in saturated fats and rich in fruits, vegetables, whole grains, nuts, legumes, fish, and poultry is associated with longevity and a 30% or greater reduction in the risk of CVD (243, 368–370). However, traditional diets based on local staples, including fruits, vegetables, and grains, are gradually being replaced in many regions of the world with increasing intake of fat, animal products, sweeteners, and processed foods (371–373). Many nutritional factors contribute to the development of CVD, including elevated total and LDL cholesterol, depressed HDL cholesterol, and elevated triglycerides. Compounding these dietary issues is a global increase in physical inactivity.

In its 2009 report on global health risks, WHO determined the distribution of deaths attributable to 19 leading risk factors worldwide. Of these 19 leading risk factors, more than half were nutrition-related: blood pressure, often caused by overconsumption of sodium; cholesterol, linked to high intake of saturated fats and oils; both underweight and overweight or obesity; fruit and vegetable intake; physical inactivity, which misaligns the energy balance of 'calories in vs. calories out'; and deficiencies of iron, zinc, and vitamin A (see Chapter 1).

With high BMI often correlating with high blood pressure and cholesterol and underweight linked to micronutrient deficiencies, there is a need to focus on food intake using these weight measures as indicators. WHO estimates that in 2005 more than 1 billion people were overweight and 300 million obese, with projections of 1.5 billion people overweight by 2015. In contrast, two billion persons suffer from micronutrient deficiencies with almost another billion persons falling victim to hunger and famine (374, 375).

This dual nutritional burden of feast and famine that exists in low- and middle-income countries and transitional economies can lead to chronic health issues. A nutrient-poor diet that is calorie-dense and rich in saturated fats can result in a combination of stunting or micronutrient malnutrition with obesity, especially in women (376, 377). In both young children and adults, these health conditions increase the risk for high blood pressure and type 2 diabetes, and contribute to the rising prevalence of other chronic diseases (378–381).

Globally, 7–41% of the burden of some cancers can be attributed to overweight and obesity alone (382), while according to Yach et al., 'overweight and obesity have become to diabetes what tobacco is to lung cancer' (4). There are potential pharmaceutical and surgical solutions to the overweight and obesity issue. However, scientists argue that anti-obesity drugs and medical procedures such as gastric bypass focus too much on weight loss and not enough on behavioural causes of overconsumption, often resulting in weight gain after the intervention has been completed (383). Instead, public health personnel should focus on prevention of obesity, CVD, and other chronic diseases through healthy dietary choices and nutrition education.

The rapid pace of industrialization, urbanization, and globalization has led to the current state of the modern food industry that has made foods, snacks, and beverages readily available in most high- and middle-income countries and many low-income countries (384). Until recent years, the majority of these products have tended to be energy-dense with relatively little emphasis on nutritional quality. Yet at the same time, the availability of a safe and predictable food supply has positively transformed how people can live. Fortification of foods, for example, is one successful strategy for addressing micronutrient deficiencies (385). Chile has one of the lowest incidences of anaemia among developing countries due to wheat flour fortifications of B complex vitamins, ferrous sulphate, and folic acid that began in 1951 (386). In fact, with the exception of sub-Saharan Africa, many regions of the world have actually seen increases in life expectancy. The US Centers for Disease Control and Prevention (CDC) reported in 2009 that nationally, life expectancy in 2007 had increased 1.4 years since 1997 and that life expectancy was listed as an all-time high for both men and women (75.3 years and 80.4 years, respectively). The death rate fell to a new low of 760.3 deaths per 100,000 people, 2.1% lower than it was in 2006 and half of what it was 60 years ago. Death rates for eight of the leading 15 causes of death, including heart disease, stroke, high blood pressure, and cancer also dropped between 2006 and 2007 (387).

Finally, according to an analysis of Medicare data, the rate of US hospital admissions for heart attack in 2007 was 23% lower than in 2002. This roughly equals out to 87,000 fewer heart-attack admissions in 2007 than would have been expected had the rate remained constant (388). Experts believe that these results are in part due to a variety of prevention initiatives and improvements in patient care such as quit-smoking campaigns, growing awareness of the importance of exercise and healthy diets, and efforts to encourage doctors and hospitals to follow evidence-based guidelines. Greater attention is being given to the health benefits of diets that feature nuts, wholegrain, vegetables, and fruits. In Finland's North Karelia, analysis of a drop in age-adjusted mortality rates of coronary heart disease between the 1970s and 1995 revealed that changes in diet accounted for part of the decline; community action and consumer demand served as effective interventions (276). Though high fat foods such as red meat are becoming more common in Japan, the country has long ranked as having one of the highest life expectancies in part due to low rates of heart disease associated with its traditional low fat diet (389).

These examples support the idea that the health of consumers can be improved, and chronic diseases prevented, if food companies alter marketing policies and product offerings to increase promotion of healthy living. If anything, gains in life expectancy highlight the triumphs of better eating and living that now need to be sustained. New age-related challenges require attention and it is important that the food industry continue to make strides in providing consumers with the tools they need to maintain a healthy lifestyle. Substantial changes in dietary practices, including changes in the types and quantities of foods and beverages consumed will be required to improve dietary outcomes and reduce CVD and other chronic disease risks associated with longer life expectancy.

The potential for increased private sector involvement

Overview of food industry

Prior to the late 19th century, virtually everyone either grew or raised all of their food and mainly ate seasonal produce. However, a heat-processing technique known as pasteurization changed consumption patterns by allowing transport of food over long distances with minimal spoilage. Developed by Louis Pasteur in 1862, this process destroyed pathogenic microorganisms and led to the development of canned, jarred, and bottled goods. The development of manufactured ice in the early 20th century also boosted the ability of rail lines to ship refrigerated foods. With these innovations, consumers could discover and eat new canned fruit, vegetable, milk, and meat products on a regular basis, regardless of geography. Over time, the food industry became responsible for the production and consumption of 'convenience foods'. Those products were developed in response to a consumer demand to outsource meals from their own kitchens to those of the largest multinational corporations. In 1925, the average US homemaker prepared all her meals at home. By 1965, 75–90% of all foods used were factory-processed to some degree (389).

With industrialization of food came an increase in the number of available to consumers. This was initially evident in the military community. Nearly 30 years before World War II, the UK government developed the Education (Provision of Meals) Act after the disclosure from recruiting army officials that over half of the young men eligible to fight in the Boer War were unable to do so due to malnutrition and underdevelopment (390). During World War II in the US, the military called the National Nutrition Conference for Defense as a result of the poor nutritional status of young men enlisting for service; army officials were shocked that 40% of men examined under the Selective Service Act had been found unfit for general military service. Brigadier General Lewis B. Hershey, deputy director of Selective Service, in speaking of these rejections to the Conference, said, 'Probably one-third of these are suffering from disabilities directly or indirectly connected with nutrition'.

Environmentalists and other advocates began stressing possible downsides of industrialized agriculture and modern food supply during the 1960s and 1970s. Concerns included pesticide safety, the presence of food additives, sugar and salt intakes, obesity, and heart disease links to the food supply, and concerns regarding 'artificial' foods. There were also major concerns regarding high levels of saturated fat present in diets. Influential research such as the Framingham Heart Study was published in the academic literature (391). With little known about the causes of both heart disease and stroke at that time, the objectives of the study were to identify common characteristics that contribute to CVD by following its development over a long period of time with a large group of participants. Since its inception, Framingham has led to the development and publication of hundreds of studies integral for better understanding not only CVD risk factors, but also related co-morbid disorders and other long-term health effects. Other nutrition-related research has also provided strong evidence of the carcinogenic role of alcohol and ethanol in alcoholic beverages and of vitamin D in reducing all causes of mortality. A study following adult men and women in Finland found that the frequency of acute coronary events increased with rising sodium excretion. Sodium also predicted mortality in overweight males (392).

The emergence of new food company products and practices

There is a broad spectrum of approaches and processes the food industry could embrace in order to improve dietary outcomes and reduce chronic disease and CVD risk. The private sector includes a range of entities from agriculture suppliers to retailers, all of which should play a role in health initiatives. For example, many inner city neighbourhoods in the US are rife with convenience stores, fast food restaurants, and dollar stores but lack healthy food options (393). Supermarkets and related retailers' policies should consider how to improve community access to more nutritional products. This recommendation relates to the idea that business models should marry performance and profitability with the deliberate purpose or goal of contributing to the solution of relevant social and environmental challenges.

Muhammad Yunus, founder of Grameen Bank and 2007 Nobel Prize recipient, and Bill Gates, founder of Microsoft, have each called for the development of 'social business entrepreneurs' and a new form of 'creative capitalism', respectively. Grameen Group backed this call by working with multinational food corporation Groupe Danone in 2006 to provide nutrition to low-income populations. This projected 10-year joint venture aims to create at least 50 plants that manufacture yogurt with micronutrients for Bangladeshi children. The partnership also hopes to contribute to environment sustainability by using solar and biogas energy during production and packing with self-degradable materials (254, 394). The CEO of PepsiCo, Indra Nooyi, also defines a 'good business' as one that addresses health and environmental needs in addition to financial success. The resulting phrase, 'Performance with Purpose' (PwP) means delivering sustainable growth through investments in the environment, health and nutrition (human sustainability), and the workforce. Larry Thompson, PepsiCo's Legal Counsel has argued that PwP is a business imperative and critical to the long-term growth of companies (L. Thompson, personal communication, March 21, 2010).

The food industry can and should play an important role in addressing issues of CVD and other chronic diseases (367, 395, 396). This is done through a uniquely acquired understanding of and adaptation to consumer needs, combined with technological capabilities and business acumen. After two Johns Hopkins University scientists stumbled across a non-caloric coal-tar derivate called saccharin in 1879, food companies capitalized on consumer interest in sugar substitutes by creating products such as Sweet 'n Low, Equal, and NutraSweet (397). The major global dairies responded to the growing market for healthy and convenient products by introducing low-fat and skimmed milk into their portfolios. Fad and crash diets in the 1990s provided a market for dietary trend products under the low-carb Atkins and South Beach names. Food companies created brands such as Lean Cuisine, Healthier Choice, and Smart Ones. Products available in smaller portion sizes were also introduced, in particular controlled snack foods and the 100-calorie snack pack.

Along with the informal sector, players at the local and national levels dominate the provision of food. Their role in addressing chronic disease cannot be emphasized enough. Yet multinational food companies are in a unique position to greatly influence the nutritional quality of the food they manufacture and the range of consumers they serve. The scale and reach of the world's 10 leading food and beverage companies is unparalleled. Top multinational companies—Ferrero, General Mills, Grupo Bimbo, Kellogg's, Kraft Foods, Mars, Nestlé, PepsiCo, The Coca-Cola Company, and Unilever—account for around 80% of the global advertising spend in the food and beverage industry and collectively have revenues in excess of $350 billion annually. Combined with a collective presence in more than 200 countries, these resources provide tremendous capabilities for global nourishment. Specific changes in food industry policies can positively impact dietary practices and nutritional status, and therefore contribute to reductions in the risk of CVD and chronic disease in both the medium and long term. These changes focus on product reformulation and the promotion of physical activity and healthy lifestyles.

Product reformulation

At present, the food industry typically applies three crucial approaches in product reformulation:

1　Reduce sodium, saturated fats, trans fats, and added sugars.
2　Enhance potentially healthy ingredients such as healthier oils, whole grains, fibre, nuts, fruits and vegetables, and omega-3 fatty acids.
3　Reduce total calories.

In addition, the industry invests in research and development to identify and deliver new products that have strong scientific evidence for reducing cardiovascular risk. The use of smaller-sized packaging to offer portion control options, as well as provide simple, clear, and consistent nutritional information for reducing chronic disease and CVD risk would also be essential. Food companies also regularly take actions to protect the public against mycotoxins (aflatoxins and mycotoxins), persistent organic pollutants, arsenic and carcinogens, radionuclide, and cyanide in cassava and process contaminants (398).

Promoting physical activity and healthy lifestyles

Advertising and marketing practices should encourage balanced nutrition and physical activity, especially amongst children. Food industry support of programmes that promote lifelong physical activity coupled with product reformulation aligns with the concept of energy balance, or 'calories in vs. calories out'. Adherence to this idea contributes to overall improvements in dietary outcomes, as well as successful control of overweight and obesity and the related phenomena of insulin resistance, metabolic syndrome, type 2 diabetes mellitus, and CVD.

Promotion of physical activity and healthy lifestyles can start within the food companies themselves. Considerable progress has been made in introducing effective workplace wellness programmes aimed at addressing chronic diseases, initially in developed countries and increasingly worldwide (399). For example, in 2005 the National Institutes of Health (NIH) provided grants to seven institutions in the US to study ways to help prevent obesity by influencing people's dietary and activity habits at work (400). The study design included interventions such as reducing portion sizes, modifying cafeteria recipes to lower energy density, increasing availability of fruits and vegetables, increasing the accessibility of fitness equipment at the workplace, and supporting employees' access to health coaching. Corporations could also benefit from promoting employee walkathons and incentivized physical activity or nutrition programmes. Various studies on the impact of workplace wellness programmes have found that the amount of returns on investment vary, but health care expenses per employee are often lowered with positive savings for companies on programme investment (401, 402).

Multi-company initiatives

Food companies are likely to have greater impact on dietary outcomes and CVD and chronic disease risks by acting collectively rather than individually. In response to the WHO released Technical Report #916, entitled 'Diet, Nutrition and the Prevention of Chronic Diseases' in 2002 and the 'Global Strategy on Diet and Physical Activity' (WHA 57.17) adopted by governments in may 2004, CEOs of initially eight, and now ten food companies pledged to develop and market fortified nutritious products to the poorest communities. The 'Global Strategy on Diet, Physical Activity and Health' contained several recommendations for the food industry to address specific aspects of chronic disease (Table 6.1). Consequently, the International Food and Beverage Alliance (IFBA) was established which formulated a set of five global public commitments in May 2008. The commitments address: 1) food reformulation; 2) consumer information; 3) responsible marketing; 4) promotion of healthy lifestyles; and 5) public-private partnerships (403). The result is the first serious attempt by any stakeholder group to intervene simultaneously on a worldwide basis and will hopefully have a broad-based impact on chronic diseases such as CVD. More focused approaches are being developed to address obesity and the concomitant increase in type 2 diabetes.

Thirteen of the US's largest food and beverage companies, including McDonald's and Unilever, have also become a member of the Children's Food and Beverage Advertising Initiative. Launched in 2006 by the Council of Better Business Bureaus and directed at children under 12, partnership in the Initiative commits companies to:

- Include healthier dietary choices.
- Not engage in food and beverage product placement in editorial and entertainment content.
- Reduce the use of third-party licensed characters in advertising that does not meet the Initiative's product or messaging criteria.

Table 6.1 World Health Organization's Global Strategy on diet, physical activity and health, with food companies' responses and recommendations

Specific recommendation to the food industry	Food industry response
◆ Promote healthy diets and physical activity in accordance with national guidelines and international standards and the overall aims of the Global Strategy	◆ Underway through the commitments made by International Food & Beverage Alliance (IFBA) to address the areas of food reformulation, consumer information, responsible marketing, promotion of health lifestyles and public–private partnerships ◆ IFBA has also established food and beverage industry groups in over 15 countries/regions, including the 27 countries of the European Union and the 6 countries of the Cooperation Council for the Arab States of the Gulf, to allow industry to react according to the different needs and concerns of different Member States rapidly and individually as well as expand company participation at the local and regional level, to optimize the local impact, and ensure that industry efforts take into consideration regional and national differences ◆ More groups are being established in many more countries
◆ Limit the levels of saturated fats, trans fatty acids, free sugars, and salt in existing products	◆ Since the Global Strategy was launched in 2004, the steps taken by the food and beverage industry are very significant and are creating measurable improvements showing a major reduction in the marketing of products high in fat, sugar and salt to children less than 12 years of age ◆ IFBA companies have reformulated and/or introduced over 28,000 nutritionally enhanced products globally. This includes specifically reducing or eliminating trans fat in about 18,000 products. Calories were reduced and saturated fats, sugar, carbohydrates, and sodium were also eliminated or reduced in a significant number of products. At the same time, many products were fortified with vitamins, minerals, whole grains and/or fibre ◆ IFBA members are also developing product formulations that compensate for chronic micronutrient shortages sometimes found in the developing world—countries in which chronic shortages of iron, vitamin A, and iodine in particular can have far-reaching health consequences
◆ Continue to develop and provide affordable, healthy and nutritious choices to consumers	◆ See above in addition, not IFBA members have increased investments in R&D aimed at achieving this and each of the companies employ scientists, nutritionists and engineers to develop innovative foods and beverages, and have established processes for internal and external expert and scientific review of their nutrition standards which are then used to drive product innovation
◆ Provide consumers with adequate and understandable product and nutrition information	◆ Ongoing efforts continue but require closer government oversight and interaction to have impact ◆ IFBA companies have also increased the use of consumer information tools, including websites, helplines, in-store leaflets, and brochures

(continued)

Table 6.1 (Continued)

Specific recommendation to the food industry	Food industry response
◆ Practice responsible marketing that supports the Strategy, particularly with regard to the promotion and marketing of foods high in saturated fats, trans fatty acids, free sugars, or salt, especially to children	◆ Considerable progress has been made through the IFBA pledge, which is being implemented globally and is subject to external audit ◆ IFBA companies' engaged Accenture to provide a global 'snapshot' of companies' compliance with their marketing commitments. Accenture tested compliance in 12 markets around the world. Accenture reported a 98.17% compliance rate for TV advertising, 100% compliance for print advertising and found only one instance of non-compliance on the Internet
◆ Issue simple, clear and consistent food labels and evidence-based health claims that will help consumers to make informed and healthy choices with respect to the nutritional value of foods	◆ Requires clarity from WHO on optimal way forward. Many individual company efforts are underway ◆ Many IFBA companies have improved the labelling on their packaging to provide easily-understandable nutritional information, including guideline daily amounts (GDAs) or Daily Value, ingredient listings, and key nutrients. IFBA companies have also made significant progress in implementing full nutritional labelling on a voluntary basis where full nutritional labelling is not compulsory ◆ For example, 88% of companies surveyed in Kenya, South Africa, and Uganda are already exceeding the legal labelling requirements and 75% plan on adding more nutritional labelling in the next 24 months
◆ Provide information on food composition to national authorities	◆ Underway in countries whose governments have clearly stated norms

Adapted from WHA 57.17; article 61.

- Limit products shown in interactive games to healthy dietary choices or incorporate healthy lifestyle messages in games.
- Not advertise to children in elementary schools.

In the US, several other industry initiatives are under way. In response to 'Let's Move', an obesity initiative launched by First Lady Michelle Obama, beverage companies in the US announced that they would enhance the visibility of calorie labelling on products, soda fountains, and vending machines. These efforts complement industry work underway to restrict sales of products high in sugar, salt, and fat in US schools. For example, in 2006 the American Beverage Association (ABA) joined with the Alliance for a Healthier Generation, a joint initiative of the William J. Clinton Foundation and the American Heart Association. The Alliance created School Beverage Guidelines in 2006 aiming to significantly limit portion size and the number of calories in beverages available to students during the school day. Shipments of full-calorie soft drinks to schools have declined by 95% since prior to the implementation of the Guidelines (404).

Private sector case study: PepsiCo's 2010 goals and commitments

In the 1950s and 1960s, PepsiCo began introducing new products that focused on health and wellness. Company offerings ranged from Diet Pepsi with zero calories in 1964 to Tropicana's 2009 release of Trop50, an orange juice with 50% less sugar and calories, and no artificial sweeteners. PepsiCo also began developing internal nutrition criteria to guide product development, marketing, and labelling in the late 1990s. PepsiCo now has in place a diverse research and development team with the capability to support product transformation and add nutrients to address particular needs of a given population. Examples from around the globe include oat-based snacks through Gamesa-Quaker in Mexico and baked snacks in Brazil (405).

In March 2010, PepsiCo unveiled a new set of eleven goals and commitments that form the core of how PepsiCo intends to encourage people to live healthier (Table 6.2). Included are product reformulation, changes in marketing and information campaigns, and ways to improve the affordability and accessibility of products in underserved communities. PepsiCo put into place global nutrition criteria based on recommendations contained in reports from WHO, FAO, and the Institute of Medicine (IOM), as well as the US Dietary Guidelines for Americans (368, 370, 406).

The criteria build on two concepts: 1) 'nutrients to limit', those of public health concern when consumed in excess and including reduction efforts on sodium, saturated fat and sugar intake; and 2) 'nutrients and food groups to encourage', based on regional nutritional needs and including those related to micronutrient deficiencies and essential fatty acids requirements. These criteria serve as the practical translation of nutrition science and dietary recommendations for marketers and food and beverage developers. Greater attention is also being given to increasing the nutritional quality of the PepsiCo portfolio by including more nuts, wholegrain, vegetables, and fruits in products. These goals and commitments will enable PepsiCo to contribute to addressing nutrition needs.

PepsiCo drew upon the successful practices of its country offices such as PepsiCo UK to determine implementation details. For example, when the UK Food Standards Agency (FSA) set a target in 2005 for salt consumption of 6g/day in order to halve the average daily consumption by 2010, Walkers had already begun reducing sodium content in products and eventually lowered levels by 25–55%. A 34.5g pack of Walkers crisps also contains 8% and 5% of an adult's guideline daily amount for salt and saturated fat, respectively (407, 408). Walkers' success in essentially

Table 6.2 PepsiCo's goals and commitments

Products	Marketplace	Community
Provide more food and beverage choices made with wholesome ingredients that contribute to healthier eating and drinking	Encourage people to make informed choices and live healthier	Actively work with global and local partners to help address global nutrition challenges
Increase the amount of whole grains, fruits, vegetables, nuts, seeds and low-fat dairy in global product portfolio	Display calorie count and key nutrients on food and beverage packaging by 2012	Invest in business and R&D to expand offerings of more affordable, nutritionally relevant products for underserved and lower-income communities
Reduce the average amount of sodium per serving in key global food brands by 25%	Only advertise to children under 12 for products that meet global science-based nutrition standards	Expand PepsiCo Foundation and PepsiCo corporate contribution initiatives to promote healthier communities, including enhancing diet and physical activity programmes
Reduce the average amount of saturated fat per serving in key global food brands by 15%	Eliminate the direct sale of full-sugar soft drinks in primary and secondary schools around the globe by 2012	Integrate policies and actions on human health, agriculture, and the environment to make sure they support each other
Reduce the average amount of added sugar per serving in key global beverage brands by 25%	Increase the range of foods and beverages that offer solutions for managing calories, like portion sizes	

* Recommended by WHO Global Strategy.
# Recommended by NCD Alliance Proposed HLM on NCDs Outcomes.

removing 2400 metric tons of salt per year from the British diet by the end of 2008 prompted the FSA to single out Walkers as an example of a company making a positive impact.

PepsiCo UK's successful strategy with Walkers began with gradual sodium reductions by up to 20% between 2003 and 2005. Walkers then highlighted seasonings for sodium reduction and implemented a policy change by directing all suppliers to reformulate seasonings not to exceed 240mg sodium/serving. Finally, by using the minimum salt necessary to obtain maximal taste, Walkers was able to achieve another 10–20% salt reduction. PepsiCo UK's experience in shifting nutrient levels and in delivering innovative and nutritious products creates a platform for global implementation of the new goals and commitments. With scientific sources suggesting that modest reductions in population sodium intake will result in major declines in population blood pressure levels and reduction in CVD risk, PepsiCo's actions can help improve the health status of at-risk individuals (409). For example, in Finland where salt intake has been reduced by about one-third since the 1970s, both systolic and diastolic blood pressure have decreased by more than 10 mmHg (410). Accordingly, the death rates from stroke and coronary heart disease have decreased by 75–80% with a corresponding increase of 5–6 years in life expectancy. Hopefully, PepsiCo's goals will help expand these health improvements to individuals around the world.

It is important to note that PepsiCo plans to match these health commitments with complementary environment targets related to energy and water use, recycling, soil conservation, local sourcing from farmers, and reducing the carbon footprint of products. Making progress toward PepsiCo's goals depends on 'integrating . . . policies and actions on human health, agriculture and the environment to make sure they support each other'. Turning this idea into action involves the development of health and environmental impact assessment methods when considering new products and processes.

Persisting challenges and needs

Other food companies have also taken steps to change the nutrition composition of their portfolios. In March 2010 Kraft Foods revealed sodium reduction plans that, if completed, will lead to the elimination of 10 million pounds of salt from Kraft products in the US by 2012 (411). Since 2005, global food and beverage giant Unilever has been conducting an assessment of its over 22,000 item portfolio, a process that has led Unilever to plan on improving the nutritional quality of more than half of its products (412). The company announced that it removed 9100 tons of salt from its products between 2003 and 2008, and continues to aim for daily salt intake limits set by national governments (6 g of salt) and WHO (5 g of salt). Outside of the nutrition arena, sustainable development has been a cornerstone of Unilever's business practices, including investing in sustainable agriculture and developing sustainable packaging.

These successes, and the future of both PepsiCo's goals and overall industry efforts, are dependent on overcoming challenges and changing inadequate policies. Some of the most pressing needs are expanding support and capacity for nutrition science research, understanding the relationship between the environment and health issues, and addressing consumer taste needs.

Expanding support and capacity for nutrition science research

The food industry's contribution to advances in basic, clinical, and population science research in nutrition and cardiovascular health have been substantial. For example, Quaker's investments in research helped delineate the relationship between soluble fibre from certain foods (the vast majority of studies were on oats) and risk of coronary heart disease (114, 413, 414). This research identified beta-glucan as the type of soluble fibre most likely associated with lowering blood cholesterol levels and has paved the way for the first cholesterol-lowering claim for a food product in the world (414). Other food and beverage companies, including Procter and Gamble, the Kellogg Company, Cargill, and Sapporo Breweries have all sponsored research on the impact of other types of fibre on cholesterol levels (46, 114, 415–419). Together with support from academia and government, industry support of research has moved beyond the heart health relationship with fibre to the beneficial effects of phytosterols, phytostanols, and unsaturated fatty acids (420–427). Other investments in science have led to improved understanding of the role of cocoa flavanols and other antioxidant foods on heart health, as well as advances in biochemistry, endocrinology, and metabolism (428–431).

Unfortunately, support for and investment in nutrition science is weak when compared to other industries. R&D intensity is a well-established indicator of industry innovation (432). The pharmaceutical and biotechnology industry has consistently ranked highest for several years by this indicator with R&D spending at about 15–20% of sales, while the food industry is typically among the lowest spenders at 1–2% (433). Among government institutions, the NIH holds the majority of research spending on nutrition and obesity at roughly 1.4 billion and 700 million, respectively. While these areas are granted higher than average funding at NIH, they fall short of the levels provided for research related to infectious and emerging infectious diseases, bioengineering, and others (434). Further, the major outcomes of NIH nutrition and obesity research often lead to new medication or surgical solutions as opposed to sustainable food-based solutions.

This mismatch between the allocation of R&D resources contrasts with recommendations of a global and diverse set of experts, who have identified the top 20 policy and research priorities for chronic diseases (435). A significant increase in publicly financed research into food and lifestyle based solutions to chronic diseases would stimulate innovation among both the private and public sectors. The need for investment in nutrition science is most obvious in emerging economies of Asia and Africa which are both beset by dual burdens of under- and overnutrition crises. The human capacity to address these needs is weak and evident when studying nutrition research output from researchers in emerging economies through the prism of journal publications. The proportion of full length publications in leading science and medical journals (based on citation indexes) by country of the first author, nutrition topic, and year was examined from 1991–2007. For the last 2 years, only about 5% of first authors for any nutrition category were from India or China—two countries which account for 40% of the world's population (432).

Low levels of research in nutrition science create obstacles for corporate innovation, retard societal progress in the field, and could erode long-term productivity. Sports drinks including Gatorade and Accelerade require a unique understanding of human biology and exercise physiology, especially when considering the needs of athletes from different sports. Creation of products such as PureVia, a zero-calorie, all-natural sweetener derived from the stevia plant, depend on continued exploration into the many beneficial uses and nutritional aspects of natural ingredients. Considering these research needs, governments should provide more support for the development of sustainable agriculture and food-based incentives. Currently, governments in developed countries provide incentives to the pharmaceutical industry to develop medicated solutions to nutritional problems. These incentives include tax breaks for pharmaceutical companies to invest in new drug development and extensive funding of public research entities like NIH in the US and MRC in the UK. Greater support for research aimed at food-based solutions could build nutrition science capacity and transform the ability of countries to more effectively address the nutrition needs of populations.

Understanding the relationship between the environment and health

Norman Borlaug helped change the face of agriculture through the 'Green Revolution' in the 1960s and 1970s by tripling grain yields in many Latin American and Asian developing countries. However, with the world's population continuing to grow at an exponential rate, experts are questioning whether the current agriculture system has the ability to keep pace. Agriculture policies and practices have inadvertently prioritized yield, resiliency traits, appearance or shelf-life above environmental impact and nutritional outcomes. While yields of wheat, rice, and maize have increased in many countries, a US analysis of selectively bred high yield conventionally grown produce from 1950–1999 found that overall nutritional quality actually decreased, with significant loss of protein content and micronutrients (277). Fast-growing varieties are believed to have root systems that are unable to keep up with growth and take up nutrients from the soil. Furthermore, crop yields did not increase in all countries, particularly in Africa where the Green Revolution failed to take hold on a large scale due to water scarcity, low soil content, and poor governance, among others. In other regions, indiscriminate use of synthetic chemical fertilizers eventually led to soil degradation and diminished yields. Subsidized fertilizers in India—urea, in particular—have stripped soil nutrients, resulting in lowered crop yields and an increased dependence on agricultural imports. Partly in response to food prices jumping 19% in 2009, the government has announced that it will offer subsidies for fertilizers based on the nutrient content but will unfortunately also continue to allow farmers to purchase urea (436).

India's troubles appear to be only one example of health issues that are now affecting global food production. Current agricultural practices, such as nitrous oxide from fertilizer use, are also believed to contribute up to 30% of global greenhouse gas emissions. With the climate changing, plants grow faster with temperature increases and have less time to accumulate essential carbohydrates, fats, and proteins (437). Pesticides persist in produce destined for human consumption while excess fertilizers and pesticides run off agricultural land to contaminate human drinking water. Research on exposure to pesticides often results in questions of correlation versus causation, but maternal exposure to pesticide while carrying a child has been linked to child malignancies such as leukemia, non-Hodgkin's lymphoma, and cancer of the brain, among others (438). Analysis of the Agricultural Health Study, a NIH- and EPA-sponsored cohort of over 89,000 individuals, has also found that herbicides may be associated with pancreatic cancer (439). Though cohort research focused on pesticide workers and applicators with greater than average exposures, increased exposure to pesticides also correlated with higher risk for Parkinson's disease (440) and cancers of the prostrate, lung, and colon (441).

Difficult trade-offs between environmental sustainability and health will inevitably be present, as shown in the case of palm oil (see Box 6.1). Yet there are also examples of positive alignment between agriculture and nutrition. One such example is oats which are an excellent source of soluble fibre and also rich in antioxidants. Fibre has been shown to decrease low-density lipoprotein, iron, and thiamin and as already noted in relation to nutrition science research, food products made with oats have the potential to lower cholesterol (442). Growing oats also limits environmental damage typically resulting from agriculture. In North America, oats are usually planted with no soil tillage and result in little to soil erosion. In fact, the crop is often grown in areas to control damage from crops with soil erosion risks because of its fibrous and prolific root system. Commercial fertilizer additions are generally low, in the range of 50–100 pounds per acre and about the same amount as wheat or barley, but produce yields that are often twice as much per acre as those same crops. The need for pesticides is relatively low due to oats' resistance to many soil borne diseases and very little water is needed for irrigation.

Box 6.1 The case of palm oil

Palm oil has a significant impact on climate change as a result of large-scale clearing of rainforests and loss of biodiversity. It is also high in saturated fats and may contribute to CVD. Using both environmental and health criteria, the food industry should be minimizing use of palm oil. Supply chain analysis, however, reveals two barriers. Firstly, palm is by far the most productive oilseed at 3.68 tons of oil per hectare with rapeseed a distant second at 0.59 tons/hectare. Given that the world is faced with widely depleted soil and water resources, the environmental impact of production capacity should not be underestimated. Secondly, increased protective packaging would have to replace the product stability characteristics of palm oil's saturated fat content if substituted for a healthier alternative.

Food companies are actively exploring how to increasingly use alternative, healthier oils and support sustainable palm oil sources, for example through the Roundtable on Sustainable Palm Oil. Healthy oils 1) contain no commercially-introduced trans fatty acids; 2) are low in saturated fatty acids; and 3) have a high percentage of monounsaturated and polyunsaturated fatty acids. Healthy oils must also be affordable; have stability and an acceptable shelf life; and have ample and reliable supply. These requirements are at the heart of the development of special breeds of sunflower seed such as the SunSeed brand used in Europe and NuSun brand used in the US. Building a future supply of more suitable oils is especially important in countries like China and India where consumption has soared in recent decades (23).

At present, there are no global or even major regional private-public alliances to build a sustainable source of healthy oils. These alliances could represent significant gains for poor farmers and companies alike. Although the WHO and FAO have urged shifts to healthier oils, they have never issued joint plans to facilitate the transition from an agricultural supply perspective. A well-structured long-term plan is required and includes investing in a range of oils that can meet large scale supply demands; supporting research to reduce the saturated fat levels of commonly used edible oils; reviewing pricing and subsidies for oils; and shifting palm oil use from unsustainable to certified sustainable sources (443). Continued industry research is also necessary to explore biochemical 'transformation' of the abundantly available and cheap palm oil into a healthier oil (with significantly reduced levels of saturated fat). While it is possible that enzymatic changes could produce a healthier palm oil, the potential for introduction of a new, unintended, and possibly more atherogenic compound cannot be excluded. Palmolein provides a very instructive lesson. Produced by fractionation of palm oil, palmolein is more stable at high temperatures, more ideal for frying than palm oil, and a nutritionally healthier alternative to palm oil.

In an effort to increase local and global supply of healthy oils, oilseed plantation and production projects have been undertaken in various countries. The countries in which modest success has already been attained include Argentina, Brazil, Chile, France, Spain, and Turkey. For example, the Argentine/Chile agricultural programme currently produces enough healthy oil for PepsiCo's Argentina snacks business, which uses 100% high oleic sunflower oil (HOSO). HOSO contains higher oleic acid content that improves both oil stability and the shelf life of its products. In Turkey, the business unit is working with a local sunflower growers' cooperative, loosely linked to the Ministry of Agriculture. Since 2008, Cheetos in Turkey have been made with 100% HOSO. It is anticipated that potato and tortilla chips will move in stages to HOSO blend and 100% HOSO as determined by cost and supply as well as consumer acceptance of flavour change. Within the Asia, Middle East, and Africa division of PepsiCo, South Africa is exploring a local

HOSO programme through which it will grow its own supply to replace European imports. Already in pilot since 2008, it is expected to take 3–5 years to establish a sustainable supply chain. It is important to point out that not all initiatives have had success. For example, in Peru, four pilot programmes conducted in 2008 concluded that low yields and high costs make it unprofitable to grow HOSO seed (444).

Addressing consumer taste needs

Public health has tended to undervalue consumer insights in promoting healthy eating (445). Some consumers are concerned about having to compromise taste for better health or to give up something to which they are accustomed. For example, underlying science strongly supports increased intake of marine-source omega-3 fatty acids. However, food companies are challenged by the need to create encapsulation technology for successfully masking the fishy taste of this nutrient. Similar challenges persist in efforts to add more potassium to food or beverages without negatively affecting taste.

In the US and Mexico, efforts are underway on a strategy to decrease sodium in products without compromising flavour. If successful, this strategy is anticipated to result in the projected removal of 10,120 tons of salt from the US food supply by 2015. In other products, a different strategy of sodium reduction is employed by using mixtures of mineral salts or spices to enhance flavours and reduce sodium load. In PepsiCo's Asia, Middle East, and Africa division, a combination of strategies has been used with significant success such that PepsiCo International guidelines for sodium reduction have been met by 65% of the portfolio in South Africa, 54% in Saudi Arabia, and 60% in Egypt. It is anticipated that by 2012, at least 95% of the portfolio in Middle East and Africa will have sodium levels of no more than 240mg/serving. However, beyond PepsiCo's efforts there are important challenges and constraints to progress in achieving global targets for sodium reduction that can be found in the informal sector, food services, and home use of salt in food preparation. In addition, the rate at which reductions is made need to be gradual to accommodate consumer tolerance.

PepsiCo's health and wellness strategy also includes reductions in sugar. Sugar plays an important role in terms of texture, volume, and colour, especially in cookies. Plans to remove substantial amounts of added sugar from the portfolio include an initial focus on hot and ready-to-eat cereals and bars, with some of the sugar reduction achieved through replacement with natural non-nutritive sweeteners and bulking agents. However, the greatest challenge in reducing added sugars is in beverages. Some of the sugar reduction will be through replacement with Reb-A, the natural non-nutritive sweetener derived from stevia. Stevia has been approved as a food additive in the US, China, Japan, Paraguay, Korea, Brazil, Israel, Malaysia, Taiwan, Australia, and New Zealand. In 2006, the additive was listed as safe for human use by the WHO/FAO Joint Expert Committee on Food Additives and in 2008 raised its Acceptable Daily Intake (ADI) to 4 mg/kg body weight. Industry and independent research institutes should continue to collaborate and develop other natural non-caloric sweeteners, as well as gain a better understanding of the biology of sweeteners in human sensory systems. This research will be critical for creating an acceptably sweet product profile along with satiety and potential mood effects.

Building public/private trust as a prelude to alliances

The public sector has experience identifying global and national priorities based on broad health needs. The food industry has global reach and expertise in food production, processing, distribution, and invaluable customer insights (446–450). Together, public-private collaboration can foster solutions to the overweight and obesity problem, an idea that former WHO Director General, Gro

Harlem Brundtland realized when hosting the first meeting between CEOs of leading food companies and WHO. Creating trust and building partnerships on a foundation of shared values are at the heart of good business. Rosabeth Kanter Moss of the *Harvard Business Review* noted, 'When giants transform themselves from impersonal machines into human communities, they gain the ability to transform the world around them in very positive ways . . . Values turn out to be the key ingredient in the most vibrant and successful multinational (corporations)' (451). Similarly, Brownell et al. said that there is a need 'to combine personal and collective responsibility approaches in ways that best serve the public good' (445). Unfortunately, levels of mistrust often block the creation of the partnerships needed to tackle nutrition problems. Brownell and Warner call for greater transparency with respect to industry funding for scientists and research while food and beverage company lobbying is also a source of contention (452, 453).

Allowing independent auditors to examine public pledges with respect to reformulation goals, marketing restrictions to children, and labelling can remedy some of this mistrust. For example, the Healthy Weight Commitment Foundation (HWCF) is using the Robert Wood Johnson Foundation (RWJ) as an auditing body. This partnership between industry, non-profits, and educators aims to reduce obesity in the US by 2015 and will have each of its platforms independently evaluated by RWJ (454). In addition, companies are subject to many independent monitoring schemes that include the Dow Jones Sustainability Index and the Global Reporting Initiative. Their investor and business community reports create incentives for positive corporate behaviours while being critical of others.

Historical reluctance on the part of public health agencies and other public entities to develop these partnerships is slowly dissolving. In the past decade, the development of new drugs, vaccines and diagnostics for neglected diseases received a boost with the establishment of public-private partnerships such as the International AIDS Vaccine Initiative and Medicines for Malaria Venture. The National Institutes of Health and other federal public health agencies have championed successful models of such partnerships; however, they have historically involved the pharmaceutical or biotechnology industry as the partners from the private sector. For example, the Biomarkers Consortium, launched in 2006, is a public–private partnership with the goal of identifying and qualifying new biological markers and whose diverse list of members includes government entities, foundations, and industry partners, among others (455). This framework can be used to engage the food industry to help innovate and accelerate product reformulation.

An IOM 2010 report focused on reducing the global burden of cardiovascular disease stated: 'many intervention approaches . . . are more likely to succeed if public education and government policies and regulations are complemented by the voluntary collaboration of the private sector' (23). Specifically, it was suggested that the food industry increase international collaborations aiming to reduce unhealthy ingredients while also placing restrictions on marketing of unhealthy products. These recommendations support the creation of more private-public alliances and are in agreement with the steps that food companies are already taking to address chronic disease. Partnerships that have the greatest chance of succeeding will be those that are formed with a strong understanding of the practical challenges to be overcome in the communities they hope to help. Business practices, cultural nuances, and the presence or the absence of distribution systems and infrastructure affect the daily reality of bringing products and solutions to individuals. Through dialogue regarding capabilities and shared values, public–private partnerships have the potential to effectively deal with these issues (456).

Conclusions

The food industry has a vested interest in helping to improve population health. The world's 10 largest global food and beverage companies have revenues that gross in the trillions of dollars on an annual basis, not to mention manufacturers at the national and local levels and the informal sector. The changes that leaders in the food industry are making are associated with many challenges and require innovation in food processing technology and substantial investments in research and development. It would be advantageous to gather relevant parties and discuss the full spectrum of actions that industry have taken, associated costs, barriers to progress, and the impact on health in general and chronic disease in particular. The lessons to be learned from such an exercise would be invaluable.

The severity of the global nutrition crisis demands that industry create a platform of trust between the public and private sectors through acknowledgment of common values and shared goals. It is the responsibility of the private sector to develop innovative strategies that utilize and share business expertise with partners in the government, academic, research, and non-governmental arenas. For company actions to reach scale and have impact, governments and other players, including NGOs and academics, will need to take complementary actions. Governments need to step up their involvement in all aspects of promoting active living, including ensuring that school children have regular physical education. Governments and WHO need to develop norms that will apply to all companies so that multinational, medium and small food and beverage companies can operate on a level playing field. Governmental support in the form of regulatory reform, business incentives, and policy change can also accelerate product reformulation. Bold new comprehensive initiatives are necessary to address the agricultural, technological, and other scientific challenges and their associated policy implications.

Despite improvements in chronic disease treatment and prevention, increasing nutrition transitions around the world suggest there is a need for a new and innovative plan of action to enable more sustainable partnerships that would draw upon all capabilities and expertise. At the November 2009 World Economic Forum meeting in Dubai, the public-private Global Agenda Council for chronic diseases proposed development of an 'Action Coalition' to stimulate joint action and promote policy coherence across sectors and businesses. The coalition will collaborate with WHO's Global Non-communicable Disease (NCD) Network, supporting the implementation of the WHO NCD Action Plan. At the latest meeting of NCD-Net, the WHO Director General, and the Executive Chairman of the WEF expressed their support for such actions to be expedited. Many food and beverage companies are already committed and engaged in such partnerships and are hopeful that these efforts will yield beneficial health outcomes. Only through new and innovative partnerships will there be opportunity and lasting change.

Acknowledgements

This chapter draws upon several recent publications from PepsiCo staff. We thank Mehmood Khan and Dondeena Bradley from PepsiCo for use of their research.

The corporate play book, health, and democracy: The snack food and beverage industry's tactics in context

William H. Wiist

Introduction

The preceding chapter has described a variety of activities that some food and beverage corporations routinely engage in as part of their 'health and wellness' strategies. While there is little doubt that food and beverage industries can play some kind of role in public health efforts to control chronic diseases, questions remain as to what the appropriate role should be. Clearly, food products are not global 'bads' like tobacco, but there is a growing body of evidence and concern that some products, such as sugary soft drinks, are causes of obesity and diabetes, especially among children (457).

In this chapter the food industry's tactics and potentially adverse effects on public health are evaluated. Lessons from the tobacco and other industries are applied to the food industry, using material drawn from PepsiCo's proposals. Our analysis suggests that food companies may be replicating several of the tactics used by tobacco companies to promote a positive image and influence research as part of an effort to reduce the prospects for public regulation and taxation (83). A series of recommendations are offered about how public health practitioners should engage with the food industry to promote healthy transformations within industry while avoiding potential conflicts-of-interest and adverse influences on the public's health and democracy.

The food industries' public health-related practices and policies in context

In setting out their proposed global public health agenda, food companies often claim that they seek to use the results of scientific research to educate residents of developing countries, and others, about how to make healthful food and beverage choices and about physical activity, to promote sustainable economic development, and to protect the environment. However, in order to accomplish these goals, food industry corporations often seek government incentives such as tax breaks and publicly financed research to use in developing products; less regulation; more favourable policy, and freedom to set health standards. An integral part of the strategy is to seek partnerships with academia, government, NGOs, and multilateral international organizations to move their agenda forward (see Chapter 6.1). The strategies outlined in PepsiCo's chapter appear to follow the playbook used by many other industries.

On the surface, the chapter's literature review, description of activities, and proposals would seem to convey a commendable message of hope to public health professionals working to ameliorate and prevent heart disease, obesity, diabetes, and cancer. Yet, several concerned nutritionists, investors, journalists, and health advocates who monitor and report on food companies (and in particular PepsiCo's products and operations) have suggested a different perspective than set out in the previous chapter about the effects of the corporation's practices, policies and products on public health and the environment (447, 458, 459). The space allotted here does not allow for a detailed analysis of the nutritional information, claims and proposals in PepsiCo's chapter and such analyses are left to independent nutrition, physical activity and obesity scientists, as some have begun to do. Monteiro and colleagues discuss PepsiCo's snack foods (460), and Sharma and colleagues discuss PepsiCo's participation in self-regulatory partnerships with Coca-Cola, Schweppes, Burger King, Cadbury Adams, Campbell Soup, ConAgra, General Mills, Hershey, Kellogg, Kraft, Mars, McDonald's, Nestlé USA, Dannon, and Unilever (445). A few questions are raised here (Table 6.3) about the food industry's operations, testing and standards that might suggest areas for further analysis.

Corporate tactics used to influence public health policy and interventions

Perhaps of greater concern than the food industry's products and nutrition-related messages is their potential influence on global and domestic policy. Public health professionals' perceptiveness and understanding of corporate operations and policies have become more sophisticated as a result of studying such industries as the pharmaceutical industry (461, 462), the food and agriculture industry (458), and the tobacco industry. Comparisons between the tobacco and food and beverage industries (83), and tobacco and obesity (463) suggest a 'corporate play book', a list of identifiable tactics (Table 6.4) common across many corporations and industries (464). These tactics include influencing legislators (465), using scientists and science funding to raise doubts about harm (466), using a public relations firm to conduct a campaign to recruit scientists and form coalitions (159), arguing that corporate products create jobs and benefits farmers in developing countries (380); arranging authorship of scientific papers (467), and conducting a 'get government off our backs' campaign (468).

We discuss each in further detail below. As we show, in each of these regards, food companies, as shown in the preceding chapter, appear to be mimicking the tactics used by tobacco, pharmaceutical and other industries to gain credibility and influence policy.

Biasing research studies

As part of a strategy to undermine tobacco control research, the US Tobacco Institute hired scientists and established health promotion strategies to mislead the public about the harmful effects of smoking. Similar to this tactic, nutrition research publications show bias from industry funding (469). Like the tobacco industry, the food and beverage industry attempts to develop customers as young as possible (470), and one tactic for doing so may be through the development of early-childhood health promotion schemes.

Hiring top health professionals and scientists to develop 'health and wellness' programmes

The implementation of a 'health & wellness' programme is used by other food and beverage corporations (471). PepsiCo's hiring of health professionals and scientists, such as those in the preceding chapter (472), and obtaining the advisory services of Gro Harlem Brundtland, former Director-General of the WHO (473), in support of the corporation's strategy is similar to those of pharmaceutical (462), and tobacco industries (474).

Table 6.3 Questions to ask about the food and beverage industry

Corporate operations

What proportion of revenues is spent on community health promotion, education, and physical activity? What types of activities are included in making those calculations?

Since the annual revenue of soft drinks is substantial why is decreasing the sale of soft drinks not emphasized in the 'health and wellness' programme?

How much of its supply, production, marketing, and distribution chain does PepsiCo control or influence through partnerships?

What is the relationship between a corporation's stock prices and 'healthful' product initiatives?

How does the compensation for a corporation's Chief Executive Officer, and its health initiative officials compare with the average wage of production line workers?

What proportion of the statutory state tax rates did a corporation pay in states where its corporate facilities are?

How much less are corporate costs for supplies and labour outside the US compared to in the US?

How much benefit does the corporation receive each year from government subsidies or tax breaks for supplies (e.g. corn, corn syrup, sugar), marketing, compared to its charitable contributions?

What proportion of revenue does the corporation spend on R&D compared to management and marketing?

How much does the corporation spend on all types of advertisements, product, or brand promotion that are seen by children?

Products, testing, and standards

What independent scientific evidence is there that voluntarily changes in products made by the corporation have reduced mortality or morbidity, obesity, or increased physical activity and children's beverage choices?

Has independent testing been conducted that shows that all ingredients of all products are safe?

Isn't it true that scientific research showed that sodium was a health risk many years ago?

How much water (& from what sources), petroleum products (i.e. for plastic bottles) and aluminium (cans) are used in soft drink production compared to investments in 'more healthful' products?

Are internally set nutrition criteria higher or lower than outside independent recommendations?

How much sodium and sugar would a consumer ingest if she/he ate one serving per day of each of the corporation's multiple products, compared to the recommended daily allowance?

How long had the content in corporate products (e.g., sugar, corn syrup, sodium) been at higher than the recommended levels (and how much higher) prior to the corporation's reduction to meet recent standards?

What role did company representatives have in setting standards for additives (e.g. sodium, Stevia)?

What is the nutritional transition that is needed in less industrialized countries to promote health?

Why would a corporation that sells meat seek to decrease meat consumption, or one that sells infant formula promote breastfeeding?

Why emphasize 'energy balance'?

Is any food or beverage product 'bad' (unhealthful) in and of itself?

Do snack foods and soft drinks contribute to solving global malnutrition and hunger?

Table 6.4 Examples from the corporate play book

Public relations
Emphasize consumer's personal responsibility, moderation, free choice, and pleasure
Use the 'government' vs. 'personal freedom and civil liberties' and 'Get government off our backs' arguments
Vilify critics, health advocates and public health scientists as 'health police' or 'fascists' and accuse them of seeking to impose a 'nanny state'
Hire a public relations firm to develop and help carry out plans to create a positive image, combat negative reports, or repair damage to credibility or image
Try to discredit independent health institutions and organizations
Use surrogates to criticize those who disagree with corporate positions
Harass critics, whether private citizens, academicians, or celebrities, including with law suits or by pressuring funding agencies
Tout its 'Corporate Social Responsibility' programmes (while violating laws, risking worker safety and health, or damaging the natural environment)
Promote the adoption of corporate voluntary codes, without including accountability enforcement, transparency, and a full role for independent civil society groups
Set up or fund 'front groups' with consumer advocacy sounding names to promote the corporate agenda and messages
Infiltration and surveillance of opposition groups
Distortion of science
Claim that independent research that contradicts corporate research is 'junk science'
Distort their corporate research results
Withhold research data unfavourable to the corporation's product
Selectively publish and report the most favourable outcomes
Manipulate research article authorship to establish credibility and control
Manipulate research design for outcomes most favourable to the corporation
Create controversy about scientific studies unfavourable to corporate products
Use the 'junk science' argument in court against public health researchers
Divert attention from health effects of their product or practices to other matters
Publish journal articles and book chapters, make presentations at scientific meetings, host conferences and workshops for professionals that give the appearance of objective science in order to convey an image of credibility, but do not present the entire picture, or misrepresent or distort information about the corporation's harmful operations, products or policies
Pay scientists or physicians or other professionals to serve as spokespersons to represent the corporation's position

(Continued)

Table 6.4 (*Continued*)

Political influence
Contribute funds to election campaigns of politicians in positions to influence legislation favourable to the corporation and to obtain favourable rulings from the judiciary
Participate as delegates in the policy-making or standard setting process to ensure the lowest or most lenient possible standards for corporate products and operations
Use lobbying to gain competitive advantage, avoid or minimize regulation and taxation
Work to reduce government budgets for scientific, policy, and regulatory activities deemed contrary to the corporation's profit

Financial tactics
Externalize as much cost as possible (e.g. dumping chemicals into rivers; not providing employee medical coverage)
Contribute funding to community and neighbourhood organizations in order to create dependency, gain allies, and influence or manipulate the organization's agenda
Set up or fund foundations that support the corporation's agenda rather than funding priorities determined through independent democratic processes (i.e. taxes)

Legal and regulatory tactics
Work to get corporate officials or industry lobbyists appointed to governmental regulatory agencies with authority over its own industry
Shop for other judiciary venues or levels of government when rulings or decisions are undesirable
In regulatory or judicial matters, avoid as long as possible having a hearing on the facts
When deemed necessary to ensure profits, employ illegal means

Products and services
Emphasize technological solutions to health problems to generate profit rather than simple inexpensive solutions
Use both direct advertising and indirect methods such as product placement and integration into the story line of entertainment venues
Connect image of product or corporation with human emotions and values

Using public relations firms to provide strategic counsel

Food companies invest considerable resources in devising elaborate public relations campaigns to improve their image. In the case of PepsiCo, Edelman, the number one rated PR firm in the US, was hired in July 2009. In June of 2008 Edelman formed a food & nutrition advisory panel to provide strategic counsel about obesity, food policy, nutrition communications, etc. Edelman is known for its work to create a more positive image of industries, for fighting against control of second hand smoke and for fighting regulatory control related to obesity (475). This suggests that, if PepsiCo is behaving like other food companies, it could be using its public-health policies as part of its marketing strategy (which, as shown in Chapter 2, centres on 'creating demand').

Influencing political debates about public health

Tobacco companies have used elaborate tactics to influence policy decisions: through political campaign contributions and direct lobbying (476), and through philanthropy (477). These activities can disproportionately influence the democratic process and reduce the effective political influence of individuals and human citizen groups. According to US Senate Office of Public Records, PepsiCo, Inc reported spending over $9 million in 2009 to lobby the US Congress (478), the third highest in the food and beverage industry (479). Based on filings with the Federal Elections Commission, in the 2008 election cycle, the company's Political Action Committee 'Concerned Citizen Fund' alone contributed $547,700 to candidates for federal office (480). Its policy emphasizes contributions to candidates who are 'pro-business', and who have a 'commitment to improving the business climate' pending their 'position or voting record' (481).

Similar to many corporations, PepsiCo's federal tax payment record revealed the company receives significant tax breaks (the implications of lower corporate tax payments is addressed below). According to PepsiCo's December 2009 filings with the US Securities Exchange Commission, PepsiCo's provision for current US Federal taxes was at the rate of 26% ($1,238,000), rather than the statutory rate of 35%, on US revenues before taxes of $4,209,000 (482). From 1981 to 1984 PepsiCo received $136 million tax rebate on $179 million in pretax profits (a negative 7.6% rate), the fifth largest corporate rebate (483). PepsiCo also used restructuring of companies like Walkers in the UK to transfer revenue to lower-tax countries (484). In its last annual report PepsiCo reported sales of $108 billion and $3 million in Foundation distributions to academia and communities (485).

Some corporations have been accused of violating human rights (486, 486a), and at times PepsiCo has been reluctant to support human rights (487, 488), HIV/AIDS policy (489), and to disclose substances in its products (490, 491, 491a). PepsiCo expends large sums to advertise its products (at least $359 million for five products in 2008) (492) and touts its policies and plans for relief of world hunger (493, 493a), its code of conduct (494), and human rights (481), all of which are subsumed under its revenue and margin growth and reputational goals and competition (485). No systematic, completely independent monitoring and public reporting by civil society organizations of performance on those policies was reported.

The issues raised from this partial deconstruction of PepsiCo's operations illustrate a potentially even greater and more serious threat to public health than immediate concerns about the nutritional quality of PepsiCo's products or its advertising practices.

Reforming the global corporation and governance to serve the public interest

In order to assure continued growth in profits a corporation must continually expand geographically to gain new customers, develop new products or lines, or reduce costs by externalizing measures such as reducing its workforce, and by avoiding taxes. A key question today is how much profit is necessary or warranted. Not all aspects of the corporate-driven global economy benefited from neoliberal economics (495). During the past 30–35 years that the neoliberal ('neoconservative' in the North) 'free market' model has been dominant, the global benefits in wealth have been unequally distributed (1). By the mid-2000's, 1% of the US population held 22% of the wealth (496). Income inequalities have been shown to be associated with poor health and social measures such as higher levels of obesity, infant mortality, homicides, births to teenagers, mental illness, and lower spending on foreign aid, lower levels of trust, women's status, education, and more (364).

The need for partnerships with corporations and the need for corporate funds for community programmes results from corporations paying less tax. In the US in 2004, corporate income taxes amounted to 8% of tax receipts compared to 34% from personal income taxes (497). A report from the US Government's General Accountability Office (GAO) showed that from 1998–2005, 34% of foreign corporations in the US and 24% of US corporations paid no taxes for at least half of those years (498). In 2002 and 2003, 82 out of 275 most consistently profitable Fortune 500 corporations collectively paid no federal tax at least one of those years; 275 paid less than half the 35% statutory rate (499).

The reliance of independent non-profit organizations on corporate funds creates dependency, conflict of interests, co-opts the non-profit into becoming an ally (500), and results in undue corporate influence in decision-making processes and control of health standards. Such mingling of interests is not prevented by financial disclosure. Lower tax revenues from corporations result in fewer government inspectors to monitor corporate operations and enforce regulations. For example, because in 2002 corporations did not pay the statutory tax rate, the US government treasury had $172 billion less with which to operate (501).

The corporation undermines human democracy through its ability to disproportionately influence the democratic process through lobbying and election campaign contributions. In 2009 the food and beverage industry spent $56,771,216 to hire 337 outside lobbyist to influence legislation in the US Congress (502). Lobbying on behalf of corporations gives them access, including to write legislation, that the individual citizen or citizen groups do not have. Due in part to this influence consumers are not able to hold corporations accountable. In the 2008 election cycle the food and beverage industry PACs contributed $4,090,349 million to federal candidate campaigns (502).

Recent events portend increasing corporate influence on elections. The US Supreme Court's ruling in the *Citizens United v. Federal Elections Commission* on January 21, 2010 permits corporations to spend unlimited amounts of money, directly from the corporate treasury, on election campaign advertising (503). This allows corporations to wield disproportionate influence over candidates who take positions on health issues that corporations oppose (504, 504a). Underlying the *Citizens United* decision was the assumption that corporations are persons. It has been presumed that corporations hold the right of personhood through misapplications of the court reporter's head notes in an 1886 Supreme Court case (*Santa Clara v Southern Pacific Railroad*). Head notes hold no legal authority, and no court, legislation nor vote of the people have ever directly ruled that corporation's are persons under the US Constitution. Nevertheless, corporations have asserted that they are entitled to the human rights flowing from the Fourteenth Amendment (to protect rights of former slaves) (505–507).

Many corporations also gain disproportionate influence on government and democratic process through the 'revolving door' by which a corporate official or industry representative is appointed to a position of authority within the regulatory agency that oversees her/his industry, then returns to a key industry or lobbying position (507a). Or, a government official, elected representative or employee of a multi-national organization (e.g. UN, WHO) leaves that position to become a lobbyist or industry employee. In that case they take with them their network of contacts and knowledge which they then use to garner influence in favour of their client or employer, drawing those networks into industry partnerships.

Through the use of such pernicious tactics corporations have subtly taken on the authority of a global governance institution (508) while governments have retreated (509). The global food and agriculture industry is a prime illustration (510). Corporations have decentralized production across the globe to the countries with the cheapest labour and weakest restrictive requirements for worker safety and health and environment protections, while centralizing of the functions of knowledge accumulation, dissemination and management. Corporations have formed global industrial networks and partnerships with governments, multinational organizations (e.g. UN) and not-for-profits that allow them to set and control standards across nation-state boundaries for health, environment, production, and transportation, etc. Corporations play one nation-state against another for the most advantageous competitive accommodations for their operations, tariffs, and as suppliers and consumers. Economic dependencies then prevent countries from taking strong positions in opposition to the corporation. Thus there is one system in which those already rich and powerful make the rules for the process that has led to worsening inequality. If we choose to continue with those social institutions we are accountable for the future and the resulting radical inequality (511).

Global trade, and thus much of the global economy, is controlled by the corporate dominated World Trade Organization (WTO) and, despite global trade influences on health (512), WTO conducts business in secret, without the participation of civil society, and without public reporting of dispute resolution (513). In the US the trade policy development process is dominated by corporations. Of the 28 advisory committees to the US Trade Representative and their 700 members (514), corporations or industry representatives hold all positions except for about three to five held by public health. Chapter 11 of the North American Free Trade Agreement allows corporations to sue governments or lower political divisions for loss of potential future profits due to health or safety laws (515). Programmes of the World Bank, IMF, agreements of the WTO, and pro-corporate government administration's deregulation have also led to an increased privatization of public services and other problems (516, 517).

Thus nation-states have become dependent upon corporations for the health of their economies, held at the mercy of corporations for their economic well-being, in a 'golden straight jacket' unable to control their own or the global economy (508). Corporations also collude with governments to commit a variety of types of crime (518), which if pursued by the justice system often result in fines of only a small fraction of revenues (462). Undergirding these relationships is the neoliberal ideology of corporatism and consumerism in which government is viewed as a pathology and public health has no place (496). Constant exposure to corporate product advertisement and the visible comparative inequalities across neighbourhoods and countries have created an individualistic consumerism that has trumped participation in democracy (519). When citizens feel helpless to effect change in the face of oppression by the government-corporate partnership they experience what has been labelled an 'abuse syndrome' (520).

Learning lessons from tobacco and other industry initiatives

Elimination of the role of the corporation as a global governance agency will require the establishment of a global governing organization (508), including health governance (521). A requirement for such an agency would be the full and direct participation of civil society representatives who are completely independent of corporate influence. Such an organization would need to have decision-making, rule-making and enforcement power, and authority, including authority to impose and collect a tax on global corporate activity that could be distributed to the countries or regions most in need (508). In addition there are a number of divestment and international legal instruments that could be applied to control global corporate activities (521, 522, 522a), and adherence to lobbying transparency and integrity principles (523), and an end to government farm subsidies (448) such those as for corn and sugar beets in the US, key ingredients in some high calorie, high sugar and high sodium snack foods and beverages with little nutritional value, and suspected of contributing to obesity (523a).

As an interim step, the decision-making and dispute resolution processes of the WTO needs to be made more equitable across nations, include civil society participation, and make all processes transparent and accountable to the public. The US President should appoint public health representatives to the USTR Advisory Committees and establish a separate Public Health Advisory Committee. Counter-part officials in other countries should ensure that their countries include full consideration of public health in their trade agreement process. The practice of co-determination, including supervisory boards and works councils, in which workers participate in the management of corporations (524) could be adopted by all transnational corporations. The precautionary principle of requiring that corporations demonstrate that all products, chemicals, etc. are safe before they are marketed to the public should be applied globally.

A variety of reform proposals have been made to bring the corporation back under the control of human democracy (525). Such proposals received additional attention after the Supreme Court's decision in *Citizens United*, including calls for a Constitutional Amendment that would ensure that corporations do not hold the rights of personhood, and without which they could not have any role in political campaigns or lobbying (Movetoamend.org; freespeechforpeople.org). Other proposals being considered include publicly funded election campaigns, giving candidates free and equal access to mass communications media, and requiring corporate disclosure in advertisements, prior approval from investors for contributions (526).

A corporation, being a governmentally chartered institution, is a legal fiction, a piece of paper that is without human emotions, motives or other characteristics and cannot be 'responsible' or 'irresponsible'. For the most part, corporate social 'responsibility' (CSR) programmes and activities have been simply voluntary, nonbinding codes and practices without accountability, public relations tools to create and promote the public's positive impression of the corporation (526a). While touting their corporate 'social responsibility' such as 'green' programmes, alternative energy development, employee health programmes, or product safety many corporations have simultaneously been in violation of laws and fined for unsafe operations or environmental pollution (527). However, there are many actions corporations could take to truly be responsible to human citizens and the democratic governments (Table 6.5) including fulfilling human rights obligations and duties (527a, 528).

Conclusion

As illustrated in the preceding chapter, food companies appear to be using a standard repertoire of tactics that corporations use to influence health and policy (529). While this chapter has drawn examples from PepsiCo, these strategies similarly appear to be occurring with Coca-Cola, Nestle, Kraft and several other food and beverage companies (458, 459). Many of these strategies pose potential risks to public health, even when they may on the surface appear to be health-promoting in the short term.

The preceding chapter reflects the fundamental purpose, goals and operations of institution known as 'the corporation', a societal level, structural influence on health (530) that serves to establish corporations as a global quasi-governmental agency (508) with dominance over human citizens and democracy. The public health code of ethics specifies that public health's primary role is to address the fundamental societal structural causes of disease (530a). Because corporate activities are determinants of health, public health ethics therefore demands that we address corporations.

The goal and values of public health and the goal of the corporation are fundamentally different: protecting and promoting the health of the public versus making a profit to return to investors, i.e. create 'shareholder value'. 'Partners' cannot have fundamentally conflicting goals.

One sector of society does have a monopoly of what is in the public interest, the overall good of society, particularly the public's health, and that is government. While other sectors such as corporations may contribute to and have duties to society, government has the sole authority to empower, regulate, and carry out activities to protect and promote the general welfare, health and safety of the collective; to do what individuals alone cannot (531). Government's protective role is particularly important during economic crises (531a). Public health professionals must not allow corporate enticement to blur or disguise the distinction between corporate and public health purposes. The corporation has neither the mandate, nor based on their absence from the constitution, the right or authority to make decisions about what is in the public interest.

Governments and multinational organizations sometimes don't act or are slow to protect health. Within a democracy delayed action sometimes occurs to ensure consideration of diverse

Table 6.5 Examples of actions corporations could take to gain the trust of potential public health partners, governments and human citizens

1 Provide independent public health officials, scientists, and representatives of NGOs access to corporate records to conduct independent, annual evaluative audits of the corporation's health promotion, environmental, worker health and safety and human rights activities relative to the corporate goals, objectives, policies, and plans. Provide these auditors access to corporate facilities and workers, research reports, health promotion budgets, e-mails and other related corporate communication requested by the auditors in order to compare it with scientific knowledge and evidence-based best practices. The auditors must be able to provide an independent, written report to the public for immediate release at a time and means determined by the auditors. Funds for audits should be dispensed through an independent, not-for-profit organization or government public health agency, with funding provided by all corporations

2 Collectively fund independent, government public health research & development institutes that would independently dispense grants to researchers to test and report on the healthfulness and content of the corporation's products, relative to scientific evidence and corporate claims

3 Fund independently developed health promoting advertisements in amounts equivalent to the corporation's advertising budget

4 All corporate health promotion and health education programmes and activities should be free of corporate branding, including logos, corporate name, products, symbols, figures, etc.

5 Make no contributions to election campaigns or issue referenda or amendments through corporate direct donations, advertising, funding to issue organizations, or to political parties, political action committees, or through any other means

6 Publicly renounce corporate personhood, including the right of political speech

7 No industry officials accept employment or appointment to government regulatory agencies with authority for any part of their industry

8 Prohibit their corporate or industry representatives to serve on government panels or committees that review their industry's research, set product or operational standards, or that make recommendations for such standards

9 Pay the full statutory tax rate

10 Forego tax write offs, offshore accounts, and stop allocating profits to operations in countries with low tax rates while allocating charges to operations in countries with higher rates

11 Immediately publicly acknowledge all funding provided to individual scientists, professional organizations, community, consumer or industry groups or other companies

12 Adhere fully and promptly with all laws, regulations, government and multi-national standards related to product safety and efficacy, workplace safety, worker health, affirmative action, corporate finances, human rights, and worksite, product, and record inspections and reporting

13 Provide salaries and wages to non-executive employee workers that, at a minimum, meet living wage standards, and that are equitable with executive compensation, and that recognize communal contributions

14 Facilitate the right of all workers, including employees of subcontractors outside the US, to organize into and freely operate unions; to negotiate with worker representatives in good faith for a fair and living wage, and safe and healthful working conditions

15 Clearly label the entire contents of products, including any amount of any substance

16 Implement the precautionary principle by submitting all products and their contents to independent testing for safety, healthfulness, and efficacy prior to marketing to the public (including product placement, story-line integration, web sites, educational materials, video or computer games, or toys)

(*continued*)

Table 6.5 (*Continued*)

17 Make available and accessible the most efficacious, healthful, scientifically validated products (e.g. medications) at an affordable cost to the poorest, least industrialized countries where disease rates are highest and vulnerability of the natural environment is highest

18 Make the priority for product research, development, marketing and distribution the products and services that are necessities for life, health, safety, disease treatment, human rights, and a sustainable environment

19 Limit the number of internal and external hired lobbyists, for example, one individual in a nation's capital of the country where the corporate headquarters is located

20 Not accept any government subsidies or price supports for research, development, marketing, advertising, or distribution

21 Conduct all operations in a manner that protects the natural environment and promotes sustainability

22 Ensure that all operations protect, and do not infringe on the rights of, indigenous peoples' land, language, culture, livelihood, and traditional medicinal and food plants

23 Cease all patenting of biological processes, and the resultant products, and of all life forms in the commons (including microbes, plant, animal and human DNA). Make any biological process discoveries freely available and accessible to everyone

24 Return a portion of corporate revenue to the public agency that funded the original or basic research, or to the public institution that conducted the research, upon which corporate products, services and operations are based, in an proportion equitable to revenues generated

25 Not engage in 'no bid' and cost plus government contracts; fully cooperate with government contract monitors and auditors

26 Charge fees for products and services to consumers and governments based on actual costs

27 Not privatize fresh water, forests, minerals, oceans, health, social and sanitary services, public information, and public broadcast airwaves

28 Not use product placement, story-line integration, web sites, educational materials, video or computer games, toys or otherwise advertise to children or vulnerable communities

29 Submit all health, environmental and human rights policies of corporate advisory groups, boards and committees for review and recommendation by independent consumer advocacy organizations and public health scientists

30 Make information that industry has about insights into consumer preferences, awareness and literacy, etc. available to public health agencies to use in designing health promotion communications, programmes and services

31 Submit CEO compensation to shareholders for approval

32 Publicly, fully and accurately report CEO total compensation in an easily accessible and understandable format, and fully comply with the law (e.g. SEC rules and principles)

33 Implement worker co-direction of corporate management

34 Board members exert an active oversight role of management, require full reporting and hold management and the board publicly accountable for all aspects of corporate operations

35. Make health and safety product changes without initiation of lawsuits or government enforcement

36 Adhere to as binding any pledges or agreements for environmental sustainability, worker safety, human rights, etc.

37 Require consumer or trade groups or organizations to make public and readily visible the amount of any funding provided by the corporation and identify the purposes for which used

Table 6.5 (*Continued*)

38 Require that corporate-funded organizations publicly identify any board members or employees who are current or former employees of the corporation or related industries

39 Include in corporate dominated or industry organizations (e.g. WTO, International Chamber of Commerce) equal and full participation by civil society; make operations transparent and accountable to the public

40 Submit to the democratic decision-making and enforcement mechanisms of a global governance organization collectively operated by nation-states and civil society, and based on transparency and public accountability

41 Develop and manufacture solutions to health problems that are simple and affordable as a priority rather than costly technological products

viewpoints, but often delay is due to the disproportion influence of corporations seeking priority for their sole interests. What serves the corporation is not necessarily in the best interest of society, nor is serving the profit motive necessarily the best way to achieve societal goals.

Those who accept corporate financing and support partnerships with corporations may believe that the positions presented here are antiquated, mistrustful, uncompromising, and antagonistic to contemporary realities. It is important to remember that the abolitionist fight against slavery, the suffragists who gained women the vote, the civil rights movement that overthrew Jim Crow segregation, and the popular uprising that overthrew South African apartheid were out of necessity uncompromising and militantly assertive, not compromising partnerships to achieve incremental rights from those who opposed their goals.

Health professionals need to guard against complicity in furthering corporate global governance and thereby a decline in human democracy and social justice. We need real and fundamental reforms more than distracting incremental change. We have a choice to either work to strengthen the ability of the democratic processes and governments to better protect and promote health, or to work to increase corporate profits. Reliance on corporate finances subjugates the independent voice of public health to commercial goals.

Power concedes nothing without a demand. It never did and it never will.

Frederick Douglas

Recommendations

Any partnership with industry in which there is corporate remuneration or exchange creates a conflict of interest and compromises the independence of the beneficiary. It is not wise to nor do people usually 'bite the hand that feeds you' and when they do they suffer negative consequences. So, if an individual, community, or organization receives money from a corporation, they are co-opted, more easily becoming an ally of the corporation's position, more willing to compromise standards, less likely to oppose the actions and policies of the corporation, and they become dependent on those corporate funds. These are potential dangers of partnerships with food and beverage industry corporations.

Since the 1880s the corporate elite class has waged incremental war in the US through election campaign funding, lobbying, and influence on the judicial system that has significantly eroded democracy. This argument about who shall rule (elite versus the common man) was argued by the US founding fathers when writing the Constitution & Bill of Rights. Overcoming the power and influence of the corporation will require a firm, determined and uncompromising progressive populism of grass roots human beings, reminiscent of the US agrarian and labour movements of late 1800s and early 1900s. Responses of advocates and the Congressional proposals after the *Citizens United* ruling, the recent financial crisis and health insurance reform debate suggest a growing progressive populism focused on reducing corporate power.

For those to whom the concepts presented here are new, below are a few actions you can personally take to begin your contributions to reforming the corporation and restoring democracy to human beings:

- Study the websites of organizations such a POCLAD.org, CorporationsandHealthWatch.org, and MultinationalMonitor.org, and similar organizations, and the journal articles, books and websites cited in this chapter.

- Participate in organizations such as the Trade and Health Forum, International Health Section, or Occupational Health and Safety Section of the American Public Health Association, or similar public health organizations in your area.

- Participate in activities of national, state or local pro-democracy organizations such as the Center for Environmental Legal Defense Fund in the US or form your own direct democracy organization and work toward passing corporate reform laws, constitutional amendments, or local ordinances.

- Vote in every election for which you are eligible, in favour of candidates who support reforms such as elimination of corporate campaign contributions.

- Read books or take courses about globalization and health economics.

- Eliminate existing, and don't accept any personal financial ties to large corporations such as consulting fees, speaking fees, grants, or sponsorships.

- Share what you learn with colleagues and friends around the globe.

In order to retake control of the corporation, the global economy and of democracy it will take the political will of human citizens working together globally, acting individually and in coalitions, using personal and mass action and the new media to educate and to organize political action. Without a reordering of priorities to focus on the corporation as a structural influence, public health has little hope of realizing the elimination of health disparities, inequities, achieving health for all, and ensuring social justice.

Chapter 7

Comparative case studies from Brazil, China, India, Mexico, and South Africa

Karen Siegel and David Stuckler

Key policy points

1   Brazil, China, India, Mexico, and South Africa have double burdens of disease: rapidly rising chronic diseases alongside high burdens of infectious diseases.

2   Each country has experienced extremely rapid, but inequitable, economic growth that has occurred without the development of public infrastructure. Thus, the context of rising chronic diseases in these rapidly growing economies differs considerably from the historical experience of advanced industrialized economies.

3   People's diets in these countries are increasingly composed of excess fat, salt, and sugar. These dietary transformations are the early warning signs of future rises in heart attacks, strokes, diabetes, and cancer.

4   Past experience in global tobacco control highlights that while it may be relatively easy for countries to sign on to global agreements for investing in health, major challenges arise in their implementation and monitoring, especially when faced with significant barriers on the ground and from vested interests.

5   Appropriate intervention strategies to reduce chronic diseases will be home-grown and self-determined. Support (both technical and through shared experiences) provided through global institutions and research networks can strengthen strategies and facilitate greater dialogue among chronic disease researchers and interventionists around the world.

Key practice points

1   Comparative country analysis can help identify key population causes of chronic diseases as well as some non-traditional reasons for success and failure at reducing the disease burden.

2   Marked variations in chronic disease burdens, risk factors, and socioeconomic contexts may necessitate tailoring policy responses to specific local, regional, and national health challenges.

In the first few sections of the book we set out the main dimensions of the global challenge of chronic diseases, spanning epidemiology, social determinants, economics, management, and political economy. We travelled from the most basic epidemiological starting point of determining how to categorize the disease burden to analysing lessons from the civil rights movement about how to influence political processes of global health. This theoretical and technical analysis has set the stage for the important sections to follow.

Here, chronic disease experts from Brazil, China, India, Mexico, and South Africa describe these areas as they relate to their society's rapid changes and emerging challenges. Each country is at a critical phase of human development. Collectively, they are tilting the balance of power to the global South, and in the process are forming unique coalitions and bases of knowledge. Rapid economic growth is creating tremendous opportunities for human development, but is also bringing rapid and radical disruptions to their populations' traditional ways of life. While the countries' historical circumstances are unique and varied, they face a shared threat to the sustainability of their development posed by rising chronic diseases.

To learn from these experts' insights into their country's successes, failures, and opportunities, We asked that they structure their chapters similarly to allow for comparisons with each other. China offers potential insights to India; Mexico to South Africa; Brazil to China. Their people's futures are inextricably tied in today's globalized environment. Soybean subsidies in Brazil affect what a person in a Chinese slum eats for dinner or an Indian farmer chooses to harvest.

We also asked that they respond to the challenges set out in the first six chapters, to: 1) identify the impact of chronic diseases on health and development; 2) ascertain what strategies health leaders and communities are using to prevent and manage these risks; and 3) in looking to the future, diagnose what challenges remain and how a range of groups, from the private sector to public researchers, and grassroots organizations to global institutions, can support their efforts to prevent chronic disease and promote development.

To maintain the authenticity of these experts' voices and perspectives, our edits have intentionally been light, where needed providing additional clarity to the author's discussion. Before we proceed, however, as a guide to readers, we provide background information about the importance of these countries and highlight a few insights that emerge from their experiences.

Rapid economic growth but high inequalities

Each country has undergone rapid transformations of its economy and society but, as shown in Table 7.1, confronts a similar set of challenges to human development. These country case studies provide a window into understanding the key successes and failures that could potentially effect healthy changes of entire societies.

Turning first to the relative similarities of these societies, it is clear that they are at similar points in their global economic and social position. Together, their populations make up about two-fifths of the world's population, contributing to one-sixth of the world's total GDP (see Table 7.1). Their economies are among the fastest growing in the world, on track to become global superpowers in the next three decades (532). For example, between 2005 and 2009 the economies of China and India grew by more than 7% per year. Despite slowdowns in growth due to the 2008/2009 financial crisis, these five countries have recovered more quickly than the rich Western countries, enabling them to improve their market position.

Rapid economic growth has brought about significant rises in their population's average living standards, but many people appear to have been left behind. Each of these countries continues to have large populations mired in extreme poverty. In India, about one-third of the population

Table 7.1 Selected Demographic, Economic, and Health Indicators by Country

Dimension	Brazil	China	India	Mexico	South Africa
			Country		
Political system	Federal democratic republic	Communist	Federal republic, parliamentary democracy	Federal presidential republic	Constitutional democracy
Demographic and social indicators					
Population size (in millions, 2008)	192.0	1325.6	1140.0	106.4	48.7
Urbanization, % of the population living in urban areas (urban population annual growth rate, 2008)	85.6% (1.5%/yr)	43.1% (2.7%/yr)	29.5% (2.3%/yr)	77.2% (1.4%/yr)	60.7% (2.5%/yr)
Urban population without sustainable access to improved sanitation (% 2006)	16.0%	26.0%	48.0%	9.0%	34.0%
Percent of the urban population living in slums (2008)	29.0%	32.9%	34.8%	14.4%	28.7%
Economic indicators					
GDP (PPP) per capita (Int'l dollars, 2008)	$10,296	$5962	$2972	$14,495	$10,109
Economic growth rate (5-year average %, 2004–2008)	4.74%	10.8%	8.52%	3.40%	4.68%
Public spending as % of GDP (latest available of 2005–08)	25.0%	11.4%	16.2%	—	30.9%
Population living below the poverty line (% living on <$1 per day, 2004)	7.5%	9.9%	34.3%	3.0%	10.7% *
GINI Index (income inequality)	0.55	0.42	0.37	0.48	0.58
Income share held by richest 20%	59.0% +	48.0% §	45.0% §	56.0% φ	63.0% *
Openness to trade (value of imports and exports as % of GDP, 2008)	28%	63%	54%	58%	76%
Imports	14%	28%	30%	30%	40%
Exports	14%	35%	24%	28%	36%

(continued)

Table 7.1 (*Continued*)

Dimension	Country				
	Brazil	China	India	Mexico	South Africa
Population health					
Life expectancy at birth (years, both sexes, 2006)	72.0	73.0	63.0	74.0	51.0
Infant mortality rate (per 1000 live births, both sexes, 2006)	19.0	20.0	57.0	29.0	56.0
Communicable disease death rate (per 100,000 pop, age-standardized, 2004)	139.1	85.9	377.4	73.0	965.5
Chronic disease death rate (per 100,000 pop, age-standardized, 2004)	624.9	626.6	713.5	501.1	867.3
Chronic disease disability rate (per 100,000 pop, age-standardized, 2004)	13,429.0	10,828.7	13,818.8	11,138.8	15,153.9
Health resources					
Per capita total expenditure on health (PPP int. $, 2006)	$765.0	$342.0	$109.0	$756.0	$869.0
Per capita government expenditure on health (PPP int. $, 2006)	$367.0	$144.0	$21.0	$327.0	$364.0
Out-of-pocket expenditure as % of private expenditure on health (2006)	64.0%	92.9%	94.0%	92.5%	17.5%
Public health expenditure as % of GDP (2006)	4.0%	2.0%	1.0%	3.0%	4.0%
Physicians density (per 10,000 population)	12.0 *	14.0 ***	6.0 ±	20.0 *	8.0 ±

Notes: Population size, Gini index, Income share held by the lowest 20%, level of urbanization, and all Economic indicators are from the World Development Indicators database, 2009 edition. All Population Health and Health Resources indicators (except age-standardized death rates), Population living below the poverty line (%), and urban population with sustainable access to improved sanitation (%) are from WHOSIS database, available at: http://www.who.int/whosis/en/. Percentage of the urban population living in slums is from UN-HABITIT Urban Observatory 2008. Age-standardized death rates are from the WHO Global Burden of Disease Study, 2010 update. Gini coefficient is an economic measure of inequality of income distribution of income/ wealth at a particular point in time, used to compare changes in income distribution within a country or between countries. The index varies between 0 and 1.0; and 1 indicates complete inequality. (URL: http://go.worldbank.org/3SLYUTVY00 (11 April, 2010).) * 2000 data; ** 2002 data; *** 2003 data; ± 2004 data; § 2005 data; + 2007 data; φ 2008 data.

lives below the poverty line (on less than $1 per day), while about one-tenth of the populations in Brazil, China, and South Africa live in poverty.

These societies have some of the highest levels of inequality in the world, appearing to become polarized into two or more societies within one country. One measure of inequality is the Gini coefficient, which ranges from 0, perfect equality, to 1, perfect inequality. According to this measure, Brazil is the 10th most unequal society in the world (Gini = 0.51), where the richest 20% holds 58.7%% of the society's overall income and the poorest 20% of the population holds only 3.0% of the income share, second to South Africa (0.58). At the other extreme, India's Gini is 0.37, mainly because more of the population is equally poor. Levels of inequality in Mexico (Gini = 0.48) and China (Gini = 0.42) fall in between those seen at the extremes of India and South Africa.

Limited public health sector resources

In pursuit of rapid economic growth, these countries have leapt past the historical stages of state-led development in the global North which invested in substantial public infrastructure projects (533). The dominant economic strategy pursued by these countries has followed the Washington Consensus, to open borders to trade, privatize state-owned companies, deregulate the economy, and scale back public spending to make room for private sector development (see Chapter 2 for more details). This free-market economic model, most prominently applied in India and South Africa, and, to a lesser extent in Brazil, has rapidly transformed these societies' agricultural sectors to specialize in cash crops and introduce foreign-owned agricultural and mineral technologies.

Large segments of the population have lost agricultural jobs, and essentially been forced to migrate from impoverished rural settings to slum city-dwellings. This process of urbanization has been sped up by leaders of these countries, who intentionally direct public resources to urban settings (including China, India, and South Africa) to increase the pace of transformation. The downside is that this policy deprives rural areas of public health infrastructure, including doctors (leading to brain drain).

As a result of these major societal changes, in all five countries urban populations have been growing at a rate of about 1.5% per year (534). About one-third of the urban populations end up in slums (except for Mexico, where this figure is about one in six) (535). In China, for example, this pace of rural-urban flows means that about 12 million people each year move from the countryside to city slums.

Overall, this pattern of uneven development has resulted in a lack of basic amenities like modern sanitation, hygiene, and safe, paved roadways, while modern conveniences, such as cell phones, televisions, and cars, are abundant. For example, one report found that about half of India's population (560 million) were mobile phone subscribers, while only about one-third of India's population had access to proper toilets (536).

Relatively low political priority of chronic diseases

External health financing makes up only about 1% of total health spending in the five countries. Their budgetary decisions are less affected by potential donor distortions of health priorities (see Chapter 5.1). Nonetheless, one recent analysis of the budgets of two of them (Brazil and India) identified a similar misalignment in their budgets as was observed in health systems that strongly depend on donor financing. This finding reveals that donors are only one reason for the skew in budgetary allocations.

Government priorities are influenced by a combination of pressures from the global health community, pharmaceutical industry, and transnational advocacy moments, to name a few (537). Researchers analysing Brazil and India's budgetary patterns suggest that the HIV movement has led to a high budgetary priority on this one disease in particular. Overall about three-quarters of these two countries health budgets are allocated to infectious diseases (of which the vast majority goes to HIV/AIDS, followed by malaria and TB). For example, in Brazil in 2002, US$372 was spent per disability-adjusted life year lost due to HIV/AIDS as compared with $61.5 for each year lost due to CVD.

Irrespective of the reasons for a low political priority being placed on chronic diseases, the lack of public resources for health means that these governments have difficulty paying for doctors, medicines, clinics, and hospitals, and other key elements of a functioning chronic care system. Overall, the countries have very high chronic disease care needs, but few resources with which to serve their populations. An estimated 6–20 doctors work in these countries to serve 10,000 people, much lower than the number available to meet the health needs of high-income countries (where the burdens of chronic diseases are significantly lower).

Rising chronic diseases and risk factors but differing drivers between countries

Figure 7.1 shows the prevalence of the main chronic disease risk factors in the five countries. In each country, nearly all of the main risks for chronic diseases have been rising, with the exception of tobacco—reflecting the success of tobacco control measures, particularly the Framework Convention on Tobacco Control (FCTC). An estimated three out of every five Chinese men smoke, compared with less than one out of 20 women. Rates among men are much lower in the other countries, averaging about 21% in Brazil, India, and South Africa. Current rates of youth tobacco rates remain unacceptably high, on average greater than 20%. The highest rates occur in Mexico, of about 28%, and the lowest rates are in China, where 5% of adolescents between ages 13 and 15 report currently using tobacco (see Figure 1.5).

People's ways of living are becoming inactive. Humans were made for movement, but these societies are being engineered to be immobile. As measured in the World Health Survey 2003, physical inactivity levels (defined as not meeting any of the following three criteria: 3 or more days of vigorous activity of at least 20 minutes per day or 5 or more days of moderate-intensity activity or walking of at least 30 minutes per day, or 5 or more days of any combination of walking, moderate-intensity or vigorous intensity activities achieving a minimum of at least 600 MET-min/week) in the five countries range from 10.6% to 44.9% of the population. In China and India, only 10% and 12% of the population is physically inactive. People in Mexico and Brazil appear to be slightly more physically inactive. The worst physical inactivity rates occur South Africa, where nearly half of the population is physical inactive.

Diets are becoming less healthy, as markets integrate and mass quantities of Western foods flow into these countries. There is, however, considerable variation across countries, at least according to crude measures of food availability from the Food and Agricultural Organization (FAO). If all food were eaten, they would perfectly reflect consumption. Of course, this is not the case. They do, however, provide some of the only available data for assessing food trends over time. According to these data, during the period 1990–2005, dietary energy consumption (kcal per person per day) increased by 2–12% in the five countries (Figure 7.2). The portion of calories from fat rose rapidly, ranging from increases of 16% and 17% in Mexico and South Africa to 55% in China (538). In all countries, however, fruit and vegetable consumption is too low, with over 70% of the population consuming fewer than the recommended five servings of fruit and vegetables per day.

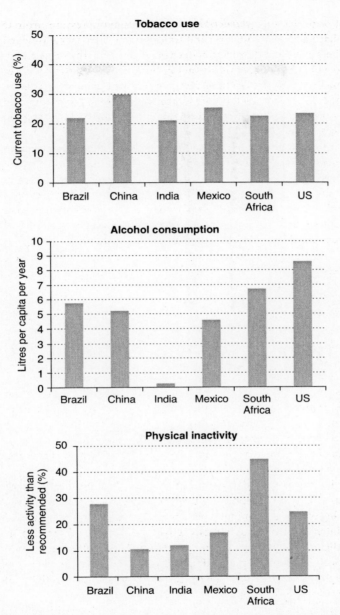

Fig. 7.1 Key risk factors by country, 2003. *Data source:* tobacco use, physical inactivity, and fruit and vegetable data are from WHO Health Survey 2003 (China data are from 2002) available at WHO Surf2 Global InfoBase (http://infobase.who.int). US data are from the WHO Statistical Surveillance System, available at http://www.who.int/whosis. Data are nationally representative. Tobacco use is defined as the percentage of the population who currently uses smoking tobacco products. Physical inactivity is defined as failing to meet any of the following three criteria: 3 or more days of vigorous activity of at least 20 minutes per day or 5 or more days of moderate-intensity activity or walking of at least 30 minutes per day or 5 or more days of any combination of walking, moderate-intensity or vigorous intensity activities achieving a minimum of at least 600 MET-min/week.

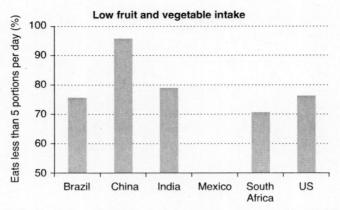

Fig. 7.1 (*Continued*) Inadequate fruit and vegetable consumption is defined as consuming less than five fruit and vegetable servings per day. Comparable data for Mexico is unavailable. Alcohol consumption refers to the per capita recorded alcohol consumption (litres of pure alcohol) among adults aged 15 years and older (2003), computed as the sum of alcohol production and imports, less alcohol exports, divided by the adult population (aged 15 years and older). Based on daily recommended allowance of 200 millilitres of pure alcohol (i.e. 2 units in the UK classification system) the yearly limit is about 7.3 litres.

However, these aggregate dietary trends mask important differences. In each chapter, the country authors reveal how these changes reflect a complex interplay of evolving trade and work patterns superimposed on historical and cultural legacies. This is highlighted by a comparison of changing dietary patterns in Mexico and China.

In both Mexico and China about one out of every 10 people have diabetes, and more than half of their populations are overweight or obese. But the main drivers of these chronic diseases are different. In Mexico, extensive trading with the US and resulting price changes has led to a situation where Coca-Cola is cheaper than milk. People drink considerable amounts of sugared beverages (especially fizzy drinks), which are proximal drivers of rising caloric intake, especially among youth. Fast-food plays an important role, albeit a less relevant one compared with the dietary changes provoked by the influx of Western supermarkets, such as 7–11 convenience stores and Walmart, alongside a sustained consumption of food from street carts and vendors.

China's dietary situation is markedly different from that of Mexico. Over the past decade, the portion of diet from fat rose to 55% (compared to 17% in Mexico), which resulted from a series of price changes that encouraged edible oils and fats (and their entry into processed foods). While people in China consume a similar amount of sugared beverages as they did a decade ago, they now eat outside of the home more frequently, and often in fast-food chains, especially Kentucky Fried Chicken and McDonald's. China's main drivers of obesity relate more greatly to fat than appears to be the case in Mexico.

At the time of writing, China has the greatest number of people living with diabetes of any country in the world (92.4 million, 60% of which are undiagnosed), followed closely by India (42 million) (539). In Mexico, diabetes has become the leading cause of death, reflecting an incredibly fast rise in obesity. In Mexico, 70% of adults are overweight adults, the second highest figure in the world only to the neighbouring US, with whom it trades food extensively. South African women have the highest rates of obesity (about 65% overweight, more than half of whom are obese; Figure 7.3), reflecting a culture that confers status and attractiveness on larger women's physiques. While rates of obesity are lower in India (about 15% overweight or obese),

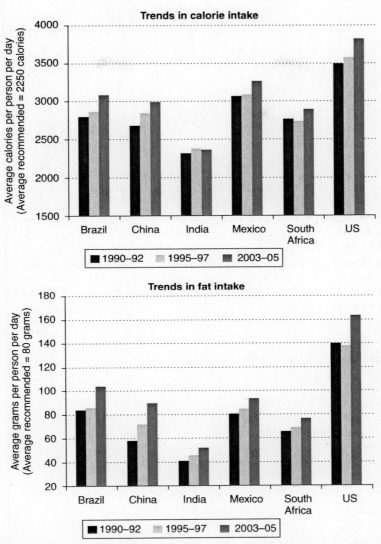

Fig. 7.2 Trends in dietary energy intake and dietary fat consumption, 1990–2005. *Note:* dietary energy and fat intake for all countries is from Food and Agriculture Organization Statistics Division, 2003–05. Dietary energy and fat intake refers to the amount of food available for human consumption as estimated by the FAO Food Balance Sheets. Actual food consumption may be lower because of food waste (e.g. uneaten foods, expired foods, fed to pets or thrown away).

about 6% have type 2 diabetes, reflecting the lower threshold of Asian populations for developing diabetes and other chronic diseases. Still, these estimates of diabetes prevalence are thought to be far too low, as in places like South Africa and India, where insulin is often unavailable, people die quickly.

These chapters are full of interesting examples that provide a sense of the commonalities, but important particularities, involved in these countries' epidemics. We encourage readers to pay careful attention to comparing and contrasting their descriptions with this in mind.

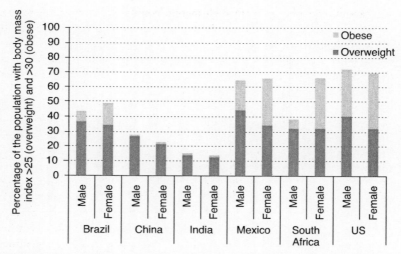

Fig. 7.3 Overweight and obesity by gender and country, 2003. *Source:* WHO Health Survey 2003 (China data is from 2002) available at WHO Surf2 Global InfoBase (http://infobase.who.int). Overweight is the prevalence of overweight (defined as ≥25 kg/m²) among individuals aged 15 years and above (2002). Obesity is the prevalence of obesity (defined as ≥30 kg/m²) among individuals aged 15 years and above (2002).

Difficulties adapting public health policies to community settings

Chapter 4 outlined promising, evidence-based intervention strategies at the individual and population level. However, since chronic diseases are deeply embedded in each of these country's social, cultural, economic, and political circumstances, we cannot simply expect a universal package of solutions to work across the board. Instead, leaders and people from these countries must be empowered to find and develop their own solutions, tailoring these evidence-based strategies to local needs and circumstances.

We spotlight one example of how a Western legal framework has helped provide scope for action, but is not sufficient to guarantee healthy development. Each of these countries is a signatory to the WHO's FCTC. Yet, despite agreeing to a framework that sets out a clear strategy of established methods for reducing tobacco use, managers of these countries have faced great difficult in implementing these policies. One common problem is that they do not account for the local context of tobacco use, production, and delivery.

In China, for example, a state-owned tobacco sector (which makes it easier to implement the FCTC's regulatory and taxation policies), appears to have maintained low smoking rates in children (about 5%, but this may be underestimated due to self-report). Nevertheless China has very high rates of adult tobacco use and relatively low taxation on cigarettes. On the other hand, Brazil's strong political leadership has enabled it to implement tobacco taxes in spite of a privately run tobacco industry and a greater reliance on tobacco farming to contribute to its exports. In all countries, the prices of cigarettes for the leading brand, typically Marlboro, is about US$1.50, which leaves considerable scope for taxation.

In India, tobacco use is very high; about one in five people smoke, and 25% of youth. The highest risks occur among the poor, who spend considerable fractions of their income on tobacco products. In this context, we might expect a tobacco tax and indoor smoking bans to be effective, as helped bring about reductions in many high-income countries. However, the most common tobacco product in India is the bidi (a hand-rolled cigarette) which is not covered by the FCTC. Even if it were, there would be little that could be done to tax these products. They are often made by local people, who sell them in carts and stalls on the streets. Their informal production and sale makes it nearly impossible to tax and regulate, making impotent the most powerful public health levers of intervention described in Chapter 4.

Similar quandaries arise in standard tools in the public health kit for addressing the much more complex issue of unhealthy diets. In Mexico, 80% of food sales are not in restaurants but from food carts, which produce fried foods very high in fat and salt content and are largely out of reach of government regulation. Additional complications arise in view of the fact that these carts are typically owned by low-income groups who rely on these foods for income. A simple strategy of trying to ban these carts would widen inequalities and poverty for many members of the population (as recently occurred in Egypt when it responded to Swine Flu outbreaks by killing pigs in cities, in so doing destroying a traditional way of living for urban pig farmers). In South Africa, about 20% of all snacks are from tax-paying food companies, creating greater potential for using a standard set of government regulations to encourage healthier dietary choices.

Combining global and local action to build capacity and raise priority

One source of fresh and innovative strategies that adapt to local needs while building on their communities' strengths and new technologies is coming from community-led interventions.

Brazil is one of the leaders in implementing community interventions to improve diet and physical activity. Their public health leaders are setting up collaborations across sectors, including health ministers, the food industry, researchers and the media to promote healthier urban-living environments. One particularly innovative community intervention, Agita São Paolo, has significantly increased physical activity (as also described in Chapter 4), while building healthier, more inclusive communities.

Much learning can be done from within these countries. Their large populations and federated structures offer the potential to identify successes and failures of their states' public health programmes. In India, Kerala and Chennai regions in particular have made significant progress in addressing chronic diseases (especially diabetes), but these successes have yet to be applied throughout the country, leaving considerable opportunities for improvement.

Raising the priority of chronic diseases and health within these countries is difficult in face of competing demands and overstretched public health practitioners. One possibility is to tap into resources available and rising interest levels from global institutions (540). These can build research networks that create opportunities for shared learning

We single out three examples: the United Healthcare/National Heart, Lung, and Blood Institute (UH/NHLBI) Collaborating Centres of Excellence, Community Interventions for Health (CIH), and the Guide to Obesity Prevention in Latin America and the US network.

In 2007, Ovations (a subsidiary of United Healthcare that services the health needs of people age 50 and older by providing health insurance and disease management services in the US) gave $15 million to set up research partnerships between high- and low-income countries (more recently, NHLBI in the US joined as a sponsor of the network). At the time of writing, there are 11 centres in Argentina, India, Pakistan, China, Kenya, South Africa, Tanzania, Tunisia, Mexico, Peru, and the Dominican Republic. As the authors note in the following chapters, the collaborating centres have begun to greatly help build local capacity for identifying and acting on certain chronic diseases, while using surveillance data to raise their political priority.

Another collaborative research network is the Oxford Health Alliance's Community Interventions for Health (CIH) programme (funded by the PepsiCo Foundation), which currently has sites in China, India, and Mexico, where local researchers are adapting evidence-based prevention strategies to local communities. CIH incorporates both research and action components, seeking to design, implement, and measure the effectiveness of interventions implemented in diverse settings across the global (see Chapter 4.2 for a more detailed discussion of CIH).

Another current international collaboration to build capacity on chronic diseases is the Guide to Obesity Prevention in Latin America and the US, a collaboration between the San Diego Prevention Research Center (SDPRC), the Mexican National Institute of Public Health (*Instituto Nacional de Salud Pública,* or INSP), and the US Centers for Disease Control and Prevention. These partnering arrangements were created to understand, assess and develop evidence-based strategies and recommendations to effectively prevent obesity in Latin-American communities and populations, living in both high- and middle-income settings.

These programmes are building research momentum. China and India are now home to the world's largest cohort studies, from randomized-controlled trials about the effects of multiple chronic disease drug interventions (the polypill) to community interventions to reduce behavioural risks of chronic diseases. One remaining challenge is to build a faster track between such academic research and its policy impact, rather than waiting decades for these research findings to be acted upon.

In closing, we note that the perspectives from these experts begin to shed light on what has been an overarching mystery of the first part of the book: why are rates of death and disability in these countries so much higher than rich countries in spite of their relatively low (albeit rapidly rising) rates of conventional risk factors such as tobacco, physical inactivity, unhealthy diet, and alcohol? As we saw in Chapter 1 in regard to COPD among women, the insights being provided by these authors force many of us to rethink our most basic approaches about how we act to address the chronic disease burden.

These countries have a critical window of opportunity before their high levels of risk manifest as additional deaths and suffering due to chronic diseases: there is still time to prevent a full-scale epidemic. In many respects, these countries cannot and should not look to the West for inspiration; in spite of some successes, their path largely reflects a model of how not to respond to the challenge of chronic disease. We look to these country experts as pioneers in developing sustainable, effective, locally responsive strategies to prevent chronic disease and promote development.

Part 1

Chronic diseases in Brazil

Victor K.R. Matsudo, Sandra M.M. Matsudo,
Tania Cavalcante, and Karen Siegel

Background

Brazil is a low-mortality, middle-income country with a population of about 192 million. Brazil has been described as three societies in one: a rich country about the size of Canada (about 40 million), a poor country whose population is about the size of Mexico (about 110 million), and a grossly impoverished country as about the size of Argentina (about 40 million) (276). The country comprises 26 socially, culturally, and ecologically diverse states including over 5000 municipalities.

Shortly after the transition back to democracy in 1985 (after alternating between dictatorship and democracy after independence in 1822), Brazil has gained economic and political stability. Poverty has fallen to about 7.5% of the population living on less than $1 per day in 2004, but inequality remains among the highest in the world. The richest quintile of Brazilians hold three-fifths of the country's income, while less than 3% goes to the poorest quintile (192).

Most of Brazil's population (70%) lives in the relatively industrialized Northeast and Southeast regions. The Northeast region is the poorest region (home to large African and indigenous populations), and contains most of Brazil's coffee-growing regions. In contrast, the Southeastern region, where 60% of industrial production occurs, is more developed, European-influenced, and slightly more affluent (541).

Brazil contains 13 mega-cities with over one million inhabitants, including São Paulo (18.8 million), Rio de Janeiro (11.4 million), and Brasilia (2.2 million). Approximately 30 million people migrated to cities between 1970 and 1990, seeking employment opportunities in the growing cities. Many did not find work, ending up in *favelas* (shanty towns, slums) (541). In 2008, 85.6% of Brazilians lived in urban areas, an estimated 29% of which (or 48 million people) resided in slums. Such a rapid increase in the amount of urban dwellers puts considerable strain on resources and infrastructure in urban areas that still persists today, while the urban population continues to grow at a rate of 1.5% per year (192). Crime, violence, and corruption are major problems, especially in these urban areas.

Brazil's economy is the largest in South America and the ninth largest in the world, and has grown at rates of up to 6.0% per year since 1992 (542). While much growth has been fuelled by the manufacturing and service sectors, the agricultural sector (consisting mainly of soy, coffee, sugar, beef, and chicken) remains an important part of the economy, accounting for 7% of GDP. Brazil is the largest sugar exporter, the second largest tobacco producer, and the largest tobacco exporter in the world.

Concurrent with these major societal changes, Brazil has experienced rapid population health changes. In 1950, about half of all deaths were among children under 15 while only one-sixth were among people 65 years or older. By 2000 the situation had reversed, so that about 17% of all deaths were among children and half were among people over age 65. Life expectancy at birth steadily improved from 51 years in 1950 to 68 years in 2000 (543).

Within the context of these transformations, this chapter describes the burden, drivers, and impacts of chronic diseases in Brazil and the responses by the health system, private sector, and government. The chapter concludes with a series of recommendations for reducing the avoidable burden of chronic diseases.

Evaluating the health burden of chronic diseases

Brazil is among only a few developing countries that has been collecting national-level surveillance data on chronic diseases for the past few decades. This section draws on these recently available national data and surveillance from the WHO to describe Brazil's chronic disease burden.

Over the past several decades chronic diseases have increased rapidly. In 2004, chronic diseases were estimated to cause 70.1% of all deaths in Brazil, approximately 30% of which were premature (366). Figure 7.4 shows the top 10 specific causes of burden of disease in Brazil. Of the chronic diseases, the leading causes of the burden (as measured in DALYs) were neuropsychiatric disorders in first place (18.6%), followed by CVDs (13.3%), chronic respiratory diseases (8.1%), muscle-skeletal diseases (5.5%), and diabetes mellitus (5.1%).

Brazil has among the highest prevalence of diabetes in Latin America. According to an international survey of adults between ages 20 and 79, about 6.0% of people in Brazil had type 2 diabetes. Forecasts suggest the current number of people living with diabetes will rise from 7.6 million to 12 million by 2030—twice the increased expected in the US.

Individual risk factors

Nearly all of the main risks of chronic diseases have risen, with the important exception of smoking. In 2005, the four leading clinical risk factors for chronic disease deaths were high blood pressure, high cholesterol, and overweight and obesity, causing 20%, 11%, and 6.5% of all deaths, respectively (182). Approximately 5–8% of the population has impaired glucose tolerance, a precursor to diabetes (544). Between 1975 and 2003, the prevalence of obesity (BMI >30 kg/m^2) increased from 2.7% to 8.8% among men and from 7.4% to 13% among women (255).

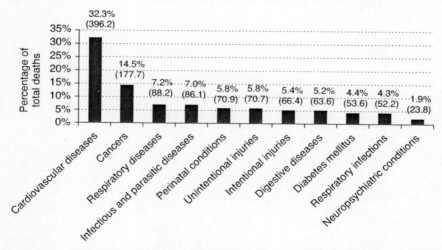

Fig. 7.4 Leading causes of death in Brazil, 2004. *Data source:* Global Burden of Disease 2009. *Note:* Data labels are percentage of total deaths (number of deaths).

Profound societal changes are also affecting children, and have significantly increased children's risk of obesity. In 2008/2009 studies of preschool and elementary students estimated the prevalence of obesity in urban areas to be 9% and 10.5%, respectively (545, 546).

Tobacco use has declined over the past two decades, from about one in three adults in 1989 to 15% in 2008. These declines have contributed to reductions in rates of cardiovascular deaths and lung cancer mortality, especially among men (547, 548). However, a delay in women's initiation of smoking has resulted in rising lung cancer rates among women (549). Reductions in tobacco have been the slowest among the rural, uneducated, and poorer segments of the population.

Physical activity levels, on the other hand, are rising. One-quarter of Brazil's population is physically inactive (as defined by IPAQ, described in the introduction to Chapter 7). One study conducted in Pelotas, Brazil, by Knuth and colleagues showed that the proportion of adults not exercising for at least 30 minutes per day, 5 times per week, increased from 41% in 2002 to 52% in 2007 (550).

Poor nutrition is a major problem in Brazil, and many are still underfed while a growing number consume an unhealthy diet high in fat, salt, and sugar (58). About 15.6 million people (9% of the population) are undernourished (551) while about four times as many are over nourished (40% of the population are overweight or obese). These conditions often coexist in the same household. One study found that 45% of households with an underweight member also had an overweight member (58).

Overall, food consumption patterns are shifting from traditional, simple diets to those higher in salt, fat, sugar, and processed foods. Between the early 1970s and 2003 a marked decline in consumption of rice and beans occurred while large increases occurred in consumption of processed foods (such as cookies and soft drinks), sugary products (including fizzy drinks), and meats (high in saturated fat) (552). Between 1998 and 2003, growth in the annual retail sales of soft drinks, breakfast cereals, and ready meals in Brazil was 5.9%, 8.9%, and 17.3%, respectively (460).

Consumption of fruits and vegetables, traditionally a core component of Brazilian diets, has also declined. The World Health Survey, conducted in 2003, found that about 40% of adults reported daily consumption of fruits and 30% reported daily consumption of vegetables (553), similar to other national surveys (554).

Air pollution is a major risk factor for chronic diseases, especially in Brazil's mega-cities. In São Paulo, for example, traffic congestion is a significant problem, and motor vehicles are estimated to cause 90% of the city's smog (541). While some of the higher income populations can afford to pay for indoor recreation facilities, poorer populations cannot, thus widening health inequalities.

Inequalities in chronic diseases and risk factors

Substantial inequalities exist in chronic disease deaths and disability rates. For instance, people living in urban areas consumed three times as many processed foods (ready-made meals and industrial mixes) as people living in rural settings.

Higher income groups also tend to have different clusters of risks than lower socioeconomic groups. Among higher-income families living in urban settings, excess calories came from higher intake of meat, dairy products, fruit, vegetables, and legumes, alcoholic beverages, condiments, and roots and tubercles. Consumption of basic foodstuffs such as rice declined markedly with rising income, while consumption of breads and cookies rose with income. Sugar consumption in the highest socioeconomic stratum was about half the level observed the lowest stratum. However, soft drink consumption rose at higher income levels. Overall, higher-income groups consumed five times as many soft drinks as the lowest-income group. Leisure-time physical activity is also strongly associated with income, particularly in urban settings: 26.3% of upper income

Table 7.2 Trends in % of foods and food groups in total calorie consumption, from household food purchase data, 1972/74 to 2003

Food groups	Survey year			
	1974/1975	1987/1988	1995/1996	2002/2003
Cereals and derivate products	37.3	34.7	35.0	35.3
White rice	19.1	16.2	16.0	14.7
Cookies	1.1	1.9	2.7	3.5
Beans and other legumes	8.1	5.9	5.7	5.7
Roots and tubercles	4.9	4.1	3.6	3.3
Meats	9.0	10.5	13.0	13.1
Beef	4.4	4.9	5.9	5.4
Poultry	1.6	2.5	3.4	3.2
Fish	0.8	0.6	0.6	0.5
Processed meats	1.1	1.5	2.5	3.0
Dairy products	5.9	8.0	8.2	8.1
Eggs	1.2	1.3	0.9	0.2
Fruit and natural juices	2.2	2.7	2.6	2.4
Vegetables and legumes	1.1	1.2	1.0	0.9
Vegetable oils and fats	11.6	14.6	12.6	13.5
Animal fats	3.0	1.0	0.8	1.1
Sugar	13.4	12.6	12.5	10.3
Soft drinks	0.4	0.9	1.4	2.1
Ready-made meals	1.3	1.6	1.5	2.3
Total calories (kcal/day per capita)	1,700	1,895	1,695	1,502

Source: adapted from (552).

urban women exercised on a weekly basis, compared to only 2.8% of lower income urban women (58, 555).

Women and men also have differing levels of risk. Results from VIGITEL, Brazil's nationally representative telephone health survey (2006), show that diabetes prevalence varies by gender (6% among women compared to 4.4% among men). Between 1989 and 1997, obesity increased significantly from 7.9% to 12.6% for low-income women, but declined from 12.8% to 9.2% (a 28% reduction) among women among high SES groups, especially in urban settings.

Obesity rates have risen more intensely in men than in women, in rural than in urban settings, and in low-income populations. Following physical activity trends, obesity has become concentrated in the poor. A particularly high rate of increase from 1975 to 1989 was noted among lower income families, with a 219% increase in numbers seen among men and a 227% increase among women. Between 1989 and 2003, obesity increased further among men (70% increase), but stayed virtually stable among the total female population, masking differences across income levels. Rising obesity have mostly occurred among low-income women, as decreases occur among higher-income women (255), consistent with patterns of a social transition observed elsewhere (see Chapter 2).

Societal determinants of chronic diseases

What are the underlying causes of these trends?

Economic drivers

In the 1990s, implementation of the Washington Consensus reforms to accelerate the deregulation, privatization and opening of the economy led to substantial transformations in Brazil's food and beverage and tobacco industries.

Subsidies and imports/exports have played a role in Brazil's evolving diet. For example, in the 1970s, policies were implemented to promote soybean production in Brazil, increasing the per capita availability of calories from soybean oil from 25.9 to 247.3 kcal per capita per day. As a result, consumption of animal fats was replaced by vegetable oils in margarines that, although healthier, led to increases in total fat content of the population's diet to close to 30% of total calories by 1988 (556).

An increase in foreign direct investment (FDI) in the food and supermarket industries is driving growing dependence on Western foods. Between 1984 and 1994, US FDI in the food processing industry doubled from $1 billion to $2 billion. An expression of this can be seen in the rising numbers of fast food chains in Brazil (including both Brazilian- and foreign-owned chains). In 1979, McDonald's opened a restaurant in Rio de Janeiro, making it the first fast-food chain to enter and remain in Brazil. Since that time sales have increased rapidly, making Brazil a key growth market. In 2002, McDonald's claimed 25% of Brazil's informal dining sector (consisting primarily of fast-food chains, hotdog vans, bakeries, cafeterias at Metro stations and other informal eateries) and was Brazil's leading private-sector employer, with 36,000 Brazilians (87% of which were under 21 years) on the payroll, and thus powerful influence, especially among adolescents (547). Burger King, KFC, Pizza Hut, Domino's, and Arby's also now have a presence throughout Brazil.

Even when people eat at home, foods are provided through foreign-owned supermarkets. In 1990, there were 14,000 supermarkets (defined as having two or more cash registers); by 2000, supermarket sales in the country's 24,000 supermarkets accounted for 75% of the country's total food retail. The five leading supermarket chains controlled 47% of supermarket sales (91% of which were foreign multinational chains, such as Ahold, Carrefour, Walmart, and the French-owned Casino) (558).

Despite being the second largest producer of tobacco leaves and the world's leading tobacco exporter, Brazil has implemented taxation of tobacco (although prices of cigarettes are still relatively low compared with the US and UK). However, tobacco smuggling is increasingly being used as a way to circumvent taxes, while policies of deregulation have weakened the state's capacity to curb this illegal activity. Thus, although legal cigarette consumption has decreased, illegal consumption (via smuggling, tax evasion, or counterfeiting) has increased (549). Youth are particularly at higher-risk of initiating smoking as a result of this illicit drug trade.

Political drivers

Despite increasing FDI, Brazil's economy is still relatively closed, with the value of imports and exports approximately 28% of GDP (only 1% lower than the US), compared to China, India, Mexico, and South Africa, where the value of imports and exports ranges from 54–76% of GDP.

Its global political engagement largely reflects the financial interests of its most powerful corporations. For example, the sugar industry exerts powerful influence on its politics, and in 2004 led the attempts to block the WHO Global Strategy on Diet and Physical Activity, which called for reducing sugar consumption as a means of preventing chronic disease (460).

The tobacco industry also exerts significant power in Brazil. In the main tobacco-producing states (in Brazil's Southern region), tobacco companies receive tax incentives from local government and election campaigns are usually financed by tobacco companies (559, 560). This leads to the significant undermining of tobacco control policies.

Social and cultural drivers

Poverty has shifted from rural to urban settings, largely due to massive migration to cities between 1970 and the 1990s. The majority of these migrants ended up in *favelas* (slums), which still remain. In major cities like Rio de Janeiro and São Paulo, 20–30% of the population live in *favelas*. About 29% of all city dwellers live in slums.

These cities also lack green space, pavements, or bike lanes. Gang violence, especially in resource-deprived areas that frequently lack sufficient police officers, prevents people from using what facilities are available. Unsurprisingly, higher-income groups report more physical activity.

Culture also plays a role. In Brazilian, thinness among women is a sign of affluence and status (in contrast to China, India, and South Africa, where being overweight is a sign of prosperity, success, and happiness). This cultural aspect may play a role in declining obesity rates among higher-educated women (561).

Social and economic consequences of chronic disease

Rising chronic diseases places high costs on resource-poor health system and threatens to undermine Brazil's economic growth.

Health system costs

Unhealthy patterns of ageing will put enormous strain on the healthcare system and on their families. The costs of caring for people with diabetes are currently estimated to be US$3.9 billion (178). From 1996 to 2005, smoking was the cause of over 1 million hospitalizations, costing approximately US$0.5 billion (549). In 2001, the burden of hospitalizations due to overweight and obesity (among adults aged 20 to 60 years) in Brazil represented 3.02% of total hospitalization costs for men and 5.83% of hospitalization costs for women, corresponding to 6.8 and 9.3% of all hospitalization (562)

Labour market costs

People living in Brazil who suffer from chronic conditions are less productive at work, more likely to take sick leave, and at risk of dying prematurely during prime working years. One study estimated that these risks would cost about International $49.2 billion of Brazil's national income (2.5% of GDP) will be lost as a result of disability and premature death from heart disease, stroke, and diabetes from 2005–2015. Rises in CVD projected to be highly concentrated in working age-groups will pose a threat to Brazil's economic productivity (563).

Management and prevention of chronic disease

How is the government responding to the risks of chronic diseases?

Health system capacity for chronic disease prevention and control

Brazil's national health system, the Unified Health System ('Sistema Único de Saúde'), was established through the Federal Constitution in 1988. The system is based on decentralized universal access, with municipalities financed by the states and the federal government in order to provide comprehensive and free care to all individuals, either through public providers or private providers

Table 7.3 Brazil's budgetary allocations for health form 2001 to 2006

		Budgetary allocations					
	DALYs	2001	2002	2003	2004	2005	2006
Neuropsychiatric disease	4,337	0.89	14.4	19.7	0.49	0.24	0.11
Cardiovascular disease	2,537	23	22.3	61.5	n/a	n/a	n/a
Unintentional injury	1,542	7.0	7.1	7.7	8.9	9.6	n/a
HIV/AIDs	229	353.7	433.5	372.2	475.5	508.6	705.9
TB	164	n/a	10.8	9.5	16.2	24.3	26
Malaria	22	42.2	21.4	40.7	37.5	36.8	35.4

Source: (537). Note: Numbers are in millions of $US, and do not comprise the government's total budgetary allocations for health. DALYs are disability-adjusted life years in 2001 (WHO).

reimbursed by the government. In 2008, about three-quarters of the population received care from the system (564). The annual overall government health budget is US$23 billion; around US$3.5 billion are allocated to primary health care.

Yet, despite their large burden, chronic diseases receive low priority. A 2010 study revealed that the federal government of Brazil gives a low priority to chronic diseases, which receive the lowest amounts of federal funding despite contributing the most to the disease burden (537) (Table 7.3).

There are signs of progress. In 2001, a national screening campaign for hypertension and diabetes, run jointly by public health, primary care medical professionals, and the media, occurred (564). During the campaign, 73% of the Brazilian adult population 40 years or older (22.1 million individuals) were screened. The national screening in itself served as an effective communication tool, raising awareness of diabetes and hypertension via a mass media campaign. The government's nutritional guidelines were also incorporated into a self-reported questionnaire for evaluating diet. More recently, the Brazilian Ministry of Health (MOH) and the World Bank have together provided approximately $500 million for public health infrastructure work of the last decade.

Fiscal and regulatory interventions

Brazil has been a leader in implementing tobacco bans and regulating false information. In 2001 Brazil was the first country to ban the use of misleading descriptors such as 'light' and 'mild' from cigarette packages. It also implemented a law requiring cigarette manufacturers to cover at least 100% of one of the two main sides of a cigarette package with warnings showing graphic images of advanced stages of tobacco-related illnesses (565). Public health education campaigns in schools and workplaces nationwide have helped raise awareness of the adverse health effects of smoking. Clinics offer free treatment for nicotine dependence in the public health system. Advertising in mass media, sponsorship of arts and sport events by tobacco products have also been banned, although advertising at point of sales. Smoking is also prohibited in enclosed public places, such as in schools, on public transportation, and in movie theatres, but federal legislation still allows smoking in designated areas (59).

Comprehensive tobacco control requires both supply- and demand-side policies. Despite evidence that raising price could decrease tobacco use, cigarette prices in Brazil remain low. A World Bank report found that the last steep drop in tobacco use, when consumption dropped by about one-fifth, occurred as a direct consequence of increasing the real price by 78.6% between 1991 and 1993 (justified as a strategy to raise government revenue in the 90s) (549, 565).

As mentioned above, illicit tobacco trade is a growing problem. To address problem, the Ministry of Finance, as part of the National Commission for FCTC Implementation, is working to increase cigarette taxes while simultaneously tackling the illegal cigarette market in Brazil, in collaboration with the Ministry of Justice. Since 1999, the main taxation on cigarettes increased 118% (62% of this increase was implemented in 2007 and 2008, and increased the price of cigarettes by 24%), generating approximately US$2.2 billion in government income in 2008 (549). The Ministry of Finance (in partnership with federal policy) is seeking ways to tackle the illegal tobacco market (566). Solutions include the required license of manufacturers and a national monitoring system that uses automatic counters on production lines and a digital tax-stamp system (developed in collaboration with the Brazilian Mint) that uniquely codes each cigarette package and easily distinguishes fake cigarettes (567).

In 2000 Brazil implemented the national food and nutrition policy, bringing together the MOH, Brazilian civil society and relevant governmental organizations, such as economic, agricultural, education, and law sectors (568). Through the policy, new food guidelines were implemented in 2000/2001, focusing on an easy, step-by-step approach to healthy eating with the goal of 'promoting, protecting, and supporting eating practices and lifestyles conducive to optimum nutritional and health status for all'.

The nutrition labelling and claims regulation mandates all packaged foods in Brazil to display calories, protein, carbohydrates, total fats, saturated fats, cholesterol, calcium, iron, sodium, and dietary fibre in 'standardized, consumer-friendly tables' (568). The regulation also introduced 'nutritionally adequate serving sizes,' for the first time in the world, as an effective way of reinforcing unbalanced eating patterns. A recent survey found that consumers appreciate the labelling and were able to use it effectively to make healthier choices. Currently, the MOH is reviewing legislation in regards to food advertisements directed at children, a first and mandatory step in establishing nutrition claims, codes for marketing unhealthy foods, and encouraging consumers to make better food choices (568).

Another part of the national programme mandated that 'a minimum of 70% of the [school food] program's annual budget of about US$500 million is spent on fresh vegetables, fruits and minimally processed foods, preferably purchased from local producers and cooperatives of small farmers' (568).

To support these efforts, the MOH has created a national TV channel to train elementary school teachers in a broad range of topics such as healthy eating and proper nutrition. Videos, aimed at schoolchildren and emphasizing regional food culture in Brazil, are broadcast every two months and reach approximately 37 million schoolchildren (568). A manual entitled *Brazilian Regional Foods* was released by the MOH in November 2001, and included descriptions and photographs of various plants found throughout Brazil, with the specific aim of reintroducing traditional foods into diets.

Urban planning and transportation policies

City planning has also taken proactive steps to increase walking and bicycling. As described in Chapter 4, city planners in Curitiba developed a groundbreaking plan in 1965 to build an efficient system of express buses and minibuses. As a result, petrol use is about 30% lower per capita than the rest of Brazil, despite high levels of car ownership. Curitiba's strategy is viewed as an international model for increasing public transport, reducing auto use, and increasing walking through active transport.

Community Interventions

Community health workers play a key role in interventions to promote health.

One example of Brazil's community health promotion strategy is the Family Health Programme, launched in 1994. About 60% of the government's primary health care budget is used to support it. The programme utilizes 27,000 teams of community health workers (Family Health teams comprised of *agents de saúde*) who each provide a range of health care to up to 2000 families (about 10,000 people) in their homes, clinics, and at hospitals in nearly all 5560 of Brazil's municipalities. These family health teams include doctors, nurses, dentists, and other health workers who try to ensure that the poor use and benefit from the services offered through the health system. Community participation is central to the health system's success; the decentralized, state and federally-funded system allows individual municipalities to transform their health services depending on patient needs.

Local communities are also working to encourage healthy eating and physical activity. One such example is Healthy Rio, which encourages physical activity by closing certain streets to traffic each night so that people may exercise safely in the streets. The municipality of Rio de Janeiro passed an innovative law in 1998 to establish 'healthy streets', as selected by local communities. Traffic is interrupted on healthy streets and public security provided so that people can exercise in safe conditions (568). Healthy Rio also promotes healthful cooking among professional chefs in collaboration with the MOH and some of the finest restaurants in Rio de Janeiro.

One major population-level physical activity intervention in Brazil is Agita São Paulo, which was the first consistent mass intervention to increase physical activity and reduce obesity in Brazil (292). The programme, launched in 1997, is a comprehensive intervention targeting schools (particularly elementary schools), worksites (including white and blue collar workers), older adults, and involving 350 partner organizations and communities across the state of São Paulo. The main goal is to increase physical activity by 30 minutes of moderate physical activity at least five times per week, through leisure time physical activity, active transportation (walking, cycling, and taking the stairs), and in the home (during chores and gardening). Key aspects included a research centre leading the process, scientific and institutional partnerships, community empowerment and inclusion, media and social marketing, and strong links to Brazilian culture (292) (see Chapter 4 for additional information and details).

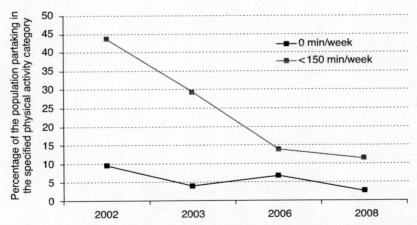

Fig. 7.5 Trends in physical inactivity categories in the state of Sao Paulo, Brazil (2002–2008). *Source:* authors. *Note:* Physical activity was measured using the short version of the International Physical Activity Questionnaire (IPAQ) and includes leisure-time and work-related physical activity. Separate weekly scores of walking, moderate- and vigorous-intensity physical activity practice were generated; cut-off points of 0 and 150 minutes/week were used.

To date, Agita has inspired physical activity programmes at the national and international level, and is now recognized as a model for promoting physical activity around the world. Agita assumes the strategic role of continental (Physical Activity Network of Americas—RAFA/PANA) and world (Agita Mundo) networks. The Agita Mundo network comprises over 270 institutions in 72 countries in the five continents, and celebrates yearly the World Day for Physical Activity in April, which involves around 2500 events every year.

Similarly, a municipal experiment to increase physical activity (Academia da Cidade, ACP) is underway in Recife, a large port city in Northeast Brazil. The programme encourages physical activity through counselling and increased knowledge about its importance, and also offers programmes for physical activity in communities during key hours like early morning and evening. A 2009 evaluation of the programme found it to be an effective public health strategy to increase population-level physical activity in urban developing settings (569). Similar community-level physical activity efforts are underway in Aracaju, Vitoria, and Curitiba.

Role of the private sector

Tobacco companies in Brazil continue to thwart anti-tobacco legislation. As mentioned above, national legislation to ban designated smoking areas in public places has been proposed. Several states and municipalities, while waiting for a court decision, passed bans on designated smoking areas at the local level. Now, the tobacco industry (and more recently the hospitality industry) is pursuing legal action against the state laws, arguing that they undermine Brazil's Federal Constitution since they are more restrictive than national policy. Defendants of state legislation argue that, in health and environment matters, state or municipal law can be more restrictive than the federal law.

Similar tactics to avoid formal control are currently being used by the food industry. Although the Brazilian food trade association responded positively to the recent MOH proposal to regulate advertising and marketing of food and non-alcoholic drinks, the industry later claimed that any statutory regulation would be illegal, infringing upon commercial freedom principles, and have threatened to appeal to the Brazilian Supreme Court if the government persists in enacting such legislation (460).

According to a 2009 audit, transnational companies are not following their own voluntary codes in Brazil. For example, nine out of 12 companies (Burger King, Cadbury Adams, Coca-Cola, Danone, Ferrero, Kraft Foods, McDonald's, Nestlé, and PepsiCo) that were monitored were found to not be following their own codes (460).

Still, there are some positive signs of food industry engagement. For example, the food industry has collaborated with the MOH on the nutrition labelling regulation in 2000 in 'the most participatory and co-operative processes involving government and the private sector ever accomplished' (568).

The media has also been instrumental in transforming health in Brazil, mainly by helping to disseminate information about healthy eating. Newspapers, magazines, and television programmes have dedicated a time and a space for 'services to the public', and studies have found that these messages are well-received by the public, making it easy to forge new partnerships between health officials, government, and the commercial media sector (568).

Recommendations

Brazil is undergoing profound societal transformations that are changing the ways in which people live and eat, and resulting in a rapid increase in chronic diseases. Although the government has responded more strongly and in a more coordinated way than many countries, there is still more that can be done to ensure its future sustainability both in economic and human development. Concerted efforts and multipronged approaches from many different sectors of society, both nationally and internationally, are required to turn the tide of escalating chronic disease rates.

Global government has a role to play in ensuring that trade policies and investments seek to promote health as much as possible. As Brazil's economy continues to grow, increased trade, investment, and communications are flowing into and out of the country, exposing the population mainly to unhealthy foods and lifestyles. Efforts could be made to ensure that Brazil's policies of trade openness and market integration seek to promote, rather than harm, health.

National government has a role to play in seeing that efforts to promote physical activity—and healthy eating—are more equitably distributed throughout the population. For example the Family Farming Food Acquisition Programme (implemented as part of the Zero Hunger Programme), encourages the government to purchase food produced by family farms. The programme ensures food supplies for poor families, school meals, and public hospitals, while at the same time creating a market for the small farming sector (556). The programme has had a reported large impact in the poorest regions in Northeastern Brazil, but could be expanded to encourage more healthy fruit and vegetable consumption.

The private sector was a partner in Brazil's national food and nutrition policy in 2000, but more recent action has highlighted persisting barriers to full engagement. In addition to the ongoing educational and informational food and nutrition interventions, better dietary habits could be achieved through greater availability, accessibility, and affordability of healthier foods lower in fats, salt and sugars. While some voluntary private sector action has occurred, legislation could help to encourage the food industry to do more in Brazil.

Brazil's government has already taken important steps towards preventing and controlling chronic diseases through national policy efforts and awareness campaigns. Significant capacity exists for preventing and controlling chronic diseases through the MOH, IGBE, the National Cancer Institute (INCA), a growing body of chronic disease researchers, and the private sector. As noted above, a 2010 study revealed a misalignment in government funding and those diseases placing the largest burden (537). Brazil is relatively donor-independent, receiving a small amount of external resources for health (only 0.24% of total health expenditure, on average, from 1995–2006); this suggests that the federal government has a role to play in scaling-up funding for chronic diseases. Brazil is a country long associated with powerful social movements and sustainable development (it hosted the first Earth Summit in 1992 and convened first World Social Forum in 2001), indicating the potential for increased prioritization through engaging with civil society and with the environmental movement on many drivers of chronic disease.

Summary points

1 Rapid social and economic transformations have led to lifestyle changes that are driving increasing rates of obesity and chronic diseases, especially among resource-deprived populations.

2 Overall rates of obesity are rising, but rates are rising fastest among the poor, among men, and among rural populations.

3 Traditional diets (primarily composed of beans and rice) are being replaced with diets high in fat, sugar, and salt, especially among high-income persons living in urban areas.

4 Physical activity rates are declining, with evidence showing that physical activity levels are declining at a faster rate among the poor, in accordance with obesity rates.

5 Most national policy interventions have focused on changing individual behaviours through education and information campaigns.

6 The most successful interventions have been population-wide, such as Agita São Paulo, but they have as yet failed to reach the lower socioeconomic groups to the same extent as richer populations.

7 Tobacco control policies that include a set of measures targeting individual level, social, and public policy level have decreased national smoking prevalence and mortality from lung cancer, but challenges still remain for reaching rural areas and lower socioeconomic groups, increasing cigarette prices, and protecting the policy from tobacco industry interference.

8 Despite being a major tobacco exporter, Brazil has successfully implemented comprehensive tobacco regulation resulting in marked reductions in tobacco use. Nonetheless, cigarette prices remain relatively low (about US$1.04 per pack of Marlboro), indicating scope for further raising taxes.

Acknowledgements

The authors would like to express the gratitude to the collaboration of Timoteo Leandro Araujo, Luis Carlos de Oliveira, José da Silva Guedes, Glaucia Braggion, Rosemeire Villamarin, Leonardo da Silva, and Mauricio dos Santos.

Part 2

Chronic diseases in China

Lijing L. Yan, Yubei Huang, Chen Ying, and
Yangfeng Wu

Background

The People's Republic of China (PRC) contains one-sixth of the world's population (over 1.3 billion people). The majority of the population is Han Chinese (92%) and there are other 55 ethnic groups; the official language is Mandarin Chinese (570).

China's economy combines planned and market elements, a 'dual-track' system with greater fractions of state ownership of enterprises. In 1978, a gradual process of reform began to transform and open the economy to trade and foreign investment, allowing village-township enterprises to earn profits. The transition process continued in the 1990s, when government agencies dismantled the 'iron rice bowl' system that provided employment benefits and guarantees for most urban dwellers. As a result of these and other reforms, China has recorded the world's fastest rates of economic growth over the past two decades, averaging over 10% per year. By 2008, GDP (PPP) per capita reached International $5962, making China the fourth largest economy in the world (532).

These free-market reforms helped lift an estimated 400 million people out of poverty (571). However, in 2004, 9.9% of the population was still living below the poverty line (on less than $1 per day) (192). Geographically, the poorest members of the population tend to be concentrated in the relatively rural western provinces, while the wealthy tend to live along coastal regions. Individuals living in rural areas still have relatively low income, literacy, education, and access to healthcare compared to urban residents.

Driving massive flows of people to the cities, China's economy is shifting from agrarian production to manufacturing. In 2008, the shrinking agricultural sector composed 11% of the economy, while the growing service and manufacturing sectors contributed 40% and 48% (570). Previously nearly self-sufficient in agriculture, China now relies increasingly on imports of grains, edible oils, and other resources to feed its large population (572).

From 1955–1978, China reversed its image of being the 'sick man of Asia' in part by developing a system of basic healthcare that covered 90% of the population (573). Citizens are living longer as mortality rates continue to fall. Before 1949, life expectancy at birth was only 35 years; today, it is 73 years (574). Despite continuing problems to control TB, hepatitis, HIV/AIDS, and some childhood conditions, the burden of disease in China is now dominated by premature adult mortality from chronic diseases.

This chapter highlights the escalating burden of chronic diseases in China as it undergoes these societal, economic, and political changes and discusses the responses by the health system, private sector, and government. The chapter concludes with recommendations for reducing the avoidable burden of chronic diseases.

Evaluating the health burden of chronic diseases

Marked changes in socioeconomic, environment, lifestyle, nutrition, and healthcare situation have also resulted in rising risks of NCDs (239, 570, 575). In this section, the most recent national data available are used, although quality of data varies and not all series of data are comparable across different time periods.

Over the past several decades chronic diseases have increased at a rate faster than in Western countries. In 2008, chronic diseases account for an estimated four out of five deaths in China each year (Figure 7.6), amounting to approximately 7 million deaths. Approximately 20% of these are estimated to have been premature (i.e. before age 70). Figure 7.7 shows data on morbidity rate and hospitalization rate (per 1000 individuals) by major disease categories from the most recent National Health Services Surveys—1993, 1998, 2003, and 2008. While morbidity and hospitalization rates due to infectious diseases dropped, rates for all other major NCDs rose significantly (with the exception of morbidity due to COPD, possibly due to declining smoking rates and improved living conditions) (576).

The most recent national survey in 2007–08 reported (539) that 9.7% of adults 20 years or older (92 million individuals) now have diabetes, an increase from 2.6% in adults over 18 years in 2002 (577). Although incomparable methodologies may in part explain this difference, there is no question that diabetes is increasing rapidly in China, especially in cities.

According to a projection published in 2010, annual cardiovascular events in Chinese adults aged 35–84 years will increase by >50% between 2010 and 2030, based on population ageing and growth alone. Projected trends in risk factors (increases in blood pressure, total cholesterol, and diabetes, and decline in smoking) would increase annual events by an additional 23%, an increase of approximately 21.3 million cardiovascular events and 7.7 million cardiovascular deaths (578).

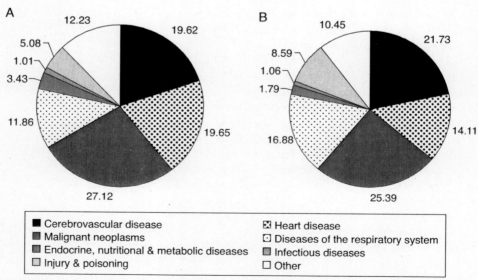

Fig. 7.6 Proportion of major causes of death among urban areas (A) and rural areas (B) in China, 2008. *Source: China Health Statistics Yearbook, 2009.*

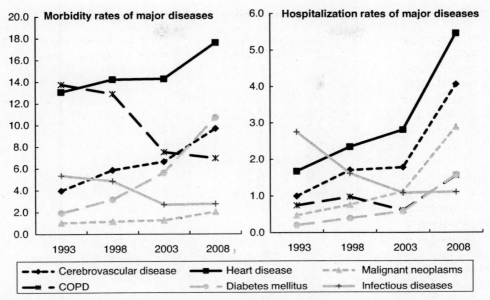

Fig. 7.7 Morbidity rates of major diseases (1/1000) and hospitalization rates of major diseases (1/1000) in China, 1983–2008.
Note: Morbidity rates of NCDs are defined as the ratio of the total number of being any NCDs half of year before investigation to the total number of the investigated population. Hospitalization rates are defined as the ratio of total number of hospitalization per year to the total number of the investigated population. *Sources:* China National Health Service Survey, 1993, 1998, 2003, 2008.

Individual risk factors

The main individual causes of rising chronic diseases are a combination of unhealthy diet (excess fat, salt), physical inactivity, tobacco use, and air pollution. Nearly all of these main risks of chronic diseases have risen, with the important exception of smoking. Between 2002 and 2006 there was a 20% increase recorded in the amount of people with hypertension, dyslipidaemia, overweight/obesity, or diabetes (Figure 7.8). Part of this rise could result from improvements in diagnostic capabilities that enable more precise measurements and thus more cases identified, but at most, this detection is likely to account for a small fraction of the changes.

In less than 20 years, the prevalence of overweight and obesity among school-aged children (aged 7–18 years) has increased more than tenfold. Between 1985 and 2002 prevalence of overweight increased from 1.2% to 16.7% among males and from 1.4% to 9.6% among females, while prevalence of obesity increased from 0.2% to 9.6% among males and from 0.1% to 6.5% among females.

Smoking prevalence has declined from 35.8% in 2002 to 25.1% in 2008. Nonetheless, it remains heavily concentrated in men, as in 2008, 48.0% of men and 2.6% of women smoked. Concerns remain that increases in prevalence of tobacco use will soon occur among women. In 2005, an estimated 673,000 deaths were attributable to smoking in China: 538,000 among men and 135,000 among women (579). But this number may greatly underestimate the deaths attributable to smoking in China comparing to the number of 1 million deaths per year estimated by Liu, and nearly another 0.1 million deaths caused by passive smoking (580, 581).

Diets have shifted from traditional Chinese staples to a more modern, complex diet, as shown in Table 7.4. From 1982 to 2002, energy intake from cereal and vegetable/fruit decreased slightly

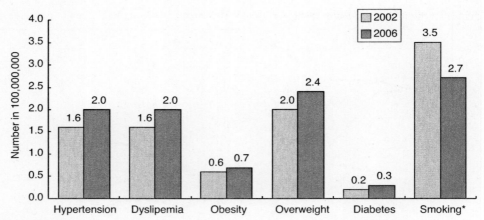

Fig. 7.8 Number of people affected by key risk factors in China, 2002–2006. *Source: Report on Chronic Disease in China* (2006). Data of the smoking were for year 2002 (China's 'Smoking & Health' Report, 2006) and 2008 (An Analysis Report of National Health Services Survey in China, 2008). *Note:* hypertension is defined as having a systolic blood pressures ≥140 mmHg and a diastolic blood pressure ≥90 mmHg. Dyslipaemia is defined as that there is any one of following three syndromes, including high total cholesterol (high TC—defined as a total cholesterol ≥5.72 mmol/L), high triglyceride (high TG—defined as a triglyceride ≥1.70 mmol/L) and low high-density lipoprotein (low HDL—defined as high density lipoprotein ≤0.91 mmol/L). Overweight is defined as having a BMI ≥24 kg/m² and <28 kg/m². Obesity is defined as having a BMI ≥28 kg/m². Diabetes is defined as having any one of the following: fasting glucose ≥7.0 mmol/L; 2-hour glucose level in the oral glucose-tolerance test ≥11.1 mmol/L; diagnosed as diabetes in a city (or higher-tier) hospital and being in treatment. Impaired fasting glucose is defined as having a fasting glucose ≥6.1 mmol/L but <7.0 mmol/L. Smoking status is defined as having at least one cigarette every day for at least 6 months for persons aged ≥20 years, and at least one cigarette every week for at least 3 months for persons aged 15–19 years.

while intake of milk, bean, egg, meat, and oils more than doubled (239). These increases occurred in both urban and rural areas but were more pronounced in urban areas. Despite a small decrease in average salt consumption, levels are still double the recommended amount of daily intake (12.0 g/day).

Physical activity has dropped, especially in rural areas (582). In 2002, only 15.1% of urban Chinese adults exercised regularly (239). Among Chinese adults aged 18 and over, average time spent on sedentary activities was 2.5 hours/day, higher in men (2.7 hours/day) than in women (2.4 hours/day), and higher in urban residents (3.2 hours/day) than in rural ones (2.2 hours/day) (583).

Inequalities in chronic diseases and risk factors

In China, marked health inequalities exist across urban/rural areas, by gender, education, and occupation level, suggesting their social causation, and that they are thus avoidable.

In the 1980s, rural areas had lower rates of major chronic diseases except respiratory disease. Age-standardized mortality rates per 100,000 individuals in 1990 and 2008 clearly reveal that in less than 20 years, a dramatic shift has occurred (Table 7.5), most likely due to a more rapid shift toward unhealthy lifestyle in rural areas. In 2008, the rates of all four major categories of chronic diseases in rural areas surpassed those of urban areas for both men and women. This likely reflects

Table 7.4 Average food intakes (in grams) in China, 1982–2002

	Urban			Rural			Total		
	1982	1992	2002	1982	1992	2002	1982	1992	2002
Cereal	459.0	405.4	366.0	531.0	485.8	416.1	509.7	439.9	402.1
Vegetable and fruit	370.3	399.4	321.3	346.4	338.7	321.2	353.5	359.5	321.2
Milk, bean, egg products	31.5	67.8	101.6	21.2	16.6	36.2	24.3	34.2	54.4
Meat	83.6	144.7	149.4	29.1	56.8	92.4	45.3	86.4	108.2
Edible oil	25.8	36.9	44.0	14.9	25.6	40.7	18.2	29.5	41.6
Starch and sugar*	10.7	7.7	5.2	3.1	3.0	4.1	5.4	4.7	4.4
Overall energy intake†	2450.0	2394.6	2134.0	2509.0	2294.0	2295.5	2491.3	2328.3	2250.5
Salt	11.4	13.3	10.9	13.2	13.9	12.4	12.7	13.9	12.0

Source: 1982 China National Nutrition Survey (1982 CNNS), 1992 China National Nutrition Survey (1992 CNNS) and 2002 China National Nutrition and Health Survey (2002 CNNHS).
Note: *, Gram per person per day; †, kcal per person per day. And the average overall energy intake in 1959 is 2060 kcal per person per day, coming from 1996 Chinese Health Statistical Digest.

Table 7.5 Age-standardized mortality rate per 100,000 population of major chronic diseases by gender and residence, China, 1990 and 2008

	1990		2008	
	Male	Female	Male	Female
Urban areas				
Cerebrovascular disease	102.07	76.66	131.81	94.78
Heart disease	73.66	60.39	130.13	99.90
Malignant neoplasms	122.12	73.64	201.48	111.37
Diseases of the respiratory system	81.78	57.76	91.87	52.85
Endocrine, nutritional, and metabolic diseases	7.16	8.90	1.99	1.50
Infectious diseases	22.09	10.78	8.15	3.53
Injury and poisoning	41.04	28.55	38.09	21.75
Rural areas				
Cerebrovascular disease	91.31	64.35	217.07	143.61
Heart disease	58.46	46.49	140.35	98.41
Malignant neoplasms	123.92	64.05	267.83	121.22
Diseases of the respiratory system	145.97	105.73	182.95	111.10
Endocrine, nutritional, and metabolic diseases	4.41	5.45	1.43	1.05
Infectious diseases	39.21	22.13	11.29	4.69
Injury and poisoning	73.68	53.18	78.37	41.79

Source: China Health Statistics Yearbook, 2009.

inequalities in healthcare access as well as a larger change from a relatively healthier, traditional Chinese diet before to a less healthy one.

Women generally have lower rates of chronic diseases than men. Rates of chronic diseases are increasing for both men and women, but they have risen faster among men, leading to a widening gender gap difference. Men continue to have greater rates of hypertension, dyslipaemia, high triglyceride (high TG), low high-density lipoprotein (low HDL), overweight and smoking. Women, on the other hand, have greater prevalence of high total cholesterol (high TC), obesity, and diabetes (239).

Societal determinants of chronic diseases

A combination of social, cultural, economic, political, and environmental transformations have increased risks of chronic diseases.

Social drivers

With rapid development in medical technology and implementation of the One-Child Policy, China is experiencing a dramatic rise in the number and proportion of the elderly. In 1953, 4.4% of the population was 65 years or older; this increased to 8.3% by 2008 (584). Current trends suggest it could reach 20% by 2040 (239).

Chinese economic strategists encourage planners to accelerate urbanization as a means to economic growth, a strategy also being applied in India and South Africa (see Chapters 7.3 and 7.5). From 1978–2008, the percentage of people living in urban areas in China increased from 17.9% to 43.1% (584) and it is estimated to jump to 59.5% by 2030 (585). As described in Chapter 2, cities increase exposure to chronic disease risks. In China in particular, the city-centred economy encourages a faster lifestyle revolving around a work-life, in which people choose fast-food over healthier sit-down meals, and lack time to be physically active.

Cultural drivers

Data shows a rapid shift in food and nutrient intake in the Chinese population (Table 7.4). This is accompanied by equally profound changes in meal and cooking patterns. More meals are being consumed outside of the home, more snacks are being consumed between meals, and cooking practices are shifting away from steaming and boiling and towards frying, which is less healthy.

Trade liberalization and FDI have increased China's exposure to—and popularity of—fast food chains that serve foods high in fat and salt and low in nutrition, especially in urban areas. Traditional Chinese restaurants are also using more oil, salt, and sugar in food preparation.

Culture also plays a role. Especially among the oldest generation, fatness symbolizes health and blessing. As a result, parents and grandparents (who often lacked sufficient food when they were growing up) tend to overfeed the child, which can lead to obesity (586). Some of these cultural norms are beginning to change with the influx of Western culture, depicting beauty as being thin and muscular. Alcohol and tobacco represent ideal gifts during social gatherings and official conferences, excessive drinking and smoking are regarded as necessary for establishing rapport.

Economic drivers

Tobacco consumption is determined in part by the State Tobacco Monopoly Administration, which provides technical assistance to and guarantees purchase from tobacco farmers. Since China became a member of WTO in December 2001, tariffs on tobacco leaf and cigarette products have gradually been reduced from 64% (1999) to 25% (2003). Correspondingly, China's cigarette imports increased by 37%, from 68.51 million packs in 2002 to 93.92 million packs in 2003 (168). The government levies 67% of the producer price on cigarette manufacturers, which is only 38% of average retail prices, relatively lower than the cigarette tax rates around the world with a median rate of about 60%.

Concurrently, rapid economic changes have shifted occupational structures and reduced energy expenditure due to technological advances, leading to a decline in work-related physical activity (587). The booming automobile and telecommunication industries and rise of modern transportation have reduced leisure-time physical activities.

Trade liberalization has greatly affected the Chinese market, with the largest influences seen in the food and beverage industry. Since re-entering China in 1979, by 2009 Coca-Cola China opened 39 bottling plants with over 30,000 employees and invested over US$2 billion (588). China is the third largest market of Coca-Cola globally, although 'healthier' product offerings such as Diet Coke lag behind American and European markets.

Importation of edible oils in China began in 1990 and 1991, following major taxation and import regulation changes. One of the most common oils consumed in China is soybean oil, whose importation increased from negligible levels in 1989 to more than fourteen million metric tons per year (78 kcal per person per day) by 2006. Economic shifts have led to the excessive use of edible oils by all social classes with the most rapid increases witnessed among the poor (589).

FDI by food and drink companies (such as McDonalds and Yum! Brands, which includes KFC and Pizza Hut) is increasing, and domestic productions of processed and packaged foods have skyrocketed. China is experiencing the world's fastest growth in supermarkets and convenience stores (587). Together, these changes have meant an increase in overall energy intake and consumption of food with higher fat, salt, and sugar content.

Environmental drivers

In 2002, 16 of the 20 most polluted cities in the world were in China (590) and in 2003, 27% of the 340 Chinese cities under surveillance were 'severely polluted' (581). This is partly caused by motor vehicle emissions, which have worsened in major cities (571). Air pollution is considered one of the main causes of respiratory diseases (591, 592). Changes to the physical environment are one major cause of the decline in physical activity level. Bicycle lanes in China give way to electronic bikes, motorcycles, and automobiles; open space for kids to run and play and adults for leisure-time activities has turned into commercial and residential complexes.

Social and economic consequences of chronic disease

Chronic diseases cause suffering that extends beyond the health of individuals, impacting the family, community, and societal levels. The healthcare system, already operating at full capacity, is under increased stress from the heavy chronic disease burden.

Labour market costs

Because chronic diseases affect people during their prime working years, they create losses of economic productivity (50). China's population aged 35–64 years lost 6.7 million years of productive life due to CVD in 2000, a figure projected to rise to 10.5 million by 2030 (585). Family members often care for chronic disease patients, causing conceivably large indirect costs related to transportation, care giving, and lost productivity (however, no comprehensive cost estimates are available).

However, the strength of these economic arguments in affecting priority of chronic diseases is likely to be low as compared with other countries (such as South Africa). Since the economy is already growing at 10% per year, anything faster is considered to be counter-productive by the government.

Health system costs

The direct cost of hospital admissions for patients with ischemic stroke was approximately US$1.3 billion in 2003, with total expenditures of US$2.5 billion accounting for 3.0% of national health expenditures (50). Data from 2002 show that the average inpatient costs for treatment of hypertension, diabetes, coronary heart diseases, stroke, and cancer ranged from 4000–10,000 yuan (the average annual income is 9422 yuan in urban areas, and 2936 yuan in rural areas) (155). As with the labour market costs, the extent and relevance of these costs to the government could be questioned, as many people fail to actually receive this care.

Management and prevention of chronic disease

Healthcare system

Healthcare in China is not well suited to face the challenge of increasing burden of chronic diseases. The system is based on a traditional acute care-oriented three-tier public provision system, including community clinics, community health care centres, district hospitals, and city hospitals in urban areas, and village clinics, township health centres, and county hospitals in rural areas (593). Provincial and central hospitals provide high-level referral care. However, access to healthcare is a more pressing problem for people living with chronic diseases, and integration of services and proper follow-ups are lacking.

Healthcare quality is generally lower in rural and in community clinics and healthcare centres due to lack of adequate training and monitoring for the majority of healthcare professionals and long-term problems such as supplier-induced demand and over-prescription of medication. Patients typically do not trust the lower-level community or township health centres with limited clinical capacity, and individuals who can afford to often seek care in large tertiary care hospitals. As a result, large urban hospitals are often crowded with long waiting times.

Within a few years after market reforms, a majority of the population (90% in rural areas) lost insurance (573). Today, whether a person gets care is greatly determined by their income and medical insurance. The proportion of out-of-pocket expenses has been extremely high—over 60% in most of the past few decades and until recently, inequality in access to healthcare had increased over time. A reliance on out-of-pocket spending has been exacerbated by rising medical costs as doctors and hospitals strived to generate profits, reducing the ability of citizens to afford services.

Recent healthcare system reform has started to address the problem. Currently, there are three parallel but vastly different social medical insurance schemes for urban employees since 1998, urban residents since 2007, and rural residents since 2004 as well as a medical assistance programme for low-income families.

The current situation represents an important achievement. However, lack of insurance is still a serious social problem for certain population groups such as urban residents and migrant workers from rural to urban areas. Although currently over 90% of rural residents are covered by the New Rural Cooperative Medical Scheme, the benefit levels remain very low. Under-insurance has led to the high proportion of patients not seeking care when ill or undergoing catastrophic medical spending, especially low-income families.

Chronic disease control

The government agency directly responsible for chronic disease control is the Division of Chronic Disease, Bureau of Disease Control in the Ministry of Health (MOH), established in 1997. Its technical counterpart is the China Centre for Disease Control and Prevention (CDC). The National Centre for Chronic and Non-communicable Disease Prevention and Control, under the leadership of the China CDC, was established in 2002 and is responsible for the National Disease Surveillance Points System (239). The National Office for Cancer Prevention and Control (founded in 1969) and the National Centre for Cardiovascular Diseases (founded in 2004) are two other key chronic disease prevention and control institutions, both directly under leadership of the MOH.

National efforts in chronic disease prevention and control began in the 1990s, although progress has been slow until the past few years when more support has been devoted to chronic diseases. Although there is reason to believe that government funding for chronic diseases has increased in line with this elevated support, the amount of government spending on chronic disease prevention and control in China is largely unknown, as a 2010 study highlighted the lack of available data to assess how much budgetary allocations are given to any specific type of disease in China (537).

To date, the MOH has launched three types of national strategies to reduce chronic diseases: 1) development of 10-year national plans, clinical guidelines, and health policies, 2) health education and health promotion, and 3) implementation and community capacity building. In the medical reform act in April 2009, all five priorities were directly related to the rising need of better prevention, care, and management of chronic diseases: 1) expand the coverage of basic medical insurance system; 2) establish a basic drug formulary system; 3) improve medical services at grass-root level; 4) promote equality in public health services; and 5) start to pilot the reform of public hospitals.

In 2008, the 'Healthy China 2020' strategic programme was launched by the MOH and specifically includes cost-effective interventions for chronic diseases (594). In 2009, the State Council revealed the long-awaited and hotly debated healthcare system reform act, highlighting the importance of chronic disease prevention and control. In the past decade, clinical guidelines on hypertension, diabetes, and dyslipidaemia prevention and control, as well as guidelines for the general public on diet, physical activity, overweight and obesity have been publicized; however, most of them have not been widely promoted among clinicians and the public.

The MOH has also organized several health education and promotion programmes. Beginning in 2000, the National Sports Administration, backed by an annual fund of about US$40 million from the China Sports Lottery Fund, installed exercise equipment in urban communities across the country. This has led to increased physical activity, especially among retired people and children. 'Health for 900 million farmers', a national rural health programme, was publicized with chronic disease risk factor prevention as an integral part of the programme. In September 2007, the National Initiative on Healthy Lifestyle for All was launched with a focus on balanced diet and physical activity and the slogan of 'Be Active, Be Healthy, Be Happy'. Another recent initiative, promoted by the Ministry and the local governments of large cities such as Beijing and Shanghai, is the free distribution of simple tools such as BMI calculators (paper wheel), retractable plastic waist circumference rulers, salt-controlling spoons and cans, and oil dispensers with portion control (49). However, most of these programmes lack mechanisms for sustainability and evaluation.

Fiscal and regulatory interventions

This section provides a brief overview of government regulations regarding tobacco, food and beverage, and alcohols.

Marketing/advertising/labelling

Five national laws explicitly prohibit tobacco advertising through mass media press or in public places. Selling cigarettes to minors is also banned (595). The Chinese government has previously had modest requirements for food labelling, although recent actions suggest this may be changing. In May 2008, the MOH passed legislation that encourages food manufacturers to identify nutrition facts, nutrition claims, and nutrition functional claims on packaged products with nutrition claims. There are no specific requirements on marketing to children, although a general provision in the Advertisement Law mandates that all advertisements should not include contents inappropriate for children. National laws prohibit the sale of alcohol to minors, but store sales persons rarely check identification cards for age or receive penalty for selling alcohol products to children. Capacity to implement these laws on the ground is weak.

Regulations regarding schools and public places

Reacting to the WHO's FCTC, by 2008 five of China's cities (Beijing, Yinchuan, Shanghai, Hangzhou, and Guangzhou) had implemented smoking bans in public places. Following this, citywide and regional bans on smoking in public places were implemented in Beijing (partly due to the 2008 Olympic Games), in Shanghai (in preparation for the 2010 World Exposition), and in Hangzhou in 2010, where significant progress in tobacco control has occurred. In particular, a 1987 law on the protection of minors stipulates that no one should smoke in schools or other places where children convene (581). These regulations are generally supported by the public, but enforcement has not been effective.

There are national regulations on physical education in primary and secondary schools as well as regional programmes in promoting physical activities at school. For example, a programme called 'Happy 10 minutes' provides schoolteachers with training and guidance to engage in 10 minutes of physical activities (indoor or outdoor) with their students each day. General feedback is positive but no formal evaluation has been conducted (596).

In many urban areas, there are local regulations on the hygiene, safety standard, and nutritional requirements for school meals. School lunches are usually made by school cafeterias or contracted to external companies meeting regulatory requirements.

Community interventions

One example of integrated health and physical education programmes in schools was the 'Health Promotion School Project' in Zhejiang province launched in 2000 (597, 598). Students were trained to plan and prepare nutritious meals, learned and disseminated information on nutrition, and shared their knowledge with their families and the wider community. These activities were supplemented with improvements in health-related school policies and the physical environment, including renovations of school facilities and playgrounds. Survey results revealed large improvements in nutritional knowledge, attitudes and behaviours among all target groups, including 7500 students and their families and 800 teachers and school staff personnel.

Cancer has led the way in community-based chronic disease prevention and control initiatives. In 2003, the MOH implemented a national cancer control plan, 'Program of Cancer Prevention and Control in China (2004–2010)', in which several key strategies in the prevention and control of common cancers were initiated, including screening and early detection of cervical cancer and breast cancer among women aged 35–59 years (599). Large-scale community-based national programmes on hypertension management have also been implemented, in which primary care physicians in community healthcare centres were equipped with electronic tools to manage hypertensive patients. As early as 1997, the China MOH and the CDC established 32 demonstration sites for chronic disease prevention and control. Main strategies and activities include community screening, community mobilization, lifestyle interventions (smoking cessation, healthy diet, and physical activity), and training programmes for community healthcare centres for hypertension and diabetes management (239).

Role of the private sector

The private sector has the goal of profit making, which can create tension and conflict with the goal of promoting public health in collaboration with the public sector. This section briefly discusses the roles of tobacco, food, and pharmaceutical industries in China's burden of chronic diseases.

Tobacco industries: fortune or burden?

China is the largest tobacco grower and consumer in the world. Though strictly speaking, the Chinese National Tobacco Corporation (CNTC) is not a private industry, certain elements of the process such as tobacco farming and cigarette retails are. For example, in 1995, Philip Morris Incorporated entered the Chinese market, reaching an agreement with CNTC for the licensed manufacture of Marlboro cigarettes in China (600). Aggressive regulations (such as graphic warning signs on cigarette packages and tobacco taxes) are strongly resisted in China, because of the jobs and taxes generated by tobacco companies.

Food industries: 'responsibility' or just 'lip service'?

In recent years, some multinational companies as well as domestic ones have made health promotion claims and commitments, under the aegis of corporate social responsibility. For example, Coca-Cola China has committed 'to develop and create programmes that support a healthy lifestyle, in particular through physical activity and nutritional education programmes in collaboration with governmental agencies and health experts' (601). PepsiCo claims to 'promote healthier lifestyles through a combination of health assessments, personalized coaching, tobacco cessation, fitness and nutrition programmes, online tools and worksite wellness initiatives' (602). It remains to be seen whether these claims and commitments demonstrate corporate social responsibility or are simply 'lip service' (see the two competing views about the role of the private sector in Chapter 6).

Pharmaceutical industries: benefit the public or just themselves?

While contributing to the rising healthcare costs, there is strong evidence showing the contribution of medical advances including pharmaceutical products in improving health outcomes for millions of patients. In China, many multinational pharmaceutical companies have been the forerunners in sponsoring research, training, and public campaigns on chronic disease prevention and control, such as the Chinese health knowledge dissemination initiative received sponsorship from Roche (2006), Pfizer (2005 and 2007), and Eli Lilly (2008). The initiative was generally considered successful in raising public awareness on chronic disease issues such as hypertension, diabetes, and healthy weight with benefits in branding and public relations for the pharmaceutical companies too. The thousands of large and small Chinese pharmaceutical companies have generally not been involved in philanthropic activities so far, suggesting that large international pharmaceutical companies are the main forces in chronic disease prevention and control efforts in the private sector.

Recommendations

Addressing the challenge of chronic disease requires concerted commitment and actions from all sectors of the society, domestically and internationally.

Global organizations such as the UN, WHO, and World Bank have contributed significantly to poverty reduction, under nutrition improvement, and infectious disease prevention and control. In light of the fast growing and enormous economic and health consequences of chronic disease, resources devoted to chronic disease prevention and control are far from optimal. Awareness of the problem and commitment from the top to fight the challenge of chronic disease is the necessary first step. These organizations, as well as major global players such as the Gates Foundation and the World Heart Federation, are expected to facilitate cross-country technical and expertise transfer. They are also well-poised to influence political atmosphere and to coordinate cross-national surveillance and other disease prevention and control programmes.

At the national level, Chinese government should take step-wise actions to prevent and control chronic disease. This could include: 1) a unifying national framework for chronic disease prevention and control; 2) intersectional actions at all stages of policy formulation and implementation; 3) policies and plans focusing on common risk factors that cut across specific diseases; 4) combining population-wide and individual approaches; 5) implementation of immediately feasible interventions with greatest impact; and 6) locally relevant and explicit milestones set for each step (52).

Specifically, such a framework should clarify the role and position of chronic disease prevention and control with clear and measurable goals achievable within a specific amount of time, such as those set in *Healthy China 2020*. Intersectoral collaboration (involving the finance, education, industry and information, and communications sectors) across many governmental agencies and levels is necessary. Efforts must be underway to clarify functions across the different government levels and within the ministries and high-level institutions that share health-related responsibilities (571). These goals and priorities need to be communicated from the highest level of governmental authorities to local and community governmental agencies. Dramatic measures such as including health outcomes in performance evaluation for government officials could be implemented when possible. Publicity and transparency of health policies and actions should serve to instil trust and strengthen the position of the government as its role in the health system evolves.

Prevention instead of treatment of chronic disease must be emphasized for the fight against chronic disease to be successful. National priority programmes that are multipronged and comprehensive are needed. Population-wide and macro-level strategies that change the environment people live in should be emphasized such as evidence-based health policies and legislations on tobacco taxes, graphic warning signs on cigarette packages, responsible food marketing, and limit on the amount of harmful food ingredients such as saturated fat and salt. Tobacco control, universal salt reduction, and obesity prevention, especially among children and adolescents, should be given the highest priority. Prevention should focus on combating these major risk factors in an integrated manner at the national, regional, community, and individual levels to tackle deeply entrenched economical, social, and cultural factors.

All prevention strategies should be supported by public policies and social mobilization, including transportation reform (to address the dramatic growth in automobile use and less friendly environments for cycling and pedestrians); education (to enhance comprehensive school-based health education and promotion); fiscal policy (e.g. to increase tobacco taxes or providing economic incentives to promote physical activity); regulatory actions (e.g. to ensure lower salt content in processed and packaged food; to prohibit smoking in public places); and urban design (to provide parks, green spaces, and paths for bicycles and walkers to promote physical activities) (575). Social medical insurance should shift away from the almost exclusive focus on curative care to reimburse antihypertensive medications, including in rural areas.

Reform of healthcare systems must be in line with the need to address the challenges of chronic disease to shift away from a fragmented acute care-oriented model. Integration of primary, secondary, and tertiary care services should be a priority to channel prevention and treatment of chronic diseases to the most cost-efficient levels of the healthcare system. It is not cost-effective or feasible to rely on tertiary care for long-term chronic disease prevention and control. Therefore, strengthening the current weak primary care and community healthcare services is urgently needed, and has been an important part of the new healthcare reform in China announced in April 2009. Limited resources (financial and technical support) should be better allocated to provide access to basic healthcare and improve quality of care to urban poor and vulnerable populations in rural China to reduce health disparities (603). The new healthcare reform in China has started to strengthen the role and capacity of community healthcare centres and workers, which is expected to make a positive impact on chronic disease prevention and control.

The private sector plays a vital role in reducing the burden of chronic disease. Their main con-tributions include 1) reformulating old products and creating new products toward healthier varieties and 2) working in partnership with governmental and non-governmental organizations in responsible marketing, health education, and health promotion. Specific examples for the food and beverage industry are to: 1) remove trans fatty acids from the food supply; 2) reduce the levels of salt, sugar, and saturated fat in their products; 3) increase the availability of products based on fruit, vegetables, nuts, grains, and legumes; and 4) use their marketing excellence to promote more physical activity and fruit and vegetable consumption, and less use of salt, especially among children. Other roles for the private sector include information and experience sharing. The private sector possesses essential and specialized skills that are valuable for chronic disease prevention and control. For example, expertise in marketing, advertising and brand promotion could be offered to strengthen public awareness and education campaigns (367).

Academic and professional training should better prepare and equip future researchers, physicians, nurses, community healthcare workers, and other health professionals to address the problem of chronic diseases. Researchers should strive to conduct not only academic studies to produce scientific evidences but also to find effective and sustainable ways to translate such evidence into practices and policies. Lastly, involvement and support of media, communications, and non-governmental organizations is an essential part of shaping public opinions, disseminating public health knowledge regarding chronic disease, and changing the sociophysical environment that make it easier for individuals to make healthier lifestyle choices.

Summary points

1 Massive urban-rural inequalities exist in chronic disease risks and resources available to address the challenge of chronic disease.

2 Rapid economic growth has been accompanied by marked increases in the economic and health consequences of chronic disease.

3 Recognition of the major health challenge of chronic disease is still lacking in all levels of government agencies.

4 A unifying national framework to position chronic disease prevention and control as a national priority is a necessary prerequisite for successfully addressing the burden.

5 Focusing on prevention of chronic disease, instead of clinical management, must be emphasized.

6 Prevention strategies should include public policy and social mobilization to address macro-environmental factors as opposed to individual programmes; tobacco control, salt reduction, and obesity prevention (especially among children and adolescents) are recommended as priorities of population-wide prevention programmes.

7 Reform the current healthcare system and channel limited resources to strengthen primary and community health care services can help to effectively and sustainably prevent and control chronic diseases.

8 Intergovernmental collaborations, as well as involvement and contributions from the private and media sectors, academia, and NGOs, are needed.

Part 3

Chronic diseases in India

Dorairaj Prabhakaran, V.S. Ajay, V. Mohan,
K.R. Thankappan, Karen Siegel, K.M. Venkat Narayan,
and K.S. Reddy

Background

India is home to one-sixth of the world's population (about 1.1 billion people), making it the second most populous country (after China) and the largest democracy in the world. The country has great diversity among its 28 self-governing states, reflected in 18 constitutionally-recognized languages and 1600 dialects (its two official languages are English and Hindi).

Since achieving independence from British Rule in 1947, the Indian government has prioritized economic growth.[1] In the post-war period, the country's model of development focused on self-sufficiency (requiring all companies to be owned and operated by Indians). This lasted until 1991, when a series of market reforms opened India's borders to international trade and business, import controls were removed and customs and duties lowered, and multinationals returned. Economic growth has averaged 6% annually over the past decade, making it the second fastest growing economy, after China.

One reason for the rising influx of multinationals is the relatively inexpensive, albeit skilled and English-speaking, labour force. The economy has transformed from being agricultural-dependent to fuelled by service industries. Although agriculture continues to employ the greatest number of workers (63% of the population), most of whom live in rural settings, this sector only contributes to one-fifth of India's economy and is shrinking, whereas the growing service sector (including the growing number of call centres, outsourcing from the US and information technology (IT) hubs) now makes up about half of India's economy.

Declining agricultural production has led to a loss of rural jobs and, as a result, mass migration to the cities. While the majority of the population (70%) still lives in and around the country's 650,000 rural villages, the remaining 30% lives in these cities (a population that grows by 2.3% per year). The southern states tend to be more urbanized (and more affluent) than the north but overall, migration to cities has strained the limited resources and infrastructure, such that one-third (34.8%) of the urban population lives in slums, and 48% lack sustainable access to improved sanitation (604). Three of India's cities are megacities—Mumbai (16.4 million), Kolkata (13.2 million), and Delhi (12.8 million).

These profound social transformations have altered the risks to health. Life expectancy (63 years at birth in 2008) is increasing while birth rates are declining. Literacy rates have increased since 1950, from 18.33% (27.16% for males and 8.86% for females) to 65.38% (75.85% males, 54.16% females) in 2001 (605). Although poverty rates are declining, one quarter of India's population still earns less than US$1 per day. Two-thirds of all children are malnourished or underweight (606). At the same time, up to 50% of adults are overweight or obese, trends that are increasingly being observed in children.

In this chapter, we describe the rising burden, drivers, and impact of NCDs in India, the country's efforts to prevent and control NCDs, the current and future roles of the private sector and government, and conclude with a series of policy options that could help reduce the NCD burden.

Evaluating the health burden of chronic diseases

Macro-level changes described above have resulted in an increasing burden of chronic disease and their risk factors. The data that exists on chronic disease burden and risk factors is largely regional and urban, and generally does not use standardized definitions for reporting of results. Prevalence estimates and epidemiological data come from a few studies, and may not be applicable to the country as a whole. However, they do illustrate the themes and trends in the NCD burden across the country. This section draws upon these data, as well as WHO estimates.

Chronic diseases are the leading cause of death and disability in India. In 2005, chronic diseases caused 53% of all deaths (5.2 million deaths out of 10.3 million deaths) in India, approximately 30% of which were premature (before age 60) (607). By 2030, chronic diseases are estimated to account for 67% of all deaths in India (563). With over 50 million individuals with diabetes, India has been referred to as the 'diabetes capital of the world', a burden that is expected to nearly double by 2030 (608). The prevalence of coronary heart disease is reported to be 7–13% in urban India and 2–7% in rural India (69).

About 800,000 new cases of cancer are estimated to occur every year. In men, the most common cancers are tobacco-related (lung, oral cavity, larynx, oesophagus, and pharynx). In women, the leading cancer sites include those related to tobacco (oral cavity, oesophagus, and lung), and cervix, breast, and ovary cancer. India has the largest number of oral cancers in the world, due to widespread tobacco chewing.

Community-based studies have estimated that the prevalence of chronic obstructive pulmonary disease varies from as high as 9% (men) in the rural areas of Uttar Pradesh to as low as 2.5% (women) in rural Tamil Nadu. Data from recent large, multisite studies carried out in urban cities such as Delhi, Bangalore, Chandigarh, and Kanpur show that 5% of men and 3.2% women above the age of 35 suffer from COPD (609) associated with smoking, as well as with indoor and outdoor air pollution.

Individual risk factors

The main individual risks of chronic diseases are rising. Hypertension is present in an estimated 25% of urban and 10% of rural Indians (69). India's prevalence of IGT and IFG totalled 85.6 million in 2003—the largest in the world—and is expected to increase to 132 million in 2025 (298).

The prevalence of overweight and obesity is rising, although it is important to note that despite a relatively high prevalence of diabetes and CVD, obesity prevalence is much lower in India than in the other countries presented (see Figure 7.3). This is due to a relatively lower threshold for CVD and diabetes risk among South Asian populations (610).

Over the past decade, the prevalence of overweight and obesity has increased slightly at the national level, and more rapidly in urban and high-socio-economic groups. The National Family Health Survey (NHFS-3, conducted in 2005-06) found the national prevalence of overweight (BMI ≥ 25 kg/m^2) to be 11.4%, while national prevalence of obesity (BMI ≥ 30 kg/m^2) was only 2.2% (611). In contrast, between 1995 and 2005, the prevalence of overweight (defined as having a BMI ≥ 25 kg/m^2) in urban areas nearly doubled, from 20% to 36% (612).

Tobacco use, unhealthy diet, and physical inactivity contribute significantly to the NCD burden in India. Tobacco use (all forms) in India has increased over a 7-year period from 1998–2005, particularly among the younger (from 19% to 40%), richer (from 27% to 46%), and urban (from 34% to 50%) populations (613). Approximately 60% of men and 11% of women in India aged 15–49 years used some kind of tobacco in the year 2005–06 (611).

A significant proportion of the Indian population is physically inactive. The World Health Survey (2003) reported that 29% of the Indian population had inadequate amounts of recommended physical activity (work-related and leisure-time) (614).

Despite having the largest burden of under nutrition in the world (251.5 million individuals in 2004–06) (615), over nutrition is increasingly a public health issue in India. Dietary trends are characterized by a shift away from traditional diets high in complex carbohydrates and low in fat to modern diets that have high contributions of energy from fats, lower contribution of energy from complex carbohydrates, and lower overall nutritional quality (332). During 1979–2001, energy and fat intake greatly increased, and consumption of meat products, milk, sugars, and vegetable oils increased by 50%, 60%, 25%, and 100%, respectively (616) (see Table 7.6)

Fruit and vegetable consumption tends to be low except among urban affluent populations (605). In the NHFS-3, only a small proportion of men and women (13%) ate fruits daily (information on recommended daily consumption not available), while 64% women and 59% men reported eating dark leafy vegetables daily (611). In urban areas, 90% of the population consumes less than the WHO/FAO recommended intake of fruit and vegetables (617).

Perhaps the most significant dietary change is the consumption of edible oils. Per capita consumption of edible oils increased by 30% from 1993–94 to 2004–05 (298). Although peanut, rapeseed and cottonseed oils were traditionally consumed most frequently (being produced domestically), the Indian population has shifted to mostly-imported palm and soybean oil, which account for approximately 38% and 21% of total oil consumption, respectively (618).

Air pollution (both indoor and outdoor) also contributes to increasing NCD rates. Recent studies from India suggest that indoor air pollution is a major cause of lung disease, particularly among rural women (7) (see Chapters 1 and 4).

Inequalities in NCDs and risk factors

Chronic diseases are more prevalent in urban areas than in rural areas (69). For example, diabetes prevalence is higher among urban populations (5–15%) than populations in semi-urban (4–6%) or rural (2–5%) settings (69, 619). However, the situation is changing unevenly across Indian

Table 7.6 Food consumption trends for selected items in India: 1979–2001

Product	1979–81		1999–2001	
	Average calories/ capita/day	% of total daily calories	Average calories/ capita/day	% of total daily calories
Meat products	16	0.77	22	0.9
Animal fats	23	1.1	47	1.9
Sugar and sweeteners	193	9.3	247	10.1
Vegetable oils	127	6.1	239	9.8
Fruits (excluding wine)	31	1.5	51	2.1
Vegetables	32	1.5	45	1.8
Total calories	2080		2440	
Fat (in grams)	30		50+	

Source: FAOSTAT 2004, adapted from Pingali et al. (616) and Siegel et al. (641).

states; one 2010 report from the state of Kerala (in the late phase of epidemiological transition) found diabetes prevalence to be 20.6% in rural areas as compared to 14.8% in urban areas (620).

Chronic diseases and risk factors are higher in the south than in the north. The National Urban Diabetes Study (NUDS) found that prevalence of diabetes was higher in three southern cities (Hyderabad, Chennai, and Bangalore) compared to three northern cities (Delhi, Calcutta, and Mumbai) (298, 617). Studies have also reported higher prevalence of CVD in southern India compared to northern India (621).

While diabetes prevalence is negatively associated with increasing socioeconomic status (SES) in high-income countries, a positive association has been seen between affluence and diabetes in India, especially in recent years (622). Tobacco use, however, shows a strong socioeconomic gradient—data from the 1998-9 Indian Family Health Survey (among adults over age 18 in all Indian states) reported that 45.5% of the population in the lowest income group used tobacco, compared to only 18% in the highest income group (623).

Societal determinants of chronic diseases

With rising longevity and falling infant mortality, the total population and the proportion of the population over age 60 is expected to double to 13.3% by 2025 (from 1991), increasing the overall prevalence of chronic disease (624). Nonetheless, an ageing population must be exposed to unhealthy societal drivers in order to yield such rapidly increasing chronic disease rates (see Chapter 2). The following section outlines economic, political, environment, and social/cultural drivers of the increasing chronic disease burden in India.

Economic and political drivers

Since 1991, trade liberalization has increased availability of pre-packaged and processed foods from multinational food and beverage corporations and junk food outlets, and rising incomes have increased their accessibility. The proliferation of massive advertising campaigns has increased their desirability. Together, these factors have resulted in increased consumption of sugar, oil, milk, and animal products (298). Poor regulatory capacity has resulted in a food market with ample unhealthy dietary choices (high saturated fats/oils, refined carbohydrates, low fibre products; junk foods like biscuits, fried food products in reheated oils) due to their relatively low cost as compared to healthy foods such as fruits and vegetables. Local foods, generally high in salt or sugar, increasingly offered in larger portions, and fried using cheap oils (mustard oil, palm oil, and vanaspati is used in the north, while coconut oil is most common in the south), also continue to play a role.

Availability, affordability, and accessibility of healthy food options are low, particularly among poorer populations. Sharp rises in the price of food commodities, particularly fruits and vegetables, have resulted in a negative impact on consumption patterns particularly among the poor, who tend to reduce consumption of expensive vegetables and fruits in favour of the cheaper foods high in saturated fats (as described in Chapter 2) (69). Moreover, a large amount of fruits and vegetables is produced in India (123.1 million tons in 2000), but remains inaccessible and unaffordable to most of the population. This is especially true in rural areas, where nearly 10–15% of grains and 25% of fruit and vegetables perish due to India's hot climate and poor warehouse infrastructure (625).

India is the world's leading importer of edible oils, largely due to elimination of state monopolies on imports in the mid-1990s, and resulting increased market access. Between 1989 and 2002, availability of calories from vegetable oils (mainly palm oil) increased by 50% (from 158 to 231 calories/cap/day) (115). These shifts in edible oil availability and consumption in India are intertwined with government policies in Brazil that resulted in a 67% increase in soybean oil production between 1990 and 2004 and a more than doubling of low-priced exports (see Brazil, Chapter 7.1). More recently, in an effort to contain inflation rates, Indian import duties on palm oil were abolished in 2009. Healthier oils are thus relatively more expensive than soybean and palm oil. India is the world's second largest producer of sugar (after Brazil), although this does not appear to have had an effect on domestic sugar consumption (yet).

Rising incomes, combined with government policies and economic incentives to develop the automobile industry, are increasing private car and motorcycle ownership, and lowering physical activity rates. The government prioritizes roadway expansion, and has recently budgeted about $10 billion for improvements (79). Between 1981 and 2002, total number of motorized two-wheelers rose from less than 3 million to 42 million—a 14-fold increase (79). Indian and foreign-owned car companies are developing small, cheap cars (targeted specifically at India's growing middle class).

Environmental drivers

Between 1901 and 2000, the proportion of the population living in urban areas in India tripled (from 10% to 27%) and is projected to rise to nearly 50% by 2030 (624). The more affluent southern states are urbanizing much faster than the northern ones. For example, Punjab (in the north) is expected to be 44.8% urban by 2021 (626), while 75% of individuals in Tamil Nadu (in the south) are expected to live in urban areas by 2025 (627).

Rapid migration to cities strains urban infrastructure. Individuals living in slums (30% of the urban population, and growing) are particularly at high risk for NCDs, due to environmental tobacco smoke, indoor stoves, and unhealthy diets, along with psychosocial stress (113).

Urbanization, especially when cities are built around car use, contributes to physical inactivity and poor air quality. India has three of the ten most polluted cities in the world (Delhi, Mumbai, and Chennai). A 2010 study found that living in an urban environment confers a great risk for obesity and diabetes (628). In particular migration to urban areas was associated with increased fat intake and reduced physical activity.

Decreased walking and cycling are typically found in larger cities, because these methods of active transportation do not receive adequate funding, legal rights, or traffic priority (64% of all accidents in India involve pedestrians/cyclists) (629). Separate bike lanes and paths are not available for cyclists in any Indian city except the planned city of Chandigarh.

Growth in India's technology industry has encouraged the development of suburbs that are generally unplanned and lack adequate public transport services. Virtually every large city has a technology park on the fringe, contributing to suburban sprawl. Longer commuting distances make cycling and walking less feasible, driving the trend from non-motorized to motorized modes (590).

Social and cultural drivers

In the past, food was not as plentiful as it is now, and families frequently had no food to eat (and often, food that was available was rancid). As a result, in contemporary Indian society where good food is abundant, parents and grandparents encourage children to eat more.

Cultural and religious practices also play a role. Sweets are an essential part of social occasions or visits to people's homes, a sign that visitors are welcome. Sociocultural and religious practices pose a threat to proper foot care in India; customs of walking barefoot can lead to costly diabetic foot complications (neuropathy, caused by poorly controlled diabetes and which can lead to high costs, is present in 70% of diabetics in India) (630).

Status plays a role in discouraging active transport among the middle and upper classes, as described above. Currently, only the poorest individuals in urban areas tend to cycle or walk because they can't afford to use public transport.

Economic changes have increased the availability (and appeal) of relatively lucrative and highly-valued management jobs in multinational corporations or at call centres. Increasingly, young Indians are moving to major cities to work in these jobs that require sedentary work habits that, combined with a more stressful work life, can increase risk of NCDs. Additionally, a changing labour force that includes women has important consequences for the family diet; as traditional roles erode and women have less time to prepare fresh and healthy meals, consumption of highly processed foods increases and more meals are eaten outside of the home.

Social and economic consequences of chronic disease

Labour market costs

Chronic diseases affect people at younger ages in India, resulting in premature disability and subsequent economic loss due to fewer productive years (367). India suffers the highest loss in potentially productive years of life of any country in the world, due to a high number of deaths from CVD in people aged 35–64 years (about 9.2 million years lost in 2000). By 2030, this loss is expected to rise to 17.9 million years, higher than the estimated loss in China, Russia, US, Portugal, and South Africa combined (16.2 million) (563, 631). As a result of premature deaths to CVD, stroke, and diabetes, India stands to lose US$237 billion in productivity between 2005 and 2015 (367).

Health system costs

Relatively little information exists regarding the health system costs of NCDs in India, due to the lack of a comprehensive healthcare system, lack of uniform documentation of medical details, and a lack of uniform norms for diabetes management (298). Most information comes from diabetes studies.

Between 1998 and 2005, the cost of treating diabetes more than doubled (113% increase) (298). This was likely due to increases in costs of diabetes medications, laboratory tests, medical consultations, hospitalizations, and surgical procedures, particularly among urban households that have access to more expensive services. India's first national report on the cost of diabetes care, published in 2000, reported an annual diabetes cost of US$2.2 billion, most of which was out-of-pocket and represented high proportions of annual family income (632).

Complications can be even more costly. For those who develop foot ulcers, cost of care can reach nearly US$28,000 only 2 years after diagnosis (632). Another study found that those without complications had an 18% lower hospitalization cost, while those with three or more complications had a 48% higher cost (633).

Management and prevention of chronic disease

Healthcare system

India's healthcare system is the most unregulated in the world. About one-quarter of the total health expenditure comes from the government, while the remaining 75% comes from private sources, 97% of which is out-of-pocket. In 2000, approximately 60% of the total health budget was spent on five national programmes: leprosy, malaria, TB, HIV/AIDs and blindness, while the remaining 40% was spent on public health institutions, hospitals and research, indicating considerable neglect of NCDs (389).

Healthcare in India is both public and private. As stipulated in the Constitution, free healthcare is provided to the poor—although in state-run institutions that are often crowded, under-staffed, and ill-equipped. The number of private tertiary-care hospitals has grown, but facilities and services offered remain limited (632). Private health insurance is not yet popular.

Clinical care facilities (for both acute and long-term care) are concentrated in cities, and thus inaccessible to rural populations. Since independence in 1947, the government has built a network of 145,000 'sub centres', 23,000 primary health centres, and 3222 community health centres. The National Rural Health Mission (NRHM) aims to improve rural health services, and from 2005 to 2012 plans to increase public expenditure on health, reduce regional imbalances in health infrastructure, and increase community participation in the management of the health system.

Even when patients do reach a health centre, the care they receive is not always high quality. At the time of writing, there are no specific NCD treatment guidelines proposed for India or Southeast Asia by WHO, and hence there is a general lack of understanding of treatment requirements for diabetes patients. In India, family physicians are the primary point of contact for diagnosis and treatment, but are not always aware of treatments and necessary tests for diabetes patients. Unsurprisingly, only one-third of hypertensive individuals are diagnosed, and of those who are diagnosed, less than half take any kind of medication. One study conducted in 89 tertiary care hospitals showed that heart attack (myocardial infarction, MI) patients, particularly poorer individuals, receive inadequate management, and thus have greater 30-day mortality post-MI (634). Lack of health care supplies is also a problem. Insulin/syringes are available and accessible to only 33% of people with diabetes due to insufficient supplies and high costs for supplies that do exist; blood glucose test strips are even less accessible, for the same reasons (635).

Chronic disease control

Those at the highest level in India have been aware of the threat of chronic diseases since at least 1956. At the time, the Health Minister submitted the first resolution to the WHO's World Health Assembly at NCDs, calling for an urgent response to the devastating health and economic costs imposed by rising CVD.

Change has been slow to manifest, but there are signs of progress. There is an NCD cell at the Directorate General of Health Services, which oversees the implementation of the various NCD control programmes. In 2008, the government launched the National Programme for Prevention and Control of Diabetes, CVD, and Stroke (NPDCS). The programme aims to 1) assess the prevalence of risk factors for NCDs; 2) promote NCD prevention in the general population (through community-based health education and promotion on healthy diet and physical activity and school-based health initiatives to raise awareness about diabetes and cardiovascular diseases among youth); and 3) reduce risks among individuals at high risk for CVD through special clinics for early diagnosis and appropriate management of diabetes, CVD, and stroke in over 100 districts. The NPDCS has not yet been integrated with the NRHM for more effective service delivery (such as trained manpower, adequate drug supplies, laboratory and diagnostics services, and referral mechanisms in all the states). Most recently, India's cabinet committee on economic affairs approved a financial outlay of US$263 million for the National Programme for the Prevention and Control of Cancer, Diabetes, Cardiovascular Diseases and Stroke, which is expected to screen more than 70 million people for NCDs (636).

Despite signs of progress, national government funding for NCDs remains disproportionate to the disease burden. Health is constitutionally a state responsibility, but the central government continues to set health priorities, which are then executed by state governments (126, 537). Out of the proposed allocation for various national disease control programmes ($5338 million) during 2007–12, 28% of funds were earmarked for NCD control programmes (637). The remaining 72% of funds were allocated to communicable disease programmes.

Weak regulatory capacity at the national level also hampers progress. Although India has held a national level consultation workshop to formulate recommendations for key elements of a national plan for the implementation of WHO's Global Strategy on Diet and Physical Activity in 2005, a formal policy and legal framework for promoting diet and physical activity in the country is still missing. Most NCD prevention and control regulation that does exist is not comprehensive, undermining intended efforts.

Fiscal and regulatory interventions

Marketing/advertising/labelling

National tobacco control legislation since 2003 aims to reduce population exposure to second hand tobacco smoke, prohibits advertisements and sale to minors, and regulates the content of tobacco products. Other government policy measures include mandates for: heavy taxes on tobacco products; pictorial warnings on tobacco products; bans on smoking in government office and public places; and bans on the advertisement of tobacco products.

India lacks specific food policies or regulations aimed at reducing NCDs. Food labelling in India is deficient, and consumers lack vital information to make informed decisions about food choices (high rates of illiteracy compound this issue). The Food Safety and Standards Authority of India was established in 2008, as a statutory body for creating science-based standards for food and regulating manufacturing, processing, distribution, sale and import of food so it is safe and wholesome for consumption (638). The authority (which includes members of government and the food industry) is considering passing legislation to encourage self-regulation of advertising and trans-fat content of commercially available oils. Current regulation on advertisements does not address the concerns of invasive marketing of junk foods that target children and adolescents.

Despite of the ban on alcohol advertising in print and electronic media, alcohol use is on the rise in India, especially in urban areas where there has recently been a rapid proliferation of bars and nightclubs (639). Since most states derive substantial amount of revenue from alcohol taxation—the second largest source after sales tax—governments are reluctant to implement and enforce alcohol control policies. Further, the powerful alcohol industry influences political parties and alcohol advertisements on clothing and through sporting event sponsorship are common. Very few states (Gujarat) have implemented a total ban on alcohol. Certain holidays such as Independence Day, Republic Day, Gandhi Jayanti (Birthday of Mahatma Gandhi) are observed as 'Dry Days'.

Regulations regarding schools and public places

Through the 2003 tobacco control legislation and the ratification of the FCTC, smoking is banned in all public places, although implementation and enforcement has been weak. In 2005, the government of India attempted to impose ban on screening smoking in cinema, but the Delhi High court overturned the ban in 2009.

Policy-level initiatives to facilitate physical activity at workplaces and in schools have the potential to influence large sections of society. One encouraging example is the decision by Kerala's government to integrate physical education and sports into school curricula. However, such efforts at the national level do not exist.

The National Urban Renewal Mission (NURM), launched in 2005, gives the Central Government priority to construct cycle tracks and pedestrian paths to enhance safety and thereby enhance use of non-motorized vehicles. A public bicycle rental programme for bicycle use in specially designated areas is also under investigation (640). However, as with many other policies, capacity and resources is currently a main obstacle to full implementation.

In response to high consumption of junk food, in 2006 the health ministry proposed a ban on soft drinks and junk food in schools, colleges, and universities nationally and is consulting with other agencies regarding implementation (641).

Community interventions

One successful example of a community intervention comes from Chennai, where a study on community empowerment and awareness of NCDs led to significant change in the community environment and individual health behaviours (Box 7.1).

Other examples include the decision by the state of Tamil Nadu and Kerala to set-up playgrounds in all villages.

The role of the private sector

The private sector is the major provider of healthcare in India, providing 75% of specialists and 85% of technology in their facilities and accounting for 49% of all hospital beds in India (643). There are serious distributional inequalities, as most private healthcare facilities cluster around urban locations while rural areas lack high-end diagnostic and therapeutic facilities for private

Box 7.1 Community empowerment in Chennai

Between 1997 and 2004, a team of researchers used a community awareness and empowerment model to teach communities about diabetes, diabetes prevention, and the benefits of physical activity. Findings showed that after 3 years of intensive intervention (including individual counselling for those at risk for diabetes, bi-monthly mass awareness campaigns and public lectures, weekly educational videos and skits, and encouragement from a social worker who visited the community), the community came to recognize the importance of physical activity—as well as the relative lack of space for exercise in their community—and decided to take action by building a community park, complete with a path for walking. Led by unofficial colony leaders, the community raised money (US$34,000 from the government, residents, and private donors), identified land, and received local government permission to build the park. Encouraged by such a positive outcome, the community shared results with local government and other residents, resulting in the community-led construction of two additional parks in Chennai, as well as significant government investment in space for physical activity throughout Chennai. To date, more than 200 parks have been constructed or repaired throughout Tamil Nadu (642).

Measures of physical activity at baseline and follow-up (1996 and 2004) show statistically significant increases in physical activity levels. Resident participants reported a 313% increase in some form of exercise more than three times a week—from 14.2% at baseline to 58.7% at follow-up. Similarly, the number of participants who walked more than three times a week increased from 13.8% at baselines to 52.1% at follow-up. These results were particularly impressive given the decrease in occupations requiring physical labour during the same time period as the study.

providers. Although there are several public–private partnerships initiated by the Government of India to improve community participation and service delivery for communicable diseases control, such models rarely address chronic diseases. Lack of government intervention in the market to regulate the retail price of drugs and diagnostics for chronic diseases is a major deterrent to chronic disease control efforts.

Unhealthy diets in India are mainly driven by locally-prepared and -sold foods high in salt, trans fats, and sugar (biscuits, namkeens, sweets) and by traditional cooking methods using palm and coconut oils high in trans fat content. Since processed, packaged foods are a minor problem in India (as compared to countries like the US or the UK), there has been no substantial activity on the food industry. Consultations on food labelling and voluntary regulation have occurred, but to date, there has been no resulting action.

Recommendations

Over the past few years, there have been several 'calls to action' to address the issue of NCDs. Yet, the global response, especially from multilateral organizations, rich and poor country governments, major funders such as Gates Foundation, and other NGOs, has not kept pace with the growing prevalence of NCDs (see Chapter 6.1). Rising attention to and action on NCDs from the global community as well as local champions has helped to increase the awareness of NCDs among policymakers in India, although much less than the focus on under nutrition, HIV, malaria, and tuberculosis.

In this context, UN organizations and multilateral agencies can help support NCD prevention in India by setting up global frameworks for action. One such example includes enforcement in FCTC-signatory countries, facilitating the adoption of tobacco control policies in India (albeit on the ground implementation remains questionable). Similarly, these agencies can advocate to domestic policymakers to improve the outcomes and performance of the Indian health system as well as help identify and create cross-governmental and intersectoral linkages to feature chronic disease control strategies in India's development programmes. For example, increasing awareness of exposure to indoor air pollution from burning biomass fuels is relevant to India because of the need to balance environmental protection to prevent climate change and availability of clean fuels to the rural population of India, which is largely dependent on biomass fuels.

The central and state governments have the responsibility to support their citizens in pursuit of health and optimal life expectancy (644). The current health system is inefficient in dealing with prevention and management of chronic conditions as is evident from the continued growth in burdens. Successful chronic disease control programmes require a combination of high-risk (e.g. reorientation of the healthcare system to deliver efficient, and comprehensive preventative and curative care for people with NCD risk factors) and population-wide approaches (e.g. integrated, multisectoral prevention strategies).

Priorities include improving the outreach and scale of chronic disease services by developing multidisciplinary health teams and building relationships among primary, secondary, and tertiary levels of care for referrals and continuity of care. According to the World Health Report 2006, India has been identified as a country with a critical shortage of health care workforce (physicians, nurses and midwifes) imposing serious impediments to health care delivery (particularly in Chattisgarh, Madhya Pradesh, and Jharkhand states) (645). The Ministry of Health and Family Welfare, in tandem with the Ministry of Human Resource Development, need to actively engage universities across the country for coordination, planning, and implementation of various medical and health education programmes in all branches of health sciences. Further, the curricula for healthcare work force training need to be integrated and should undergo periodic revision as per the changing requirements of the health system and developments in health research. Academic institutions, especially the national medical bodies, should focus on changing medical curricula from sign-based teaching to holistic teaching methods.

As mentioned, the private sector is the major provider of chronic disease services in India. Measures to ensure standardization and quality of chronic disease services along with price controls can improve accountability of the private sector for the services they provide. Screening, surveillance and referral care are some of the areas for engaging the private sector and fostering public–private partnerships in chronic disease services. Also the research and development of drugs, devices, and medical equipment is in its infancy and the private sector needs to invest and innovate towards making them more widely available at affordable costs.

The most important areas for action are better implementation of tobacco control policies, policies aimed at population wide salt reduction, agricultural policies aimed at promoting growth of healthy foods and remodelling the built environment and improvements in public transport to improve physical activity and reduce indoor air pollution.

Summary points

1 Trade liberalization and rapid economic growth in India have contributed to rising population consumption of unhealthy food and tobacco.

2 Loss of traditional farming in rural areas has led people to seek new job opportunities, leading to large-scale flows of people into mega-cities has further increased exposure to unhealthy diets and reduced levels of physical activity.

3 India's population holds both the largest number of malnourished individuals in the world (251.5 million) and the second-largest population of individuals with diabetes (50 million), reflecting an extremely high double-burden of disease.

4 Surveillance of NCDs and their risk factors is particularly poor—most data comes from regional and urban studies that are often sporadic and lack standardized definitions and results.

5 There is some evidence of NCD action at the national level, but most efforts are state-led and fragmented. There are no unifying policies for NCD prevention and control across the country. State-specific successes, such as the TamilNadu NCD programme, provide lessons in designing future programmes to combat NCD.

Part 4

Chronic diseases in Mexico

Rebecca Kanter, Simon Barquera, Barry Popkin,
and Karen Siegel

Background

Mexico, a Federal Constitutional Republic located in North America south of the United States, is comprised of 31 states and a Federal District (Mexico City) and 106 million people (534). Mexico has stark socioeconomic inequalities: the richest 20% of the population holds 56% of the nation's income (534). The more affluent tend to live in the north or in Mexico City, while the poor tend to live in the south. 97% of the population speaks Spanish and 7% speak an indigenous language.

The Mexican economy is closely linked to the US and Canada. In 1994, the North American Free Trade Agreement (NAFTA), an economic union between the three countries, was the first trade agreement to unite two rich countries with a significantly poorer one. Prior to NAFTA, 60% of Mexico's land was used to cultivate corn, a source of livelihood for 3 million producers (8% of the Mexican population) (646). Liberalization of food markets after NAFTA's passage resulted in a more than 15% decline in Mexican agricultural producer prices (especially corn) between 1993 and 2004 as Mexican farmers were and are unable to compete with the flood of US corn and other staple crops into Mexico (5). Consequently, approximately 1.3 million of the poorest Mexicans lost their farms and moved to cities. By 2008, 77.2% of all Mexicans resided in urban areas, a population that grows at 1.4% per year (534).

Meanwhile, Mexico has experienced significant improvements in living conditions and public health (647). Part of this attributes to expanding programmes for water sanitation, birth control, vaccination, diarrhoeal diseases, and recent targeted health and nutrition programmes (648). Infant and under-5 mortality (649) and under nutrition (648) have declined sharply in Mexico over the last 20–40 years. In turn, demographic and epidemiological transitions occurred as more people lived to acquire chronic diseases and simultaneously, as described above and below, the environment has been altered to encourage unhealthier behaviours over healthier ones (284).

Evaluating the health burden of chronic diseases

In 1950, deaths due to communicable diseases, reproductive diseases, and undernutrition comprised nearly half (49.8%) of total mortality, while deaths from chronic diseases contributed 43.7%; by 2008, chronic diseases caused 75% of all adult deaths, approximately one-third of which were premature (prior to age 60) (648). Table 7.7 shows the specific leading causes of death in Mexico in 2005.

Chronic diseases also contribute significantly to the burden of disease in Mexico (Table 7.8). In 2008, chronic diseases caused 68% of disability-adjusted life years. Although diabetes is increasingly prevalent in Mexico (9.5%, or 5.5 million adults in 2006), there is evidence that CVDs are declining. Between 2000 and 2006, the incidence of both ischaemic heart disease and

Table 7.7 Main causes of death by disease in Mexico in 2005 (Percentage of total deaths)

	Men*	Women*	Both sexes (2004)**
Diabetes mellitus	11.3	16.3	9.7
Ischaemic heart disease	10.9	10.6	13.0
Cirrhosis and other chronic liver diseases	7.6	3.0	5.5
Cerebrovascular disease	4.7	6.5	6.0
Chronic obstructive pulmonary disease	4.1	4.1	4.0
Homicides	3.2	—	—
Motor vehicle accidents (occupant)	3.1	1.1	4.4
Lower respiratory infections	2.9	3.2	3.9
Nephritis and nephrosis	2.2	2.4	2.6
Birth asphyxia and birth trauma	2.0	1.9	3.0
Hypertensive heart disease	2.0	3.4	3.2
Lung cancer	1.8	—	—
Prostate cancer	1.8	—	—
Breast cancer	—	1.9	—
Protein-energy malnutrition	1.5	1.9	—
Motor vehicle accident (pedestrian)	1.5	—	—
Uterine cancer	—	1.9	—
Liver cancer	—	1.1	—
Stomach cancer	—	1.1	—

Source: *From: Secretaría de Salud. Programa nacional de salud 2007–2012. por un mexico sano: Construyendo alianzas para una mejor salud* [Spanish]. Mexico: Secretaria de Salud, 2007.
From: Stevens G, Dias RH, Thomas KJA, et al. Characterizing the epidemiological transition in Mexico: National and subnational burden of diseases, injuries, and risk factors. *PLos Medicine* 2008; **5(6):e125.

cerebrovascular disease declined in Mexico; from 60.4 to 54.1 cases per 100,000 inhabitants for ischaemic heart disease and from 34.3 to 30.9 cases per 100,000 inhabitants for cerebrovascular disease.

Individual risk factors

The main causes of chronic diseases are: unhealthy diets (high in fat, salt, and sugar), physical inactivity, and tobacco use (see Chapters 1 and 2). These behaviour risks interact to cause and magnify chronic health problems—mainly obesity, hypertension (high blood pressure), and hypercholesterolemia (high cholesterol). Table 7.9 shows the risk factors that cause the most death in Mexico: high blood glucose (hyperglycaemia), overweight and obesity (i.e. BMI ≥25), hypertension, and alcohol use.

Since the 1980s, overweight and obesity prevalence has increased dramatically among both sexes and across all socioeconomic strata and geographic regions, and these trends are expected to continue. Currently an estimated 52.2 million Mexicans (70% of adults) are now overweight or obese.

Children and adolescents are also increasingly overweight and obese. In 2006, 16.5% of boys and 18.1% of girls (aged 5–11 years) were overweight; while 9.4% and 8.7% were obese. The prevalence of overweight is higher among adolescents (12–19 years) than among children (21.2% in males and 23.3% in females) while the prevalence of obesity is similar (10% and 9.2%).

Table 7.8 Main causes of disease burden by disease and risk factor in Mexico in 2004 (percentage of total DALYs)

Disease	Men	Women	Both sexes
Unipolar depressive disorders	4.2	8.6	6.2
Road traffic collisions	6.5	2.4	4.6
Birth asphyxia and birth trauma	4.6	4.0	4.3
Diabetes mellitus	3.0	4.2	3.5
Ischaemic heart disease	3.6	2.6	3.1
Cirrhosis of the liver	4.4	0.0	3.0
Violence (homicide)	4.6	0.0	2.9
Asthma	2.3	2.5	2.4
Alcohol use disorders	3.6	0.0	2.4
Lower respiratory infections	2.4	2.3	2.3
Risk factor			
Alcohol use	11.4	2.4	7.3
High BMI	4.3	6.0	5.1
High blood glucose	4.5	5.6	5.0
High blood pressure	2.4	2.3	2.4
Unsafe sex	1.9	1.7	1.8
Low fruit and vegetable intake	1.6	1.2	1.4
High cholesterol	1.3	1.1	1.2
Physical inactivity	1.1	1.3	1.2
Childhood and maternal underweight	1.1	1.1	1.1
Tobacco smoking	1.4	0.6	1.1

Source: Adapted from Stevens G, Dias RH, Thomas KJA, et al. Characterizing the epidemiological transition in Mexico: National and subnational burden of diseases, injuries, and risk factors. *PLos Medicine* 2008; **5**(6):e125.

Table 7.9 Main causes of death by risk factor in Mexico in 2004 (percentage of total deaths)

Risk factor	Men	Women	Both sexes
High blood glucose	11.6	17.3	14.1
High BMI	9.9	15.1	12.2
High blood pressure	8.8	11.4	9.9
Alcohol use	12.1	3.3	8.3
Tobacco smoking	6.0	4.3	5.2
Low fruit and vegetable intake	4.6	4.5	4.6
Physical inactivity	3.8	5.0	4.4
High cholesterol	3.1	4.1	3.5
Urban air pollution	1.5	1.7	1.6
Unsafe sex	1.5	.4	1.0

Source: adapted from Stevens G, Dias RH, Thomas KJA, et al. Characterizing the epidemiological transition in Mexico: National and subnational burden of diseases, injuries, and risk factors. *PLos Medicine* 2008; **5**(6):e125.

Tobacco use is another key risk factor for chronic disease. Compared to the other countries presented (Brazil, China, India, South Africa), in Mexico, the smoking prevalence among adults is slightly lower at 25.2% (30.4% for men and 9.5% for women), but is relatively high among youth (28%), portending a high future burden of tobacco-related illnesses.

Leisure-time physical activity levels in Mexico are low, and have decreased over time. In 2004, only 17.7% of Mexican adults performed the recommended amount of physical activity (as defined in Chapter 7.1) (650). Mexican women are more sedentary than Mexican men, and physical inactivity increases with age for both genders. In 2006, only 38.3% of adolescent (10–19 years) males and 32.9% of adolescent females reported being physically active for 7 or more hours per week (651).

Poor nutrition remains a substantial problem, and underweight and overweight currently coexist. Although stunting has declined significantly (from 26.9% in 1988 to 15.5% in 2006), prevalence remains high in the rural south (30.1%) where many indigenous people live (648, 652).

For the majority of the population, however, dietary habits increasingly reflect those of high-income countries that consume nearly half of their dietary intake from added sugars and fat. Between 1984 and 1998, purchases of high-energy dense carbohydrates and soda rose by 6.3% and 37.2% (648). Consumption of wheat-based instant noodles is now higher than the consumption of rice and beans.

In particular, sugar-sweetened beverage consumption is increasing. Mexicans now drink more Coca-Cola than milk (653). Between 1992 and 2002, consumption of sugar-sweetened beverages (mainly Coca-Cola) in Mexico rose from 275 8oz servings per person per year to 487 servings per person per year in 2002, surpassing that of the US (654). This increase in soda consumption is associated with a decrease in whole milk consumption (648).

At the same time, fruit and vegetable consumption is decreasing. Between 1984 and 1998, fruit and vegetable purchases decreased by approximately 29% (648).

Inequalities in chronic diseases and risk factors

Inequalities exist in chronic disease prevalence. For example, diabetes prevalence varies by gender, area, and by geographic region. Prevalence is slightly higher in women than men, urban than rural areas (8.1% versus 6.5%), those with a family history of diabetes (11.4% versus 5.6%), and in the Northern and Mexico City regions (655).

Obesity prevalence varies substantially by gender and socioeconomic level. There is a greater combined prevalence of overweight and obesity among females, compared to males, in both urban (73% versus 68.8%) and rural (67.9% versus 58.9%) areas (652). However, while the prevalence is highest among the middle and highest groups (72.3% and 71.5%, respectively, compared to 63.9% among those of low SES), overweight and obesity rates are increasing most rapidly in the lowest SES quintile, rising nearly 400% from 1988 to 2006 compared to 55% in the highest SES quintile.

Societal determinants of chronic diseases

Economic drivers

Mexico's proximity to the US and the passage of NAFTA in 1994 has catalysed recent dietary changes. For example, NAFTA has resulted in the significant growth of supermarkets and large retailers and increased the availability and consumption of high-calorie food (646). Fresh markets no longer dominate Mexico's food system, having been replaced by Walmart and domestic clones (558, 656). Three out of every 10 pesos spent in Mexico on food are spent in Walmart (646).

It is important to note that while NAFTA is seen as a major force in Mexico's changing dietary landscape, many dimensions of globalization—from the introduction of large supermarket chains such as Chedraui and Walmart to modern food processing and agribusiness controls over the food supply—have happened concurrently across all of the Americas.

Nonetheless, NAFTA has had a large impact on Mexico's agricultural sector. Most significantly, the trade agreement has resulted in a diminished number of Mexican farmers. Between 1995 and 2003, 500,000 Mexican farmers (half of which were subsistence producers and half of which grew and sold corn, beans and other staples in local and regional markets), lost their jobs (5).

Remaining farmers have been forced to change their crops. With one of the highest per capita soda consumption in the word, sugar cane has become one of the most cultivated crops in Mexico; an economy that involves about a half-a-million workers (657, 658). The government has also subsidized certain crops, but subsidies mainly affect crops used to produce high-energy dense foods, rather than fruits and vegetables. In 2002, the Secretary of Agriculture, Livestock, Rural Development, Fishing, and Food passed a package of agricultural programmes and policies called Agri-food Armor (659). Within Agri-food Armor is a Target Income Subprogram that guarantees a target income for producers of certain grains (corn, wheat, feed wheat, sorghum, rice, triticale) and oilseeds (safflower, canola, cotton, soybeans) but not fruits and vegetables (659).

Some former farmers who left agricultural work altogether have migrated to Mexican cities (or to the US) in search of employment opportunities. Declining physical activity trends are driven in part by this shift away from rural agricultural labour to urban, more sedentary, service sector jobs (660). As of 2009, only 15.1% of Mexicans were employed in the agricultural sector, but 25.7% and 59% were employed in the industry and service sectors, respectively, suggesting that employment is no longer a significant source of physical activity in Mexico (661). Women are also adversely affected by these changes; factory labour is often the only opportunity for uneducated, working-class women to earn wages (662).

Environmental drivers

Urbanization is occurring in Mexico, although at a relatively slower rate than in China, India, and South Africa. As described in Chapter 2, cities increase the likelihood of developing lifestyle habits that contribute to chronic disease risk. Between 1950 and 2000, the number of cities in Mexico grew from 84 to 369; 77.2% of Mexicans now live in urban areas, a population that grows at 1.4% per year. Approximately 15% of the urban population lives in slums (535). Although this is approximately half the percentage of slum dwellers found in urban areas in Brazil, China, India, and South Africa, it still represents a large segment of the Mexican population that resides in conditions that contribute significantly to ill health (both infectious and chronic).

Cities in Mexico are not the only source of chronic disease risks. Small towns and rural areas are gaining increasing availability of unhealthy food products. In these areas, small 'tiendas' (convenience stores) are the predominant food source and how most transnational and domestic food companies sell their foods (115). Over 90% of all sales of Coca-Cola and PepsiCo (which sell soda in 3-litre bottles in Mexico) come from tiendas (115).

Another source of energy-dense foods in Mexico comes from 'street foods' sold along streets and in schools (663). While there is little data about the nutritional quality of these foods, the increased use of cooking oil and decrease in vegetables in Mexican food is apparent, as previously un-fried street foods have become fried.

Notably, school environments in particular encourage unhealthy food consumption, putting students at risk for obesity and chronic disease. One study found that within the 4.5-hour school day there were many eating opportunities for students, mainly at informal, unregulated, concession stands (including those on school grounds) that sell snacks high in sugar, fat, and salt (663, 664). Even in urban areas, most schools lack formal cafeterias or kitchens, and so most food provided to children is sold through informal 'cooperativas', often run by parents of children at the school. These cooperativas tend to serve foods that are fried or high in salt or sugar, and often help to generate additional revenue for the school. Schools often lack access to potable drinking water, exacerbating students' consumption of sugar-sweetened beverages.

In addition to access to high-energy dense foods, students have only two opportunities for physical activity in school: recess and physical education class. During the 30-minute recess, little or no physical activity (ranging from 5–12 minutes) is achieved; instead students spend time purchasing and consuming unhealthy foods.

Social and cultural drivers

Female participation in the workplace affects dietary patterns of Mexican families by decreasing the time a mother has to cook, promoting a greater proportion of food consumed and/or purchased outside the home. Furthermore, among very low-income rural households, women working outside the home were more likely to have consumed caloric beverages (sugar sweetened- and alcoholic beverages) than housewives in the past week, even when controlling for SES. Furthermore, men and women of the highest occupational grade were more likely to consume soda than those in lower occupations (665).

Increased food consumption outside of the home is driving dietary changes in Mexico. By 2002, food expenditures outside the home accounted for nearly a quarter (25.4%) of total food expenditures and have likely continued to increase. Food expenditures outside the home were more than twice as large within the highest income quintile as those in the lowest income quintile (648).

Technological advances have increased the affordability of modern conveniences, such as cars and televisions. For example, between 1990 and 2000, motor vehicle growth (38%) significantly outpaced population growth (17%) (663). The pervasiveness of television sets in Mexican households among all socioeconomic sectors also likely effects sedentary behaviour, particularly among children and adolescents (663). Women who watched television frequently were more inactive (30.9%) compared to men (20.5%) who watched television frequently (650). Adolescent males spent more time (≥21 hours per week) in front of a screen (33.5%) than females (20.8%) (651).

Parents' perception of a child's nutritional status (influenced by household SES or by the parent's nutritional status) may also affect that child's risk of becoming overweight or obese. This association has been noted in Mexico. For example, one study in the state of Veracruz showed that many parents of obese children did not identify their children as having any weight problem (663).

Social and economic consequences of chronic disease

Labour market costs

The social and educational impacts of chronic diseases are not well documented in Mexico. However, education and health have been highlighted as 'precious public goods' that are indispensable for Mexico's sustainable development (666). Between 2000 and 2008, the indirect costs of lost productivity in the workforce increased at an average annual rate of 13.5% (666).

The economic burden of chronic diseases falls heaviest on the uninsured; approximately half of all Mexican healthcare expenditures used to come from regressive out-of pocket spending. Nearly all (95%) of Mexico's private healthcare expenditures comes from out-of-pocket spending (647). Until 2007, when the Mexican healthcare system grew to include Popular Healthcare Insurance (Seguro Popular), every trimester nearly 1.5 million Mexican households fell either below the poverty-line or further into poverty due to out-of-pocket healthcare costs (284). Half of all diabetes spending in Mexico comes directly out of individual or household income (667).

Health system costs

Chronic diseases are an immense economic burden on Mexico's healthcare system. In 2006, 43.6% of total hospital expenses (public and private) were due to chronic diseases (666). From 2000 to 2008, healthcare costs associated with the medical attention of those with diseases attributable to overweight and obesity increased by 61%.[2] In 2008, these healthcare costs represented 33.2% of federal (public) spending on health services budgeted per person over the fiscal year and are predicted to increase to between 60.5% and 79.5% by 2017.

Diabetes and associated complications contribute significantly to healthcare costs. In 2005, diabetes-related healthcare costs were a third (34%) of all Mexican government-sponsored healthcare expenditures (655). By 2010, the total costs due to diabetes were US$778 million; $343 million in direct costs for drugs and treating diabetic neuropathy and US$435 million in indirect costs (667). Mexico's Secretary of Health (SoH) worries that, 'if we do not implement sound diabetes interventions, diabetes could bring about an economic collapse and saturation of health services in the country' (655).

Management and prevention of chronic disease

Healthcare system

Prior to 2004, Mexico's healthcare system was divided between a public government health insurance system (i.e. social security), other government healthcare programmes (i.e. public assistance), and private health insurance providers; and was not initially designed nor financed to address the dual-burden of disease facing Mexico (284).

Established in 1943, the government-sponsored health insurance system originally provided insurance to individuals who worked as a salaried or government worker (284, 668, 669). Those unemployed, self-employed, or day labourers were classified as uninsured, but eligible for some government and state healthcare services. In 2004 the Mexican healthcare system began a gradual reformation to cover the uninsured (~50 million Mexicans) through the Popular Health Insurance programme (Seguro Popular [SPS]), financed primarily through state government resources (284). By 2007, over 90% of Mexicans received some form of government healthcare; 48% had government health insurance, the uninsured 42% received some form of government healthcare services, and the remaining 10% had private health insurance (669). Ideally, universal (government-sponsored) health coverage will occur (284).

From 2004 to 2006 (after the implementation of Seguro Popular) government healthcare spending increased by 12.3% per year. As of 2007, public health expenditures constituted 46% of total healthcare spending and had increased at a faster rate than private health expenditures. Within the healthcare system for salaried non-government workers (IMSS) is a prevention component: Preven-IMSS, which also includes television and radio advertisements that encourage healthy lifestyles, and a nationally circulated health promotion and disease prevention magazine sold in public newsstands (663). There is evidence that this renewed emphasis on disease prevention has positively impacted both sides of the double-burden of disease in Mexico, with decreases seen in mortality due to TB, infant mortality, and prevalence of some chronic disease risk factors (284).

Chronic disease control

The Mexican government has prioritized obesity and chronic diseases, encouraging their prevention and control through a multisectoral approach coordinated by the SoH. For the first time, the National Health Plan includes explicit objectives related to obesity. In February 2007, President Calderon signed the National Strategy for Promotion and Prevention of Better Health, nested within the 2007–2012 national health programme (el Programa Nacional de Salud 2007–2012 [PRONASA]), which calls for broad-based chronic disease prevention and control (647).

At the forefront of the national health programme is a long-term vision (Vision 2030) that focuses on health promotion and disease prevention through ten overarching strategies. The SoH proposes one inter-institutional programme that consolidates the health promotion and prevention and control of overweight, obesity, CVD risks, and diabetes. The main goals are to have 45% of all diabetic and hypertensive patients under control and enrolled in at least one support group at a public health centre, to increase by 15% the detection of CVD risk and diabetes in those greater than 20 years of age, to decrease mortality due to heart disease by 15% in those under 65 years of age, and to reduce by 20% the rate of increase in deaths due to diabetes seen between 1995 and 2006 (647). For example, to better control hypertension, the SoH is promoting physical activity, weight control, case detection and improved patient treatment.

Obesity prevention has been a particular focus. Funds are allocated for an intersectoral national obesity policy that aims to decelerate and detain overweight and obesity prevalence by promoting myriad changes at all societal levels—increasing consumption of drinking water, working with industry to reduce the amount of sugar, salt and fats (and eliminate trans fats) in processed foods, and decreasing portion sizes in restaurants (666). In January 2010, the President—and members of government, industry, and academia—signed an agreement supporting a national multisector strategy for the prevention of overweight and obesity, based on the WHO Global Strategy for Diet and Physical Activity.

The Secretary of Health is also modifying its chronic disease control strategies to include 'diabetes literacy', weight management, and self-healthcare. Health services are also being updated to incorporate gender-specific health issues into health promotion programmes, disease prevention, and medical attention. Support groups for people who are overweight, have hypertension, diabetes, or dislipidaemias has been created by the SoH. So far, these groups have shown modest results (647).

The Secretary of Health has also committed to constructing a new, innovative health culture through public policies. To accomplish this, the government has appointed a sub-secretary of health prevention and promotion. In 2009, the Secretary of Health launched the 'Five Steps for Health for a Better Life' programme, which aims to prevent overweight and obesity from infancy through adulthood by encouraging people to: 1) move, 2) drink water, 3) eat vegetables and fruits [sic], 4) measure yourself (i.e. monitor health status and lifestyle) and; 5) share (i.e. enjoy all the 5 steps with your loved ones).

A final example of the focus on chronic disease prevention is the Secretary of Health's Beverage Guidance Panel (648). Following its report, beverages provided by government welfare programmes were changed. Soft drinks were excluded and over 20 million people were shifted from whole full fat- to 1.5%-milk. Congress has been working on beverage taxes and many other beverage-related changes are underway in Mexico.

Fiscal and regulatory interventions

Marketing/advertising/labelling

Advertising and mass-media regulation falls largely under Mexican federal law (663). The government institutions responsible for regulating children's advertising are the Attorney General for Consumer Protection, the Secretary of the Interior, and the Secretary of Health. Mexico's constitution protects consumers under age 18, stating that children are entitled to the satisfaction of their needs for food, health, education and recreation in a manner that guarantees their overall development (670). The Federal Law on Radio and Television prohibits advertising that promotes the consumption of alcohol, tobacco, or illegal drugs. The Federal Health Code imposes regulations on the advertising of alcohol and tobacco products as well as restrictions on the advertising of pharmaceutical products. Alcohol and tobacco advertisements are banned from broadcasting periods suitable for all audiences (e.g. 5am to 8pm) and from within 200 metres of schools (as well as school materials, such as notebooks), hospitals, parks, sports, among other sites.

There are currently no special regulations for children's advertising of other food and beverage products. Food marketing to children and adolescents is self-regulated by a recently approved industry code called *Self-regulatory Code of Food and Non-alcoholic Beverage Marketing to Infants* (*Código PABI*) which is in the process of evaluation. However, as television advertising is the main medium by which food and beverage advertising is conveyed to the Mexican population, greater efforts are needed to determine how television advertising affects children's food and beverage preferences and subsequent household food acquisitions.

Mexico has a set of policies, norms, and guidelines for food labelling. One set of policy criteria provides voluntary recommendations for the population, including the consumption of certain foods for nutritional benefits (such as eating beans and legumes), and reading food labels (671). It also establishes general dietary guidelines, and categorizes the diet into three basic food groups (vegetables and fruits; cereals and tubers; legumes and foods of animal origin). The 2007–2012 national health programme aims to strengthen food labelling regulation to both inform and orient consumers towards an integral diet; and to design intersectoral actions to regulate advertising, especially of foods and sugar-sweetened beverages to infants (647). In 2009, Mexico began discussing how best to label food and beverage products; currently, dietary guidelines based on a plate rather than food pyramid model exist, but its inclusion on food packaging is voluntary.

In 2004, Mexico became the first Latin American country to ratify the WHO's FCTC (672). As of 2009, taxes encompassed 65% of the retail price of cigarettes in Mexico (673). Deceitful terms are banned from Mexico's tobacco packaging, and new cigarette package warnings were effective in 2010. These include a picture based message on the top 30% of the package and text-only messages on 100% of the back and 100% of one of the side panels and a front/back/side matching picture and text message.

Regulations regarding schools and public places

Mexico banned smoking in all government offices and healthcare facilities in 2000, but these policies were ignored. In 2008, four years after Mexico signed the FCTC, a comprehensive smoke-free law passed, further prohibiting smoking in enclosed public spaces (e.g. restaurants and bars) and workplaces in Mexico City. Efforts are underway to replicate this throughout all of Mexico.

Responding to a considerable lack of physical activity among children (especially during the school day), a PE programme of two 50-minute PE sessions per week has been implemented in all elementary schools, but evidence suggests that this PE policy is not implemented as designed; moreover, 30–50 minutes of exercise twice a week is not sufficient for weight-gain prevention in children. There are no PE mandates by the Secretary of Education for secondary or preparatory schools. Mexican schools do not have healthy meal programmes and most do not serve lunch.

The Secretary of Health and Sub-Secretary for Health Prevention and Promotion has proposed a Schools and Health Programme to modify health determinants through integral health promotion actions (e.g. through improving physical activity and mental health programmes). Ideally, this programme will be carried out through the health and education sectors between 2007 and 2012 in collaboration with federal, state, and municipal governments. The Ministry of Education is also working to remove most high-calorie beverages and energy-dense snacks (high in sodium, fat, and sugar) from schools.

Community interventions

Another initiative to prevent, control, and monitor chronic disease is the national programme of 'health caravans', a programme affiliated with Seguro Popular (647). The goal was to have caravans in all states by 2010 to attend to the 20 million localities that are still lacking health services. These caravans will offer health promotion and prevention services as well as ambulatory medical attention; supported by a medical doctor, nurse, and health promoter and the use of various mobile units (e.g. dentistry, ultrasound, telemedicine).

Similar to Brazil, public physical activity initiatives have been implemented in Mexico, although to a lesser extent and mainly concentrated in major cities. For example, in Mexico City, central streets are closed on alternate weekends during the month, allowing and encouraging people to walk or cycle freely throughout the city. Mexico City also has a 'Ciclovía de la Ciudad de Mexico' (cycling and walking path) that extends across the entire city from the North to the South. The path is supported by the Mexico City government and the Secretary of the Environment and free for use by the public.

The role of the private sector

The Secretary of Health has close interactions with the food the industry, but resistance to product modifications is common. In 2008, an expert panel for recommendations on healthier beverage intake was established. Similar efforts have been made for food labelling and advertising to children and adolescents; and, for the reduction of fat, sugar and sodium in foods. In all cases, industry has proposed alternatives rather than changing their own practices. Fearing modifications will harm product sales, new products compliant with healthy recommendations are instead developed. Physical activity and nutrition education are also promoted rather than any form of product regulation.

Many food companies, such as Kellogg's, Bimbo, Danone, Nestle, Pepsico and Coca-Cola, are propelled in part by growing pressure from society, government, academia; and following a global trend have launched nutrition or health institutes, foundations, physical activity programmes and research grants in Mexico as a strategy to improve public perception of their company and products. One of the most significant achievements of the current administration, involving a great deal of negotiations between various actors and groups, was getting food industry representatives to sign the 10 objectives for obesity and chronic disease prevention in Mexico.

In Mexico, industrialized food comprises a large part of the population's diet, and awareness of its health impact is increasing. In this context, the trend towards cooperation and partnership observed in developed countries is likely to be observed in the near future in Mexico. The sooner the country overcomes resistance to change in implementing effective actions to reduce sugar, fat, sodium, total energy, and portion sizes, the better chronic diseases will be controlled. Currently the Mexican Secretary of Health, Secretary of Finance, and Food Standards Agency along with the

INSP are working to finalize front-of-pack food profiling standards. The Secretary of Health also aims to modify food policies by working with the food industry to eliminate trans fats, reduce sodium, saturated fats and sugars in foods; on regulating advertising to children to help prevent and control chronic diseases; and to promote 'the beverage recommendations for a healthy lifestyle' (655).

Recommendations

Many of Mexico's problems are global. Mexico's economy is deeply intertwined with the economies of the US and Canada. This has led to declining traditional agricultural practices and increasing exposure to processed, packaged foods.

The government recognizes the devastating role obesity and diabetes play now and in the future, and is attempting to implement regulations, taxation policies, and programmes that address poor diets. The beverage guidance panel and multisectoral work to promote healthier beverage consumption is one major initiative; the work to reduce sodium, trans fats, saturated fats, and added sugars in all processed foods and for front-of-pack labelling are others. Regulations of food and tobacco media and advertising in Mexico will become a main policy issue. There is a lack of experience and understanding in how to address the informal street food sector. Diabetes treatment receives little attention, yet is rapidly becoming a major health issue.

As described above, NAFTA has resulted in the availability and consumption of foods high in fat, salt, sugar, and total calories. Government support for healthier food crops (e.g. beans) and ways to shift tortilla consumption to healthier products are critical. Removing corn and beans from NAFTA will not solve agricultural sector problems; non-medical institutions need to work with the government and WTO to help protect small Mexican farm-holders from low-priced imports (5, 556). However, these actions are unlikely to occur as these are key aspects of Mexico's free trade structure. More trade liberalization will exacerbate rural poverty; greater regulation of both exports and imports is critical for rural poverty reduction.

Mexico's desire to shift towards healthier beverages and front-of-pack labelling are key dimensions of its need to collaborate with the food industry. Global and local food companies, the major international and domestic food distributors, and the government (e.g. Walmart) need to work together to reduce added salt, sugar and saturated fats from products.

The programmatic and policy role of academic institutions, such as the Mexican National Institute of Public Health (INSP), is critical. Its capacity for technical and scientific support, while remaining the country's key public health research body, should be strengthened. There is currently limited funding provided for the collection of dietary data and subsequent studies of dietary patterns and their shifts. Absence of a Mexican panel to follow the array of government changes as they affect diet, activity, obesity, and diabetes is notable. There is a need to link INSP with other major Mexican universities to do collaborative research on poor diets, activity patterns, smoking, pollution and other causes of the major preventable chronic diseases affecting the Mexican population.

As myriad sectors in Mexico work further to change and improve the environment to be more conducive towards mitigating, rather than perpetuating, chronic diseases and their risks, their progress to date should be acknowledged. Greater awareness and attention must be paid to Mexico's rich dietary history. The reclamation and re-incorporation of these diverse diets, composed of many vegetable and protein sources, are both powerful and imperative towards ensuring future sound health and cultural well-being in Mexico.

Summary points

1 Mexico has among the highest rates of overweight (>70%) and type 2 diabetes (9.5% of the adult population, or 55 million individuals) in the world.

2 Escalating overweight/obesity and chronic disease rates are mainly being driven by rapidly changing dietary patterns and by decreasing rates of physical activity.

3 Smoking rates in Mexico are relatively low among adults, but are high among youth, suggesting a future increased burden of tobacco-related illnesses.

4 Dietary changes began long ago and have been accelerated by economic policies (e.g. the NAFTA) as well as the broader globalization forces affecting all of Latin America. These changes have further disrupted agriculture and traditional farming and diets, and increased the availability and consumption of high-calorie, low-nutrient foods.

5 The Mexican government has prioritized the prevention and control of chronic diseases through health care and societal interventions. Cross-sector collaboration is beginning to occur.

6. Mexico was the first Latin American country to sign the FCTC and to later make a major city (Mexico City) smoke-free, but this needs to be scaled up at the national level.

Part 5

Chronic diseases in South Africa

Krisela Steyn, Debbie Bradshaw, Naomi Levitt,
Estelle V. Lambert, and Karen Siegel

Background

South Africa is a developing middle-income country located at the southern tip of Africa with a population of 48.7 million individuals. Often referred to as the 'Rainbow Nation', South Africa's population is demographically mixed, with approximately 79% Blacks, 10% Whites, 9% Coloureds, and 2% Indian or Asian. There are currently 11 official languages in South Africa; English is only spoken by around 10% of the population, but is most commonly used among the affluent classes and commercially.

Fifteen years into its post-apartheid democratic era, the South African population faces major challenges of inequality in terms of income and health. Both pre- and post-apartheid economic policies have resulted in a society with one of the largest income inequalities in the world (Gini coefficient of 0.58) (674).

The country is undergoing social, political, and economic changes that are resulting in increased urbanization and negative impact on health behaviours. Living conditions range from traditional houses in rural settings to formal and informal settlements and suburbs in urban areas. Access to electricity has grown rapidly (58% in 1996 to 80% in 2007) and the extension of basic services has seen the proportion of households lacking toilet facilities declining from 13.6% in 2001 to 8% in 2007. Currently, 60.7% of individuals live in urban areas, a population that is growing at 2.5% per year. A relatively high 28.7% of the urban population lives in slums, where poverty is rampant and health suffers (534).

At the same time, the opening of South Africa's borders in 1994 has led to significant economic growth (averaging 4.68% in 2005–2010). Imports and exports have increased and are valued at 58% of GDP (30% for imports, 28% for exports). Together with urbanization, these trends increasingly expose the population to processed foods and sedentary lifestyles. Uneven development has left the urban poor particularly vulnerable to these unhealthy lifestyles.

South Africa is now experiencing a so-called 'quadruple burden' of disease. The HIV/AIDS pandemic has reduced life expectancy by an unprecedented 20 years—average life expectancy is now 50 years for men and 54 years for women (675). The pre-existing TB epidemic has been compounded by HIV and exacerbated by the emergence of drug resistance, ensuring that South Africa has one of the highest TB burdens in the world (676). Yet, the country also contains a burden of chronic diseases (677), displaying elements of a protracted and polarized health transition, in which different types of diseases exist in the same population and compete for resources (284).

Evaluating the health burden of chronic diseases

The distribution of mortality in South Africa's nine provinces in 2000 is shown in Figure 7.9 (678). While all provinces experience a significant chronic disease burden, those where the largest

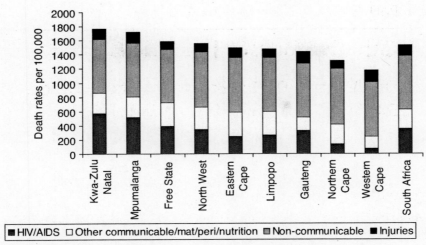

Fig. 7.9 Provincial mortality patterns in South Africa in 2000. *Data source:* (708).

proportion of the population live typical Westernized lifestyles (the Northern and Western Cape) have the lowest levels of infectious disease mortality and among the highest levels of chronic disease mortality. In contrast, the more rural and resource-deprived provinces (Kwa-Zulu Natal, Mpumalanga, Limpopo) suffer from a continued high burden of infectious disease mortality and growing chronic disease mortality rates.

Despite the continued high infectious disease burden accounting for 44% of all deaths (29% of which were due to HIV/AIDS), chronic diseases (including CVDs, diabetes, respiratory diseases, and cancers) accounted for 37% of deaths and 16% of DALYs in 2000. Chronic diseases are emerging in both rural and urban areas, but are particularly prominent among the urban poor. Premature chronic disease mortality (among individuals 15–64 years) is comparable in economically disadvantaged districts (e.g. Khayalitsha) and wealthier areas (e.g. Southern and Northern suburbs); 33% and 39%, respectively.

Individual risk factors

Through recent global and local surveillance efforts, patterns and prevalence of chronic disease risk factors in South Africa have emerged. These risk factors are common and show considerable differences by sex (Table 7.10). The risk factor profile of men is characterized by a relatively high prevalence of smoking and alcohol use, while that for women is characterized by a high proportion of overweight and obesity with low levels of physical activity. Notably, nearly half of South African women may be considered at risk on the basis of high plasma cholesterol concentrations (679).

The South African Demographic and Health Survey (SADHS) of 1998 indicated that 31.8% of women were obese and 26.7% were overweight, while only 6% of men were obese and 19.4% were overweight. For women, there were no differences between the different ethnic groups in the distribution of overweight and obesity, while for men the lowest rate of obesity was observed in black African men and the highest rate among white men. Older people and those living in urban settings were more overweight or obese compared to younger people and those residing in non-urban settings (680).

Table 7.10 Prevalence of risk factors for chronic diseases in adults

Risk factor	Men	Women	Data source
Obesity (15+ years)	6.9%	29%	1998 SADHS (673b)
	8.8%	27%	2003 SADHS (673c)
Hypertension (15+ years)	13%	16%	1998 SADHS (673b)
High cholesterol (30+ years)	45%	50%	(673d)
Tobacco smoking (12–22 years)	29%	15%	2002 Youth Risk Behaviour Survey (673e)
	26%	15%	2008 Youth Risk Behaviour Survey (673f)
Tobacco smoking (15+ years)	42%	11%	1998 SADHS (673b)
	35%	10%	2003 SADHS (673c)
Alcohol use (12–22 years)	39%	26%	2002 Youth Risk Behaviour Survey (673e)
	45%	29%	2008 Youth Risk Behaviour Survey (673f)
Alcohol use (15+ years)	58%	26%	1998 SADHS (673b)
	48%	22%	2003 SADHS (673c)
Physical inactivity (12–22 years)	31%	43%	2002 Youth Risk Behaviour Survey (673a)
	37%	46%	2008 Youth Risk Behaviour Survey (673f)
Physical inactivity (18+ years)	43%	47%	2002/3 World Health Survey (673h)
Physical inactivity (15+ years)	48%	63%	2003 SADHS (673c)
Low fruit and vegetable intake (30+ years)	80%	80%	(673g)

Following a peak in the early 1990s, tobacco consumption in South Africa has declined as a result of government tobacco control initiatives. Smoking rates dropped markedly from 32% and 34% (adults ≥18 years) in 1992 and 1995, respectively, to 25% (adults ≥15 years) in the first SADHS of 1998. Smoking prevalence has been considerably higher among men than women. Declines have been most notable among Africans, males, young adults and poorer people (681). The second SADHS (conducted in 2003) found that daily or occasional smoking prevalence among women remained unchanged at 10–11%, but decreased among men from 42% (1998) to 35% (2003), with the most significant decline among the poorest individuals. Higher income and education were associated with low prevalence of smoking, while living in urban areas was associated with higher rates. African men and women smoked significantly less than other population groups (682).

There is relatively little data on physical activity levels in South Africans. The 2003 SADHS showed that 63% of men and 49% of women were insufficiently active or inactive (defined as having less than 150 minutes of physical activity per week or less than 600 MET/minute/week). The prevalence of inactivity was greater in urban than in rural areas and, particularly in leisure time, increased with increasing age (683). To date, reported inactivity levels among South African adults are the fourth highest in the Africa region, and contribute significantly to all-cause mortality among South African adults (684). Adolescents show similar physical inactivity patterns; nearly 38% are insufficiently active, as measured by the Youth Risk Behaviour Survey in 2002, and which increased to 42% in 2008 (685, 686).

National data on dietary intake were not available prior to 1999, and as a result, FAO food balance sheets on food availability (1962, 1972, 1982, 1992, 2001) have been used to crudely measure trends in dietary intake. Over 40 years, per capita dietary energy intake has increased from 2603

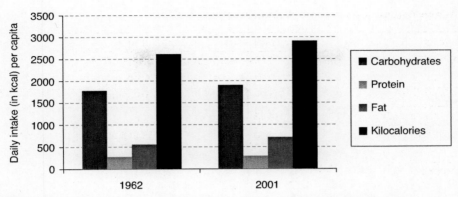

Fig. 7.10 Trends in dietary energy supplies from fat, protein, and carbohydrate (CHO). *Data source:* (533).

kilocalories per day in 1962 to 2921 kilocalories in 2001. During the same time period, fat consumption increased from 61.2 g to 79 g per day. Per capita consumption of vegetable oil and meat increased significantly, accounting for the large increases in fat and saturated fat intake (sunflower oil is the most commonly consumed vegetable oil, followed by canola oil). Fruit and vegetable consumption remained constant at approximately 205 grams per day (still less than the recommended 400 grams per day) (538). Notably, 80% of South African men and women over the age of 30 years have inadequate daily intake of fruits and vegetables (less than 600 grams per day) (687).

Only one published study has recently addressed the contribution of specific foods on the intake of sodium. The study showed, surprisingly, that respectively for black and white people living in Cape Town, the bread and cereal group of foods provided 48.6% and 54.9% of the total salt intake (688).

Unhealthy diets are also increasingly common among children. The first nationally representative dietary survey (National Food Consumption Survey, or NFCS) was performed in 1999, and included children aged 1–6 years. Results show that urban children consumed a diet with a higher energy intake, as well as more sugar, more protein, and more fat, than their rural counterparts (Table 7.11).

Table 7.11 Mean nutrient intake of children in the National Food Consumption Survey, 1999.

	Children 1–3 years (n=1308)			Children 4–6 years (n=1083)		
Nutrients	Urban	Rural	RSA	Urban	Rural	RSA
Energy# (KJ)	4403 (2043)	3992* (1790)	4200 (1933)	5614 (2375)	4963* (2283)	5271* (2349)
Energy (calories)	1048 (486)	950* (426)	1000 (460)	1337 (565)	1182* (544)	1255* (559)
CHO (g)	154 (72)	151 (71)	152 (72)	192 (80)	193 (91)	193 (86)
Added sugar# (g)	26 (23)	18 (17)	22 (21)	36 (30)	24 (34)	29 (33)
Protein# (g)	33 (18)	29 (17)	31 (18)	43 (21)	36 (19)	39 (21)
Fat (g)	29 (21)	22 (16)	25 (19)	38 (25)	42 (21)	31 (24)
Fibre (g)	9 (6)	10 (7)	9 (6)	13 (7)	13 (8)	13 (8)

Source: (709).
Significant urban rural differences (p<0.01).
* Mean intake is less than FAO/WHO (2002) required nutritional intakes.

Compared to the diet of people living in rural settings, the diet of people in urban settings was more energy rich, with a higher salt, fat, and processed sugar-based intake, while fibre and potassium intake was lower because of less fruit and vegetables. South Africans living in rural environments consumed more cereals and vegetables, while urban adults and children consume greater amounts of sugar, meat, vegetable oil, dairy, fruit, roots, tubers, and alcohol (84). Blacks and females also consume more sugar on average; the prevalence of dental caries approaches 90% in most South African adult communities—urban more than rural, and blacks (generally lower income groups) have lower fruit and vegetable intake than whites (higher income) (84).

Indoor smoke from the use of solid fuels is also a public health issue in South Africa. Exposure to indoor air pollution (smoke from solid fuels) is estimated to have caused 0.5% of all deaths and 0.4% of all DALYs with almost 99% of this burden occurring in the black African population. More than 1.1 million children under 5 years of age were exposed to indoor smoke in 2000, accounting for 1.2% of all healthy life years lost in this age group (689).

Societal determinants of chronic diseases

Social and economic drivers

During the transition to democracy in 1994, South Africa opened its borders to the rest of the world. The African National Congress's Growth, Employment, and Redistribution (GEAR) policy aims for economic growth of 4.2% per year, with a focus on deficit reduction, tight monetary policy, and trade liberalization. Restructuring of the economy has led to a further rise in male unemployment and probably an increase in the poverty rate, and the potential for the concentration of chronic disease risk factors among the poor.

Demographic change is a key driver of the chronic disease epidemic. Notwithstanding the impact of HIV/AIDS, the South African population is expected to grow. The proportion of the population that are 60 years and older (7.3% of total population in the latest census of 2001) is expected to rise almost threefold by 2025 (690).

Social mobility that has accompanied economic development is leading to increasing obesity and hypertension. Following the relaxation of the influx control mechanisms that restricted settlement of Africans into urban areas, South Africa has seen a massive movement of persons from rural to urban areas and a proliferation of informal settlements on urban fringes (509). Younger adults continue to move into cities seeking jobs, while elderly stay in rural parts, contributing to rising diabetes rates among the younger, working-age populations (691).

As part of GEAR, economic strategists have encouraged urbanization as a means to economic growth. Globalization and urbanization facilitate opportunities for transnational food companies to sell their products in developing countries. These transnational companies back free trade and discourage agricultural subsidies, consequently driving rural farmers out of business as the foods from industrialized countries become cheaper than those grown in South Africa. These cyclical trends lead to food insecurity for farmers and drive them off their farmlands to more urbanized areas, where new lifestyles can lead to development of chronic diseases (84).

FDI has increased exposure to Western fast-food chains. The first McDonalds opened in South Africa in 1995, and by the end of 2002 there were 100 branches throughout the country. A 2008 survey based on data from 85% of 531 franchised systems found 59 fast-food franchised operations and 73 restaurant chains operating in South Africa, reflecting substantial growth over the 2-year period from 2006 (from 4558 to 4633 fast food business units) (SBFF 2008). Restaurants and fast food franchises are an important source of employment with about 110,000 employees, accounting for about 28% of total employment in the franchise industry (692). These trends affect which foods are advertised and marketed most frequently in the media, furthering their appeal, particularly among children.

Increased access to modern technological advances, particularly in urban areas, is also driving declining physical activity rates. For example, in 2002 it was observed that one in four South African adolescents watch more than 3 hours of television per day—more recent data suggests this is now closer to one in three adolescents (693).

Cultural drivers

South Africans are increasingly exposed to contemporary (and unhealthy) global food trends, as described in Chapter 2. For example, trends show that approximately 70% of new food products being developed target indulgence and convenience (694). Moreover, the traditional South African diet, already heavy in starch and sugar, is contributing to increasing obesity rates through-out the country (695). Maize meal and white bread are staple foods among the urban poor, and cultural norms endorse putting 'three spoons of sugar in coffee and tea' (84).

There is considerable variation in the perception of ideal body shape amongst South Africans. In particular, black African women perceive being overweight as desirable, signifying beauty, affluence, health, and negative HIV status (696). These beliefs often start in adolescence: in one study, two-thirds of the 240 randomly selected black African adolescent girls living in Cape Town perceived fatness as a sign of happiness and wealth, and 75% of the girls associated thinness with ill health, particularly HIV/AIDS and TB. Interestingly, one-third of the girls had contradictory views about overweight/obesity due to its association with diabetes and hypertension, and with increased difficulty in finding appropriate clothing sizes (697).

Political and environmental drivers

Pollution, both indoor and outdoor, remains a problem in South Africa, although there is limited data for exposure to air pollution and adverse effects on health in the country (698). Solid fuels (wood, coal, and dung) are still commonly used for cooking and heating, although this varies considerably by population group and province. In 2000, an estimated 20% of South African households were exposed to indoor smoke from solid fuels that emit significant quantities of health-damaging pollutants and carcinogenic compounds. As noted above, this exposure has been shown to increase the risk of chronic diseases in children and adults alike. Other major sources of air pollutants are motor vehicles and industries burning dirty fossil fuels (coal, fuel oil, and diesel) in appliances that generally do not have emission control devices.

While many policies, including GEAR, contribute to the development of chronic diseases, the reduction in prevalence of tobacco use between 1990 and 2004 has mainly been driven by an impressive tobacco control policy that is focused on tobacco control legislation and rapidly increasing excise taxes, as well as the ratification of the FCTC in 2005 (84). Steep rises in excise taxes increased real cigarette prices by 115% between 1993 and 2003.

Social and economic consequences of chronic disease

There is a dearth of information on the specific impact of chronic diseases on the economy, society, the education system, or the health care system in South Africa. A single study on the economic impact of CVDs estimated that the cost to the economy was between R4.035 and 5.035 billion in 1991($0.538 and $0.671 billion) (699). This estimate excluded the costs of reha-bilitation or follow-up of patients with CVDs. It was estimated the 42% of the total cost was direct health care costs, while the remainder was indirect and intangible costs.

Management and prevention of chronic disease

The HIV/AIDS crisis and the related TB epidemic in South Africa dominates the allocation of scarce public health resources, but there is growing evidence that chronic diseases are beginning to receive government attention. Unfortunately, it is impossible to quantify the South African government's level of investment in chronic disease control, since much of the health budget allocated is not specified by disease groups (other than HIV/AIDS) and therefore no budgetary allocation data could be located. It is unlikely that the proportion of the health budget actually used for chronic diseases has decreased because of the additional funding for HIV/AIDS.

Health system

The country spends 8.7% of GDP on healthcare through parallel private and public systems with wide disparities in resources and utilization of each. Health services in South Africa are subject to the National Health Act No. 61 of 2003 which provides the framework for a structured health system for the country (321). The Department of Health (DOH) is responsible for national health policy and the public sector, while implementation of these policies and service delivery remains the responsibility of the nine provincial departments of health. Preventive services fall under local government control. The public sector primary healthcare system consists of community clinics (largely nurse-driven in non-urban areas), and district hospitals. These are complemented by secondary and tertiary hospitals, although the latter are unevenly distributed in the country, concentrated in urban areas. The DOH aims to improve access to health care for all by reducing inequity, and to improve prevention, health promotion, and delivery of care.

Approximately 15% of the population accesses the private sector through membership of health insurance schemes, and participation is proportional to income. A further 21% use the public sector for hospital care, but seek private care for acute illnesses. The remaining 64% depend entirely on the public sector for their healthcare needs. Health expenditure across the sectors differs considerably; 46% of health expenditures occur in the private sector—in 2005 the annual expenditure on medical schemes and out-of-pocket payments was approximately US$1170 per beneficiary, compared to about US$185 per person in people who access both systems, and less than US$160 per person for government primary and hospital care. The apparent inequalities in resources also extend to staffing. Approximately one-third of registered medical practitioners and specialists work in the public sector and 34% and 45% of public sector medical and nursing posts, respectively, remain vacant in 2008 (509).

Despite high levels of healthcare spending, the public sector has been chronically under-funded for many years. Furthermore, the system is traditionally geared to acute care, and is poorly equipped to handle rising numbers of chronic care patients. The HIV/AIDS epidemic has also profoundly affected healthcare resources. Major deficiencies exist in the quality and access to care for chronic diseases, and these diseases and their risk factors are diagnosed infrequently and managed inadequately (Box 7.2). Clinics are swamped by large patient numbers. Healthcare workers do not have the knowledge or skills, in particular communication skills, to optimally provide patient-centred care. Stock shortages of essential drugs, lack of access to others (e.g. lipid-lowering agents), and limited recourse to testing (e.g. glycated haemoglobin) also hinder healthcare delivery.

The principle of an integrated chronic disease care model is increasingly discussed, suggesting that South Africa and similar countries with high burdens of both chronic disease and HIV/AIDS (and other infectious diseases) need to consider new and appropriate models of care. As treatment of AIDS with antiretroviral agents becomes more common, aspects of effective chronic disease care apply equally to patients with AIDS on antiretrovirals, as they apply to patients

Box 7.2 Undiagnosis and poor control of hypertension and diabetes in South Africa

In the first SADHS conducted in 1998 of the patients with hypertension (blood pressure ≥140/90 mmHg or on antihypertensive medication) 26% of men and 51% of women were aware of their condition and 9.9% of men and 17.9% of women had well-controlled blood pressure below 140/90mmHg (700, 701). In cross-sectional prevalence studies, 50–60% of people with diabetes were undiagnosed.

A high percentage of individuals with diabetes (particularly those in rural, resource-poor areas) have also been found to be unaware of their condition. For example, in a survey in a rural black community in Kwazulu-Natal, 85% of the identified patients with diabetes were previously undiagnosed (702).

In contrast, a similar survey in the peri-urban black community Cape Town 40% of patients with diabetes were previously undiagnosed (703).

receiving chronic management for diabetes or hypertension. Successes and failures in the care of these different groups of patients requiring chronic care, can serve as models to improve care for all patients that suffer from chronic conditions and require long-term management and care.

Chronic disease control

Since 1994, a number of health policies relevant to chronic disease management, primary health-care, and community care workers have been formulated and adopted by the DOH.

In 1996, the Directorate for Chronic Diseases, Disabilities, and Geriatrics was instituted by the DOH and the first director was appointed, marking the beginning of both national and provincial government prioritization of chronic diseases. The unit's objectives are to:

1 Provide clinical management guidelines, tools, strategies, and policies which enhance quality management of such persons.

2 Support Provinces to develop, enhance, and sustain the comprehensive management of persons with chronic diseases, cancers, eye conditions, disabilities; those at risk as well as older persons.

3 Support the monitoring and evaluation of related policies, strategies, and guidelines at a Provincial level.

4 Support the capacity development, in-service training, as well as therapeutic education of health personnel providing services to the above target groups.

5 Participate in relevant intersectoral processes at National and International levels.

6 Facilitate contribution toward research in related fields.

The unit has produced several national guidelines and publications for the prevention and control of chronic diseases (including a 'Strategic Vision'), which have been widely distributed in public sector services. The guidelines include the management of hypertension, diabetes, obesity, stroke, and a National Cancer Programme. The guidelines were formulated by expert committees of various professional associations. This has resulted in some inconsistencies between the different guidelines, which may be confusing for clinicians in charge of implementation of the guidelines. The extent to which these guidelines are implemented, and their effectiveness, remains unevaluated.

Nutritional status in children (particularly stunting and underweight) has been prioritized since 1994. Although the Integrated Nutrition Programme (INP), developed by the Nutrition Directorate of the Department of Health, has primarily focused on under nutrition, specifically household food security, development, and consequences of under nutrition, recent developments suggest this may be changing. The Nutrition Directorate has supported development of strategies for nutrition-related chronic diseases, utilizing consultative processes to set objectives to 'reduce the prevalence of obesity from 9.3% in males and 30.1% in females in 2000 to 7% and 25% respectively'. Based on findings from the study by Charlton described above, the DOH has noted the need to reduce the amount of salt in the foods available to the population and is investigating the possibility to do so (688).

The most recent formulation of the DOH's Medium Term Strategic Framework for 2009–2014 does not specifically mention chronic diseases, although improvements for chronic disease care can be inferred in many of the statements included in the DOH priorities (704). The priorities include:

1 Increasing life expectancy.

2 Combating HIV and AIDS.

3 Reducing the burden of disease from TB.

4 Improving health systems effectiveness.

The activities are further specified in a '10-point plan', which has a strong emphasis on improving quality of care.

Additional developments show that political prioritization of chronic disease prevention and control may be increasing. In December 2006, the G77 (a bloc of 132 developing nations led by South Africa) encouraged the UN to adopt a declaration on diabetes. This Resolution was passed in late 2006, calling on all nations to develop national policies for the prevention, treatment, and care of diabetes in line with sustainable development of their healthcare systems, and signifying an important turning point for diabetes prevention globally.

Furthermore, the 52 African nations, including South Africa, recently drafted the Diabetes Declaration and Strategy for Africa, a 'call to action' encouraging governments to prioritize diabetes within their healthcare agendas. The declaration incorporates an overarching framework of agreed principles, goals, and strategies, with a mission is to improve access to high-quality and affordable services for prevention and care of diabetes, and provides a prototype for action (705).

Fiscal and regulatory interventions

Marketing/advertising/labelling

Tobacco control policies are prioritized in South Africa, and have resulted in the previously-mentioned declining tobacco consumption patterns between 1990 and 2004. The FCTC has been ratified and the elements are included in national legislation, which focuses on tobacco control and excise taxes (84).

In 1993, the Tobacco Products Control Act introduced health warnings on cigarette packages and advertisements in South Africa. In 1994, the government implemented a steady 50% increased excise tax on tobacco products. In 1999, the Tobacco Products Control Act was amended to ban all advertisements and the sale of tobacco products to minors. Further amendments to the Tobacco Products Bill (B7-2008) aim to close loopholes that allow the tobacco industry to target youth through advertising; to increase public awareness of the health hazards associated with cigarettes and other tobacco products; and to restrict young persons' access to cigarettes. Aggressive marketing techniques (targeting youth), distribution of free cigarettes to youth, and promotion of tobacco products at point of sale has been addressed in recent amendments to the Tobacco Products Control Amendment (706).

The regular increase of tax on tobacco products above the inflation rate will progressively make tobacco products less affordable. The tobacco industry regularly suggests that the increases in tax on tobacco products is increasing illicit trade and smuggling of these products, however no objective data exists in South Africa to indicate such a trend.

To date, food labelling efforts have been less comprehensive, although there are signs of progress. In 2005, the DOH revised food-labelling regulations, mandating that these be more informative and more detailed, and minimizing misleading food, health, and nutrition claims. To educate consumers about the new regulations, the Nutrition Directorate of the DOH is working together with the Directorate of Food control to plan and implement appropriate strategies. Furthermore, the Heart and Stroke Foundation and the Cancer Association in South Africa provide their logos on food products that meet certain health claims and nutrition standards, a practice that raises awareness of the relationship between food and health. To date, food labelling that addresses functional illiteracy (12% of the adult South African population is unable to read) has not yet received attention, but is an area for potential expansion.

Trans fatty acid content in South African foods has been largely unregulated. Recently, a few food companies have voluntarily removed trans fatty acids from packaged food products sold in South Africa. In some of the regulations recently promulgated under the Foodstuffs, Cosmetics and Disinfectant Act No. 54 of 1972, it is stated that trans fatty acids in man-made food products must be limited. However, the implementation of this act is limited.

Some formal food outlets have begun to use health awareness marketing strategies, emphasizing reduced salt and fat in their products and promoting fresh fruits and vegetables. However, such marketing and regulation efforts around food labelling and trans fat content will have limited effect in South Africa, since a large proportion of food sales comes from the informal sector, outside the reach of formal regulation that is mainly aimed at multinational food companies. For example, as much as 80% of all snacks sold in South Africa are made and distributed in the informal sector, and often contain sodium, additives, trans fats and microbial contaminant levels that are extremely high.

Regulations in schools and public places

The South African Government is a signatory of the FCTC and supports the WHO's Global Strategy for Nutrition and Physical Activity. The Tobacco Products Control Act No. 12 of 1993 and subsequent amendments in 1999 and 2008 have ensured that laws address all aspects of an effective comprehensive tobacco control programme, prohibiting smoking in all indoor public places. These regulations aim to reduce smoking prevalence by approximately one-third.

There are no regulations regarding the nutritional content of meals served in schools, or regarding the amount of physical education required in schools.

Community interventions

The Health Sector Strategic Plan (2004–2009) includes five key components, three of which are promotion of physical activity, promotion of good nutrition, and tobacco control. The 'Healthy Lifestyle Campaign' was launched in 2004, precipitated by the World Health Assembly's Resolution on Diet, Physical Activity, and Health. This campaign formed part of the plan for comprehensive health care in South Africa, and was one of the strategic priorities for the period 2004–2009. The 'Healthy Lifestyle Campaign' had five main pillars, which included: promotion of physical activity, healthy nutrition, tobacco control, responsible sexual behaviour, and combating the abuse of alcohol. In 2004–2005, the 'roll-out' of the campaign involved representatives from both the national and provincial departments of health visiting selected communities, typically those in peri-urban or rural settings. The Healthy Lifestyle 'day' was structured to begin with a 2–5-km walk within the community, lead by a representative from the National Minister of Health's office, followed by health risk screening including free blood pressure, cholesterol, random glucose, weight, height, and waist circumference measurements.

In May 2005, the 'Move for Health' campaign was launched by the DOH, in collaboration with other national agencies. The programme is focused in schools, workplaces, and community settings, and includes advocacy and social mobilization promoting mass participation in health walks, health screenings, and a national workshop that draws on international experience in health promotion (such as Agita São Paulo, described in Chapters 4 and 7.1). More than 36 organizations participated in two national workshops focused on encouraging physical activity across various sectors, and provincial health promoters have undertaken specific Vuka activities country-wide. Future plans include the development of a campaign logo, a mass media campaign, development of a 5-year National Plan, and the design of a monitoring and evaluation tool.

The Ministries of Sport and Education support these priorities, targeting 'increased mass participation' in sports and sports development, as reflected in the White Paper on Sport and Recreation in South Africa, whose theme is 'getting the nation to play'. The directorates of Health Promotion and Chronic Diseases have launched initiatives to encourage physical activity in older adults as well as youth, focusing on an intersectoral strategy aimed at the 'Promotion of Healthy Lifestyles' and 'Change from Risky Behaviour'.

Role of the private sector

The private sector remains an under-utilized partner for health promotion, primary and secondary prevention of chronic diseases, and cost-effective management. A number of private health insurance companies have implemented, but not generally evaluated, wellness programme initiatives and wellness benefits (e.g. BankMed, Discover Vitality, Oxygen Medical Scheme, etc.), in which health-seeking behaviours, in the form of health-risk assessments, gym membership, the purchase of healthy foods, opportunistic screening, chronic disease management programmes, and worksite wellness interventions, are fully or partially subsidized and in some cases, incentivized.

One example is the Vitality Healthy Food™ benefit, launched in January 2009, which reimburses health insurance scheme members 15–25% for more than 6000 healthy food items purchased in a major grocery retail chain. When members join the benefit, they automatically receive a 15% discount, while those who enrol in the 'Health Risk Appraisal' scheme receive a discount of 25% of their medical aid membership fee. The programme demonstrates that healthy food items make up about 18% of retail grocery expenditures among members of the programme, and to date, more than R150 million (approximately US$18 million) has been spent on HealthyFood™, with cash incentives paid back to members valued at R37,948,225 (approximately US$4.5 million). More importantly, the uptake of 'Health Risk Appraisals' has more than doubled since the launch in 2009 (Marieke Loubsher, personal communication, Discovery Vitality, Healthy Food Advisory Panel). This initiative may have important implications for subsidy programmes and value-added tax (VAT) exemptions for healthy foods through government channels.

The private sector may also engage in activities directed at the prevention and management of chronic diseases, through corporate social investment activities, e.g. the provision of dedicated research and training funding, the implementation or support of school- or community-based programmes promoting physical activity, healthy eating, and tobacco control, as well a social marketing campaigns focusing on healthy choices and health-seeking behaviours. For example, Unilever South Africa has removed trans fatty acids from their foods sold in South Africa, and has provided support for a variety of studies to assess the impact of blood pressure of reducing salt in commonly consumed products (707).

Recommendations

Global government (i.e. multilateral agencies such as the WHO) should develop generic evidence-based policies and therapeutic guidelines and tools that can be used to support health departments in developing countries to design, implement, and enforce appropriate chronic disease prevention and control policies. South Africa has gone some way in developing a surveillance system to guide policy. There is a need to strengthen vital registration, population based surveys and health system information systems to provide comprehensive information to review programmes. Given South Africa's past, it is essential that these data systems be able to monitor inequities in health.

The national government can respond by better embracing the demands of the dual burdens of acute and chronic diseases, and create multisectoral, integrated programmes for prevention, early diagnosis, and cost-effective treatment to optimize the use of limited resources.

The intensive role out of ART for thousands of patients with severe AIDS would result in an increased prevalence of diabetes, suggesting that healthcare provision for patients with HIV/AIDS must include integrated surveillance for diabetes, and aggressive treatment of diabetes and other related chronic disease risk factors in these patients.

As described, an estimated 80% of snacks sold in South Africa come from the informal sector, which tends to produce products high in fat and salt, but is outside of the realm of formal food and nutrition regulation. The fact that this informal sector provides significant employment (particularly for the poorer populations) requires carefully designed solutions.

Public health aspects of the prevention and care for chronic diseases need to be incorporated in the training of undergraduate health professionals. Public health students must clearly understand the dual focus of chronic disease prevention and care which includes, on the one hand, a focus on the total population for the promotion of a healthy lifestyle, and on the other hand, the early diagnosis and cost-effective treatment of patients at high risk for chronic diseases.

Summary points

1 Despite the rapid onset of AIDS and a continued high burden of injuries and maternal and child health problems, South Africa is experiencing a burgeoning epidemic of chronic diseases.

2 The chronic disease burden is mainly the result of the ageing of the population and the consequences of increasingly unhealthy diets and physical inactivity.

3 These behavioural changes are driven by economic changes—development and social mobility associated with growing consumerism—and cultural drivers.

4 The Apartheid legacy and current macroeconomic policies has resulted in different population groups being in different stages of the epidemiologic transition with poor urban Africans being highly vulnerable and experiencing multiple burdens of disease.

5 Currently, chronic disease prevention and control is a growing priority at the national level. More transparent budgetary allocations data is needed to see how much money is being invested in chronic disease prevention and control, and where it is going.

6 Impressive national-level tobacco control measures (smoking bans, advertising bans, increased tobacco taxes, education, and awareness efforts) have resulted in marked declines in tobacco use and could be used as a model for increased chronic disease efforts to tackle unhealthy diets and high levels of physical inactivity.

Endnotes

1 Between 2002 and 2007, President Kalam aspired to transform India into a 'developed' nation by 2020. The current President Patil, the first woman to serve in the office, endeavours to sustain current rates of economic growth.

2 In 1998, costs related to obesity accounted for nearly a quarter (24.9%) of total public health costs and 10.8% of total health costs in Mexico (Secretaría de Salud 2009).

Chapter 8

Responding to the global challenge of sick societies

David Stuckler and Karen Siegel

One of our daily rituals is to look in the mirror. Every morning, we wake up, take a look at ourselves, and check to make sure everything is in order. The image we see is a reflection of who we are and who we are becoming. In this book, we have held up a mirror to reveal an image of our society. Our health reflects who we are as communities and what kind of world we are building for our children.

As we gaze into this mirror, one of the first reflections we see is Suman, a morbidly obese Indian girl, who faces a lifetime of suffering and illness. While her situation is in many respects a vast improvement over what it might have been three decades ago, when she had a lower chance of surviving to her fifth birthday, one would hardly be able to describe the changes to her living conditions as development. Looking deeper into Suman's background, we can see out the power-ful ways in which her life's choices and possibilities are being developed as though by an 'invisible hand'. Prices, availability, and marketing of unhealthy products seem to conspire against her ability to freely choose a healthy, active life. As we pan our view to the global landscape, we notice that similar circumstances confront millions of children like Suman across the world.

At other times when we stare in the mirror, we behold an image of ourselves. Every day we see the same person, yet, before we realize it, we become old and grey. When we look back at pictures from decades prior, we can barely recognize the person now staring back at us. It seems hard to believe how quickly we truly changed. In global health, when we look at pictures from the past decades, we recall the gross injustice of starving, infected, and malnourished children and adults. Today, we can see how far we have come to conquer these killers that have claimed millions of lives, although we still have a long way to go. What we have great difficulty recognizing is how too many of us suffer from the same threats of poor nutrition, but in a different form: we have slowly become obese and burdened with chronic disease. Indeed, it is as though entire societies have aged quickly, and we are now old—much older than we should be for our actual age: girls like Suman are dying too young from chronic diseases.

Even though we have difficulty spotting these incremental changes, we tend to pay extra attention to the one thing we think is wrong or wish we could change. For some of us, it is wrinkles under our eyes; for others, our nose is too big, or we have stretch marks, or bad skin. While each of us can clearly see a different problem, our reactions are usually one of three: we simply learn to ignore them; we try to conceal these problems; or we try to change them. So it is in development and public health. In development, many of the problems we focus on and isolate in the image are about violations of human rights and climate change. In public health, we see the longstanding challenges related to HIV, child survival, malaria, neglected tropical diseases, mental health, and, increasingly chronic disease. Many of us turn a blind eye, learning to ignore these issues; others try to conceal the issue by throwing money and technology at a problem that they know only acts as a band-aid covering bigger issues that led us to this profoundly inequitable situation in the first place. There are those, however, who try to intervene; we hope by holding up the mirror to society with this book that this group will grow.

Returning to the river analogy of Chapter 4, we are all downstream, trying to pull different bodies out of the river. As we step back from the mirror to take a broader view, we can see how our focus on each of our individual problems overlooks the ways in which they are interconnected and deeply rooted into the ways in which we live and build our societies. This insight forces us to change our view. We can begin to ask deeper questions like: who is holding the mirror and framing our view?

For many of us the mirror will be set in a comfortable, three-bedroom house or apartment, where we go about a daily routine. Surely it is us who hold the mirror? Surely it is us that have to be happy with the image we see? But we all know people who, when they look at themselves, see a big nose or ears even though they are actually quite normal. Our impressions of who we are can be shaped by a world that shapes our vision of what is attractive or not. Analogously, in development and global health, there are a few powerful groups who set the agenda, and in so doing decide what is sexy and what is not. One day the fashionable remedy for HIV/AIDS is condom use; the next day it is antiretroviral therapy; a week later is it mass circumcision. The problem we can begin to see is that while the issues are cross-cutting and deeper, our focus has been placed on the most immediate and pressing social problems, and homes in on quick-fix, magic-bullet solutions. Our focus has been skewed.

This distortion has led some people to see rising levels of heart disease, cancer, diabetes, and other chronic diseases as a sign of success, or at the worst, growing pains that we can live with. The image that they see is of people who could have chosen to be healthy but instead chose to be sick, and as a result, they view every chronic disease death like rationally committing a slow suicide. The people who see this image are usually those who have never lived alongside, or broken bread with, people who live in poverty. They have not confronted the bereaved families of people who have died for lack of insulin, or the parents of morbidly obese children who are at their wits end about what to do. They say 'be more responsible' to children like Suman who have fatty streaks in their arteries, whose bodies have reached their fifth decade by their teenage years, ageing at five times the rate of our current generation. They blame her.

There are, however, others who see the profound social injustice revealed in this book's pages. Some of these people will claim to be realists and argue that, while chronic diseases are an issue, we have only enough resources to tackle a few causes of poor health. With so little money, they see a road ahead where we must choose who lives, who dies, and from what. Their vision is one of human sacrifice. Yet they do not confront why it is that they pour billions of dollars into preventing diseases that have as yet killed no one, or why it is that they give vast sums of money not only for the sake of others, but largely to help themselves.

But there are those who look into the mirror and see social injustice and are driven by a desire for profound change. They don't wish to simply conceal the imperfections or ignore them, but instead to make radical change. They see that poor health is concentrated among the poor, and want to walk to the head of the river and confront the killers head on. These people, who we hope are you, are those who do not want to see more bodies being thrown into the river. The following sections set out lines of attack that can be formed which we believe will change the image we see from one of sick societies to one of greater global health equality.

Restoring the public health imagination: a guide to building a global citizens movement for action on the social and economic determinants of health

Public health and medical students

Undergraduate or graduate students in public health and medicine are the future of global health. Whatever change occurs likely starts with you.

This book has repeatedly pointed to the importance of acting on the upstream determinants of health. To get started, you must overcome numerous barriers in your training, career development, and institutional networking.

Getting training

The famous public health doctor Rudolph Virchow wrote in the 19th century, 'Medicine is a social science'. Follow his prescription: master epidemiology, then learn how to do epidemiologies of entire societies. Where do you begin?

The odds are that there are few courses easily accessible to you in global chronic diseases (a reason we have penned this book). Some courses are offered in chronic disease epidemiology but most focus on a narrow set of risk factors, as described in Chapter 2. There is growing potential for studying the societal determinants of health at universities, albeit these courses mostly focus on high-income countries. Training available to you largely reflects where the money is invested in the field. As we showed in Chapters 4 and 5, thus far, there has been a focus on narrow biomedical and genetic determinants of disease and, in global health, on immunizations, vaccines, and cost-effectiveness. Finding a research group that covers all the necessary areas to uphold Virchow's tradition may be difficult.

Build your own curriculum. Take courses in sociology, political science, economics, psychology, and anthropology. Include three sets of tools:

First, develop expertise in advanced quantitative methods. At times it may seem like bitter tasting medicine, but these tools are your most powerful weapons for bringing the often unheard voices of the poor to the fore and revealing a healthier, fairer society that we can imagine. Many very good courses in biostatistics and epidemiology are available to you at medical and public health schools, but these should be complemented by econometric and demographic tools.

Second, these quantitative methods help you find answers, but are of little use in defining important questions. Many compelling hypotheses can be found in the simplest of ways: talk to people living in resource-poor communities, and listen hard. This approach draws on ethnography, a widely used method by anthropologists and sociologists. Qualitative methods are crucial to hear the voices of those who are often silenced and not detected by our inadequate surveillance systems (169).

Third, seek training in political economy that draws on rich traditions in sociology and political science (and to some extent economics). The school of health policy analysis we emphasize is simple: ask who benefits and who loses? Follow the money, power, and vested interests and you will find the root cause of many of our society's most intractable health problems. These approaches to applying scientific methods to study power and politics have yet to become mainstream in public health. Fortunately, the tools have been developed in political science and sociology. To help you get started, at the end of this book we provide resources that will give you ideas and methods for addressing the ultimate social, political, and economic determinants of health and health inequalities.

Recognizing barriers to success

Following the tradition of Virchow will not be your ticket to a boring life, nor will it be an easy path to academic success. When Virchow was asked to investigate the causes of typhus in Upper Silesia, he reported that the problems lied in the distribution of political and economic power (710). He recommended a sweeping set of reforms including land tenure and housing reform, water regulation, and other societal interventions. Outraged, the authorities responded that his report was not a medical document but a political one—and he was thrown out of the country.

So we issue a warning: these epidemiologies of modern societies can be viewed as critiques of people in power, and are frequently controversial. Whenever you seek to address the societal determinants of chronic diseases, and confront vested interests, the implications of your studies are powerful: they will hold up a mirror to people in power—showing them how their decisions either saved or killed people. But to do otherwise does not escape this problem. No study or intervention you do will be value-free and apolitical,[1] and you must be aware of this fact.

While you may not get thrown out of your country like Virchow (although there are some epidemiologists living today who have been),[2] there is a reasonable chance you will face other kinds of social and institutional backlashes. For example, you may face difficulty getting grants. Or you may see yourself bypassed by your peers who study genetic determinants of chronic diseases or do more of the same kinds of statistical studies or randomized controlled trials about individual risk factors. Pursing Virchow's tradition offers little hope of winning multimillion dollar grants that result in large laboratories, medical infrastructure projects, and huge bonuses.

Remember that grants are made, not simply awarded. Success in research is driven by merit, but also one part luck and at least another part networks. These networks reflect power. As we described in Chapter 5, the global health and medical research community is largely driven by a powerful base of pharmaceutical and food companies, along with health institutions and national development agencies that principally service economic and political objectives.

The easiest path to academic success is to create answers to questions asked by people in power that reflects what they want to hear. Virchow's approach starts in the opposite direction. People living in poverty and poor health define the questions; and researchers investigate the objectives and powerful impacts on health of the decisions made by people in powerful positions. If your research reveals critical findings, these groups will be reluctant to back your research agenda and career development.

Building a social network

Given the enormity of the challenge, and the considerable barriers you face, it would be incredible if along the way you did not begin to feel demoralized, apathetic, and fatalistic. But remember the Maniacal Dictator of Death in Chapter 5: this is the desired response by those who would prevent a social movement from arising. But you are not alone: there is a large community of people who share your concerns about sick societies and social injustices in health.

Recall that you also have a rich tradition of social medicine to fall back on. It dates to Virchow, but lives on in the traditions of Primary Health Care, liberatory medicine, and, most importantly, in the Social Determinants of Health movement. His tradition in public health is embodied by Sir Michael Marmot, Martin McKee, Nancy Krieger, and Vicente Navarro, to name but a few. The recent WHO Commission of the Social Determinants of Health, led by Marmot, concluded that 'social inequalities are killing on a grand scale'. The logical next step (which the Commission could not express for obvious political reasons) is to identify who and what decisions are perpetuating these inequalities and creating sick societies. If we seek to address the 'causes of the causes of causes' of poor health and health inequalities, we will have to engage not just the societal determinants of health, but those who determine the societal determinants of health. In Chapter 2, we have pointed to but a few of these groups; many exist, and your challenge is to find them and make the effects of their decisions visible and unmistakeable.

You can also build your own network of passionate advocates for a fairer society. The tactics to mobilize community, bottom-up movements by forging broad alliances in Chapter 5.2 apply most directly to you. In taking these steps, your work will help build a global social citizen movement in health that responds not only to the challenge of chronic disease, but to the overarching challenge of sick societies.

To get started, we have provided a list of these organizations at the end of this chapter. Get in touch with them; join forces; and start your own network. The easiest way to get plugged in is to offer to help. Work for free (if you can). Contact people.

As a final set of tips to help build a movement:

When studying: ask what you believe are the most important questions facing society. Then look for the answers, wherever this quest leads you. Do not be afraid of breaking new ground. Without a certain degree of irreverence for what has come before, progress would never be made. Keep sight of the broader human goal and purpose. Never forget to ask who wins and who loses as a result of your work. Take pleasure in the details (especially the boring financial and legal ones): they are often critical.

When publishing: avoid obscure language (something that we as authors are often guilty of). People 'muddy their waters to make them appear deep' but also, perhaps unintentionally, to hide the bases of power in society. Their language cloaks invisible hands in a complex, highly technical discourse. Keep things simple and accessible. That will help you build a broader community and create a shared dialogue with your partners and colleagues in other fields. Most importantly, simple language will allow you to share your knowledge with ordinary people who need your help. Socialize your expertise. Remember your work is a public good.

When building networks: focus on the structure. Provide a forum where people can hear the voices of the poor. Create accountability. Use expertise to support, not direct. Be open to criticism. Reveal your assumptions and core values. Speak frankly about morality.

Chronic disease academics and researchers

If you are a professor working in these areas, the most important work you can do is to help re-frame the debate. The first set of tactics in Chapter 5.2 is addressed directly to you.

As an expert you have much greater responsibility to the public. Inaction is a decision to side with those in power. As Edmund Burke famously said, 'all that is necessary for the triumph of evil is that good men do nothing'. That can possibly be excused for those who are unaware or incapable. But your education and ability to see deeper into society puts the onus on you to do more for the public good.

As noted throughout this book, the challenge of responding to chronic diseases has shifted from being mainly a technical to a political issue. Evidence is needed that can help build a social movement on global health and, within it, chronic diseases. Focus on exposing vested interests, understanding political determinants of information and public health programmes, and creating evidence about the societal causes of chronic diseases that can spur public health interventions.

Re-framing the debate

The greatest expansion of research is needed on the societal determinants of the risk factors. Often we see in our statistics that age, sex, ethnicity, and income are statistically significant risk factors. But why? These clues reveal the existences of unfair social inequalities in disease, but don't help us intervene. We need to know more about the social and institutional drivers of these socially patterned diseases and risk outcomes that manifest in our statistics. In the case of cigarettes, these drivers are tobacco companies and a series of tactics they employ, such as sophisticated marketing to children and complicity in smuggling to influence markets (72, 83, 110, 156, 706).

There is also a need to know more about the political determinants of global health. Why are rich, white men suddenly interested in global health? How do they set their priorities? What are the effects of their money on the well-being of the poor? We lack answers to these fundamental questions. We have great difficulty tracking where money comes from and where it goes in global health. The activities of private foundations such as Coca-Cola Foundation or Bill and Melinda Gates Foundation, while projecting a positive image, may also be pursuing the development of commercial products and creation of markets ('profiting on the poor'). There is a need to understand the full potential for conflicts of interest to affect the global health agenda and resolve the ethical issues they raise (308, 712). Chapter 5 has launched an initial study into the political economy of global health, but much more work needs to be done.

Transforming the private sector

The next major unresolved issue is how to engage the private sector. Unlike tobacco, food is not a global bad (although some ingredients might be). Food companies have an undeniable role to play. Yet there is too much history to believe that they will just be 'partners'. We recommend the following core principles of engagement by public health professionals:

1 The influence has to go from public to private, not the other way around.

2 Voluntary private sector action is only viable if the private sector profits (in terms of public relations or managing risk such as potential lawsuits).

  Within this framework, public health experts can act as health investment advisors:

  ◆ Helping transform portfolios and bringing poor people into markets;

  ◆ Providing scientific and technical information about healthy product development

3 In all other cases, public regulation is needed:

  ◆ Making markets work better and enforcing standards of fair competition

As noted in Chapter 6, many public health people have been hired to work on the inside of food companies as part of these companies' core business strategies. Yet, companies are complex organizational systems: they can sequester departments and restrict information flows, often distributing its bases of information across different countries. To those working in these companies, we offer a simple note of caution: be wary that you are not a cog in an elaborate public relations campaign. Work from within these companies as advocates to change unhealthy practices and promote long-term social responsibility. Or, in the case of ethical compromise, become whistleblowers to advance the global health movement.

In past cases of tobacco control, critical support came from people who worked on the inside of tobacco companies and who, feeling ethically conflicted, leaked confidential information. They did so at risk of serious reprisals to their careers and families. These people are heroes.[3]

Supporting litigation

Engaging the private sector is the most important battle public health will face. Food and beverage companies, recognizing the threats they now face, will likely seek to make the minimum changes to their products needed to avoid taxation and prevent the tide of public opinion from turning against them. To speed up this process of transforming the private sector to promote health, one of public health's most powerful tools is litigation.

Your research is needed to support lawyers who are currently bringing legal cases against companies that manufacture unhealthy products in an attempt to get access to their internal documents. One major turning point in the tobacco control movement came when the case of *State of Minnesota v Philip Morris et al* forced tobacco companies to disclose their documents (at least those that could be found before they were shredded). In almost every social movement, legal interventions played a formative role. It is likely that in the same way that tobacco ended up in the courts, junk food cases will too.

Litigation plus legislation equals real change. The achievements of litigation against the tobacco companies have likely saved more lives than any other public health intervention in the past decade. Albeit difficult and expensive, litigation can create access to vital information. In tobacco control it took five decades to get discovery of documents that led to huge awards and, ultimately, paved the way for legislation to reduce smoking. While the job is not complete in poor countries, where there are difficulties enforcing laws on the ground, we can draw lessons from past experiences to facilitate public interest litigation in those countries as well as avoiding the devastating cost of inaction (numbering more than 16 million lives in the US alone) (83).

Briefly, as summarized in Chapter 5, there are four pieces of evidence needed to build a case about junk-food or other unhealthy products that cause chronic diseases:

1　Products are addictive.[4]

2　Products have health impacts.

3　Companies know they are addictive and have health impacts (which can be found from their sponsored research studies), and

4　Companies publicly denied and distorted the record.[5]

To be most effective, focus studies on children and adolescents. These groups evoke an attractive media image, and are most susceptible cognitively and developmentally to manipulative messaging. Tobacco companies aim to hook teenagers (83, 713, 714). While we cannot say with certainty that food companies use this approach (although it is difficult to interpret their inclusion of toys with their products in any other way), as we noted in earlier sections, neuroscientists and psychologists are being hired to develop marketing and products that can get youth and adolescents to become customers for life.

Knowing industry counter-tactics will also help. Their main defences will be to argue that individuals had overindulged of their own volition. It will make individual litigation difficult. In 2002, for example, the courts dismissed an obesity-related complaint on the grounds that plaintiffs freely chose to consume fast-food.[6] Food industries also support pseudo-consumer groups who oppose the 'public health nanny states' life-saving protections, ranging from seatbelts to salt reduction.

As noted in Chapter 6, these industries will also hire scientists to develop research, potentially as part of a strategy to confound an effective public health response. Recall the cautionary tale of tobacco expressed throughout this book. As part of their public relations strategy, tobacco companies hired 'whitecoats'—their term for scientists—who they employed, often through industry pseudo-scientific front groups, to create public confusion and distort the scientific evidence base (72, 159, 252, 715). Decades later we discovered tobacco documents that revealed how many well-intentioned and respected scientists had no idea whose interests they were ultimately serving (716). It is likely that this process is continuing today through a variety of industry-fronted NGOs and grant-making foundations that have vested interests in food, beverage, and alcohol products. Much of the global research used in this book drew from industry-funded studies (mainly in Chapter 5), because industries and private foundations are some of the few major funders of chronic disease-related work in developing countries (although the sums they give is very low compared with their other global health activities).

Some industry strategies, however effective as public health measures, can also crowd out potential for successful litigation and deeper change. Nutritional labelling, for example, will make it easier for industries to argue that people are making informed choices, in the same way that airlines print advice to move around to avoid thromboses in in-flight magazines, yet squeeze so many seats in as to make movement almost impossible. Similarly, industry's decision to remove trans fats from foods gets rid of a potentially addictive and globally bad ingredient, thereby greatly reducing the scope for litigation.

The legal road with food, beverages, and alcohol will be long, difficult, and expensive. Just like the early stages of tobacco, the litigative path is considered by some to be outlandish. Yet, so far there have been early signs of success (717). For example, McDonald's was recently sued about mislabelling the nutritional content of their products, and settled for $12 million out of court. Within 24 hours their nutrition labelling changed. It is important to ensure that these companies' food products actually contain what they say they do. Recently Kraft had been sued over trans fats in Oreo cookies, but before it went to court, they voluntarily removed them. As a result of a legal case, the New York School system removed soda and snack machines from school property.

In the case of tobacco, even when litigation failed, it helped politically mobilize the society around the relevant issues, contributing to the social movement's momentum. The key is to start.

Health policymakers

If you are working in a low-income country, you are well-aware how many Westerners come to your office and want to talk about a very narrow set of diseases. Lately it has been HIV/AIDS, HIV/AIDS, HIV/AIDS. See this as a major opportunity to build up chronic care capacity. Build clinics that can jointly deliver goods for all chronic causes of poor health. Point out that people with HIV/AIDS in your country are dying from heart disease and diabetes. Tell these Westerners how unfair it is that people living with diabetes cannot get access to low-cost medicines that could easily be provided.

The strategies set out in Chapter 5 about creating and identifying political opportunities are largely directed to you. We single out three ways you can use health as an instrument to achieve political and economic goals.

Using health as a political and economic instrument

First, you can use health as a political tool. For example, by going out and exercising with people, or launching a campaign to make healthy food more affordable, or providing publicly-sponsored cafeterias with healthy food, you will help build community and deliver immediate changes that people can see and believe in. It will show that you care and help you get their support (and votes).

A second argument with a strong evidence base is that health is not just a cost to be contained, but an investment in a society's economic potential. This is especially relevant with regard to chronic diseases which affect people during their peak working years (109, 192, 718). Chapter 3 has set out the main arguments, and these are addressed to you. Investing in health can boost an economy's productive potential—increasing its labour supply and productivity. When people are sick, they save less money and their children's education can suffer; when governments pay for expensive healthcare, they forgo money that could have been invested in technological development or infrastructure. Failing to provide effective chronic disease care will only delay the expense, and can increase the cost overall. One approach to making an economic case for intervention to finance ministers is to use the models in the tables presented in Chapter 3 to calculate scenarios of how much growth your country loses each year because of chronic diseases (roughly about 0.5% per year for each 10% higher burden).

Protecting health from unfair trade in unhealthy products

A third main argument is to use health as a powerful bargaining chip to help your finance ministers achieve their trade goals, especially those who work in Brazil, China, India, Mexico, and other rapidly growing economies of the Global South. At the time of this writing, negotiations at the Doha trade round have ground to halt, resulting from a stalemate between the rich countries and growing Southern states (Brazil, India, and China). Finance ministers are concerned about how the US and Europe cheat on free-market rules (for example, by subsidizing unhealthy agricultural products), and would like to help support their domestic medium- and small-size industries, which have competitive disadvantages against gigantic Western multinational companies.

Explain to your financial ministers and other leaders how health can be used as an argument to protect economies from hazardous western imports and to control the predatory activities of multinational companies. Just as Trade Intellectual Property Rights protections are included in free-trade agreements (protecting pharmaceutical companies), include health and safety protections in these agreements (protecting people). Make Health Impact Assessment[7] a formal part of free-trade agreements—following the physician's mantra to 'first do no harm'. Of course, you will be challenged that these are non-tariff barriers to trade but, as long as your arguments are soundly based on health, you are likely to prevail.

This tactic of imbedding health into free-trade agreements would have strong support from domestic business leaders and popular constituencies (but not from those who are benefiting from contracts and kickbacks from Western companies, although here you can take advantage of the growth on anti-bribery legislation in rich countries). It would also be useful to governments coming to power in Latin America that seek to counteract the prior decisions that have locked their societies into free-trade agreements (a process that has been referred to by some observers as the 'hollowing out' of democracy).

Human rights groups

Sick societies and chronic diseases are human rights issues. They affect people's fundamental right to life and human capabilities, as outlined by human rights leader, Martha Nussbaum (603, 719, 720). For example, people in the global South are being deprived of the right to access healthy choices about food and activity. People are not being adequately nourished: the previous symptom was undernutrition, the current one is overnutrition. Chronic diseases also affect people's bodily integrity: the powerful social and economic forces documented in this book impinge on people's freedom of choice about what happens to their body and their control over their environment; tobacco and second-hand smoke is another example that is having major health consequences in resource-poor countries. Securing people's fundamental right to life will require addressing chronic diseases—its number one threat.

Building global social health protection

One starting point is to build on what already exists. A first step towards safeguarding people's rights to health has been created with the Global Fund for AIDS, TB, and Malaria. This Global Fund redistributes money from rich countries to people who are deprived of healthcare. The result is a growing network of clinics and treatment centres that provide antiretroviral therapy for people living with HIV/AIDS. These efforts have not only saved millions of lives, but established a precedent for guaranteeing human rights (145).

This global development marks a tremendous advance over the prior framework of international aid and charity that had largely failed to secure the right to care for millions of people living with HIV/AIDS. As noted above, many of us devote our lives to pulling bodies out of the river—addressing human trafficking, sexual violence, climate change, maternal health, and chronic diseases, to name a few. But if we combine our efforts to create a system of global social protection, we can achieve many of our desired goals at once. Today's truly global threats to people's rights to life, liberty, and health demand a permanent, democratic, and publicly accountable system of global social health protection. Expanding the scope of the Global Fund is a good place to start.

Climate change and alternative globalization groups

One of the leading causes of environmental degradation is methane emissions from agribusiness. Extensive consumption of meat, high in saturated fats, is causing heart disease. Both are being fuelled by unfair agricultural subsidies. Another example is palm oil, a heavily subsidized product used for cooking. Its production is hazardous for the rainforest and for people's health. Focusing on these common causes gives rise to shared goals that climate change, alternative globalization, and public health campaigns can mobilize towards.

People

This book is about you and your world. Get involved. While participation may seem difficult to fit into our busy lives, it has never been easier to do with the advent of modern social media such as Facebook and Twitter. These Internet sites even offer applications for generating interest about a cause, disseminating information, and raising money and resources.

Take a stand; believe in something; change the image you see. Traditional ways of building a better society and making your voice heard, such as voting, are still important; but you can make your votes count even more by casting them all over the world about topics that matter. You can build a global citizens movement from where you sit every day. It is that easy. As we described in Chapter 5, these campaigns have already been used to fight against unfair elections, terrorism, and human trafficking. And they work. But don't take our word for it: governments and ministries of defence all around the world are launching these sites to meet their goals.

Preventing chronic diseases and sick societies will be the defining human health challenge of our age. We hope you will join us in our global quest to promote human development.

Endnotes

1 To be clear, we are not calling for subjectivity in science. Researchers should strive to be completely objective, divorcing themselves from ideology, interests, or preferences in the data collection and analysis process. However, we can never be politically neutral in our choices about what to study, nor can the implications of our studies be apolitical and value-free.

2 One of the remaining few, Vicente Navarro, at Johns Hopkins, critiqued the unhealthy situations of Pinochet regime and Soviet government was similarly thrown out of the country. This kind of repression happens under dictatorships, but it is more subtle under democracies. See Navarro (710) for more details and the example of Virchow's social medicine approach

3 If you come across these documents, send them to public health experts at state universities or, if possible, to WikiLeaks. In the case of documents received by the University of California (state university property), the California National Guard's assistance was necessary to secure offices against the industry's lawyers. See the story of Merrell Williams, a paralegal working for a law firm, who went public with 4000 pages of documents from the British American Tobacco group detailing a 'sophisticated legal and public relations strategy to avoid liability for the diseases induced by tobacco use' (721).

4 Considerable research exists about tobacco addiction, but much less has been done regarding the addictive properties of sugar, fat, salt, and other nutrients. As one Tobacco Institute lawyer noted, 'the entire matter of addiction is the most potent weapon a prosecuting attorney can have in a lung cancer/cigarette case' (716).

5 These steps reflect key elements of the case to show duty, breach, causation, and damage.

6 However, the court did note concern about 'McFrankenstein' creations, whereby foods, through processing, had been stripped of its presumed health or character (failing to disclose manufacturing processes ingredients, linked to arguments above) (717).

7 These Health Impact Assessments must incorporate openly debated principles and avoid capture by powerful vested interests. In view of the lessons from the experiences of how tobacco companies sought to manipulate scientific guidelines and standards, this is clearly no simple task.

Appendix

Resources for action

Material in this section draws from McKee M, Gilmore A, Schwalbe N. International cooperation and health. Part 1: issues and concepts *Journal of Epidemiology and Community Health* 2005; **59**:628–31 and International cooperation and health Part 2: making a difference. *Journal of Epidemiology and Community Health* 2005; **59**:737–9.

Activists and organizations

Third World Network: a network of organizations and institutions involved in issues related to development. It conducts and publishes research on economic, social, and environmental issues and provides a platform for discussion and presentation of this work. http://www.twnside.org.sg/.

World Social Forum: a yearly gathering intended to provide a counterbalance to the World Economic Forum's Davos meeting. According to its charter of principles it is 'an open meeting place for reflective thinking, democratic debate of ideas, formulation of proposals, free exchange of experiences, and inter-linking of effective action by groups and movements of civil society that are opposed to neoliberalism and to domination of the world by capital and any form of imperialism'. http://www.forumsocialmundial.org.br/index.php?cd_language=2.

People's Health Movement and People's Health Assembly: a meeting organized by international organizations, civil society groups, NGOs, and women's groups seeking to promote the principle of 'Health for All' and to advocate greater implementation of the Alma Ata Declaration with its principles of primary health care and 'people's perspective'. The primary objective of the assembly was to 'give voice to the people and make their voices heard in decisions affecting their health and well being'. http://www.phmovement.org/.

Partners in Health: the base of social movements in HIV and TB control. As their mission statement notes, 'At its root, our mission is both medical and moral. It is based on solidarity, rather than charity alone. When a person in Peru, or Siberia, or rural Haiti falls ill, PIH uses all of the means at our disposal to make them well—from pressuring drug manufacturers, to lobbying policy makers, to providing medical care and social services. Whatever it takes. Just as we would do if a member of our own family—or we ourselves—were ill'. http://www.pih.org/who/vision.html

Young Professionals' Chronic Disease Network: The Young Professionals Chronic Disease Network is a global network promoting research, policy and advocacy work on non-communicable diseases (NCDs). It capitalizes on the energy, innovative thinking, and courage of young people to challenge the status quo. The YP-CDN participates in the local and global knowledge economy using social media to create virtual platforms for sharing knowledge and ideas. Members are students and budding experts in their fields-public health professionals, doctors, sociologists, anthropologists, philosophers, nutritionists and architects. www.ypchronic.org

Methods and tools for action

Power structure analysis

For example, to study the influence of corporations, we suggest reading alternative news media, such as DemocracyNow (http://www.democracynow.org/), Huffington Post (http://www.huffingtonpost.

com/), MultiNational Monitor (http://multinationalmonitor.org/), and Center for Media and Democracy PR Watch (http://www.prwatch.org/). Some of the most important tools and hypotheses come from investigative journalism.

For research tools, we recommend consulting the following websites: Bill Domhoff's page (http://sociology.ucsc.edu/whorulesamerica/methods/how_to_do_power_structure_research.html) and An Internet Guide to Power Structure Research (http://darkwing.uoregon.edu/~vburris/whorules/corporations.htm).

Read Z-Magazine: http://www.zcommunications.org/zmag.

Counterpunch: http://www.counterpunch.org/.

The Nation: http://www.thenation.com/.

Institute for Policy Studies: excellent information on the global economy and foreign policy. http://www.ips-dc.org/.

Corporations and health

Wiist WH. *The bottom line or public health: Tactics corporations use to influence health and health policy, and what we can do to counter them.* New York: Oxford University Press, 2010.

Tobacco Industry Documents: more than 30 million pages of industry documents are available. They provide a critical source of information that can help you to understand how industries attempt to influence public health interventions. http://legacy.library.ucsf.edu/.

Social and economic determinants of health

CSDH. *Closing the gap in a generation: Health equity through action on the social determinants of health. Final report of the Commission on Social Determinants of Health.* Geneva: World Health Organization, 2008.

Farmer P. *Pathologies of power: health, human rights, and the new war on the poor.* Los Angeles, CA: University of California Press, 2003.

Kim JY, Millen JV, Irwin A, Gershman J (eds). *Dying for Growth: global inequality and the health of the poor.* Monroe, ME: Common Courage Press, 2000.

Marmot M. *The status syndrome: how social standing directly affects your health and life expectancy.* New York: Henry Holt, 2004.

Klein N. *The shock doctrine:* Harmandsworth: Penguin, 2008.

Patel R. *Stuffed and starved: the hidden battle for the world food system.* Brooklyn, NY: Melville House, 2008.

Qualitative research

Narayan D. *Voices of the poor: can anyone hear us?* Washington, DC: World Bank, 2000.

Political determinants of scientific change

Epstein S. *Impure Science: AIDS, activism, and the politics of knowledge.* Berkeley, CA: University of California Press, 1998.

References

1. CSDH. *Closing the gap in a generation: Health equity through action on the social determinants of health. Final report of the Commission on Social Determinants of Health.* Geneva: World Health Organization; 2008. http://whqlibdoc.who.int/publications/2008/9789241563703_eng.pdf

2. Stuckler D, Basu S, McKee M. Drivers of inequality in Millennium Development Goal progress. *PLoS Medicine* 2010; **7**(3).

3. Strong K, Mathers C, Leeder S, Beaglehole R. Preventing chronic diseases: how many lives can we save? *Lancet* 2005; **366**:1578–82.

4. Yach D, Stuckler D, Brownell K. Epidemiologic and economic consequences of the global epidemics of obesity and diabetes. *Nature Medicine* 2005; **12**(1):62–6.

5. Bruce N, Perez-Padilla R, Albalak R. Indoor air pollution in developing countries: a major environmental and public health challenge. *Bulletin of the World Health Organization* 2000; **78**(9).

5a. Perez M, Schlesinger S, Wise TA. *The Promise and the Perils of Agricultural Trade Liberalization. Lessons from Latin America.* Report. Washington, D.C.: Washington Office on Latin America (WOLA) & the Global Development and Environment Institute (GDAE) at Tufts University, 2008.

6. Mishra V, Retherford RD, Smith KR. Biomass cooking fuels and prevalence of tuberculosis in India. *International Journal of Infectious Diseases* 1999; **3**(3):119–29.

7. Smith K, Samet JM, Romieuc I, Bruced N. Indoor air pollution in developing countries and acute lower respiratory infections in children. *Thorax* 2000; **55**(6):518–32.

8. World Health Organization. *Global health risks: mortality and burden of disease attributable to selected major risks.* Geneva: WHO; 2009. (See also reference 62).

9. Rose G. Sick individuals and sick populations. *Bulletin of the World Health Organization* 2001; **79**(10):32–8.

10. Murray C, Lopez AD. Alternative projections of mortality and disability by cause 1990–2020: Global Burden of Disease Study. *Lancet* 1997; **349**(9064):1498–504.

11. Murray C, Lopez AD. *Global burden of disease: A comprehensive assessment of mortality and disability from diseases, injuries and risk factors in 1990 and projected to 2020.* Cambridge: Harvard School of Public Health; 1996.

12. Nolte E, McKee M. *Caring for people with chronic conditions: A health system perspective.* Brussels: Open University Press; European Observatory on Health Systems and Policies; 2008.

13. Lynch J, Davey Smith G. A life course approach to chronic disease epidemiology. *Annual Review of Public Health* 2005; **26**:1–35.

14. Hotez P, Daar AS. The CNCDs and NTDs: blurring the lines dividing noncommunicable and communicable chronic diseases. *PLoS Neglected Tropical Diseases* 2008; **2**(10):e312.

15. Lönnroth K, Jaramillo E, Williams BG, Dye C, Raviglione M. Drivers of tuberculosis epidemics: the role of risk factors and social determinants. *Social Science & Medicine* 2009; **68**(12):2240–6.

16. Omran A. The epidemiologic transition: a theory of the epidemiology of population change. *Milbank Quarterly* 1971; **49**(4):509–38.

17. World Health Organization. *Global Burden of Disease Surveillance.* Geneva: WHO, 2004.

18. World Health Organization. *Mortality and burden of disease estimates for WHO Member States in 2004.* Geneva: WHO, 2009.

19. World Health Organization. *Noncommunicable diseases, poverty and the development agenda.* Geneva: WHO, 2009.

20. World Health Organization. *Statistical Information System (WHOSIS).* Geneva: WHO, 2009.

21. Stuckler D. Population causes and consequences of leading chronic diseases: A comparative analysis of prevailing explanations. *Milbank Quarterly* 2008; **86**(2):273–326.

22. Sydenstricker E. *The challenge of facts.* New York: The Milbank Memorial Fund, 1974.

23. Institute of Medicine. *Promoting Cardiovascular Health in the Developing World: A Critical Challenge to Achieve Global Health.* Washington, DC: IOM, 2010.

24. Leeder S, Raymond S, Greenberg H, Liu H, Esson K. *A race against time: the challenge of cardiovascular disease in developing countries.* New York: The Earth Institute at Columbia University, 2004.

25. Behera D, Balamugesh T. Lung cancer in India. *Journal of Chest Diseases* 2004; **46**(4):269–81.

26. International Diabetes Federation. *International Diabetes Federation Atlas.* Brussels: IDF, 2010.

27. Krieger N. Epidemiology and the web of causation: has anyone seen the spider? *Social Science & Medicine* 1994; **39**(7):887–903.

28. Buck C, Liopis A, Najera E, Terris M. *The challenge of epidemiology.* Washington, DC: Pan American Health Organisation, 1988.

29. Peto R, Lopez AD. Future worldwide health effects of current smoking patterns. In: Koop C, Schwarz MR, Pearson CE (eds). *Critical issues in global health,* pp. 154–61. San Francisco, CA: Wiley (Jossey-Bass), 2001.

30. Morris J, Heady JA, Raffle PAB, Roberts CG, Parks JN. Coronary heart disease and physical activity of work. *Lancet* 1953:1053–7.

31. World Health Organization. *Global status report on alcohol.* Geneva: WHO, 2004.

32. Corrao G, Bagnardi V, Zambon A, Vecchia CL. A meta-analysis of alcohol consumption and the risk of 15 diseases. *Preventive Medicine* 2004; **38**(5):613–19.

33. American Institute for Cancer Research and World Cancer Fund. *Food, nutrition, physical activity and the prevention of cancer: A global perspective.* Washington, DC: AICR, 2007.

34. World Health Organization/Food and Agricultural Organization. *Diet, Nutrition and the Prevention of Chronic Diseases.* Geneva: WHO, 2003.

35. Ben-Shlomo Y, Kuh D. A life course approach to chronic disease epidemiology: conceptual models, empirical challenges and interdisciplinary perspectives. *International Journal of Epidemiology* 2002; **31**:285–93.

36. Chiolero A, Madeleine G, Gabriel A, Burnier M, Paccaud F, Bovet P. Prevalence of elevated blood pressure and association with overweight in children of a rapidly developing country. *Journal of Human Hypertension* 2007; **21**:120–7.

37. Agyemang C, Redekop WK, Owusu-Dabo E, Bruijnzeels MA. Blood pressure patterns in rural, semi-urban and urban children in the Ashanti region of Ghana, West Africa. *BMC Public Health* 2005; **5**:114.

38. Jafar T, Islam M, Poulter N, et al. Children in South Asia have higher body mass-adjusted blood pressure levels than white children in the United States: a comparative study. *Circulation* 2005; **111**:1291–7.

39. Short K, Blackett PR, Gardner AW, Copeland KC. Vascular health in children and adolescents: effects of obesity and diabetes. *Journal of Vascular Health and Risk Management* 2009; **5**:973–90.

40. Skinner A, Steiner MJ, Henderson FW, Perrin EM. Multiple markers of inflammation and weight status: cross-sectional analysis throughout childhood. *Pediatrics* 2010; **125**(4):e801–9.

41. Eisenmann J, Welk GJ, Wickel EE, Blair SN. Stability of variables associated with the metabolic syndrome from adolescence to adulthood: the Aerobics Center Longitudinal Study. *American Journal of Human Biology* 2004; **16**:690–6.

42. Ogden C, Flegal KM, Carroll MD, Johnson CL. Prevalence and trends in overweight among US children and adolescents, 1999–2000. *Journal of the American Medical Association* 2002; **288**:1728–32.

43. Lau X. Lazy lifestyle as a weighty issue. *Beijing Review* 2004; **47**(6):28–9.

44. ADA. Type 2 diabetes in children and adolescents. *Pediatrics* 2000; **105**:671–80.

45. Cockram C. The epidemiology of diabetes mellitus in the Asia-Pacific region. *Hong Kong Medical Journal* 2000; **6**:43–52.

46. Narayan V, Boyle JP, Thompson TJ, Sorensen SW, Williamson DF. Lifetime risk for diabetes mellitus in the United States. *Journal of the American Medical Association* 2003; **290**:1884–90.

47. Olshansky S, Passaro DJ, Hershow C, et al. A potential decline in life expectancy in the United States in the 21st century. *New England Journal of Medicine* 2005; **352**:1138–45.

48. Adeyi O, Smith O, Robles S. *Public policy and the challenge of chronic non-communicable diseases.* Washington, DC: World Bank, 2007.

49. Rutstein D, Berenberg W, Chalmers TC, et al. Measuring the quality of medical care: A clinical method. *New England J of Medicine* 1976; **294**(11):582–8.

50. World Health Organization. *Preventing Chronic Diseases: A Vital Investment.* Geneva: WHO, 2005.

51. Bibbins-Domingo K, Chertow GM, Coxson PG, et al. Projected effect of dietary salt reductions on future cardiovascular disease. *New England Journal of Medicine* 2010; **362**(7):590–9.

52. Epping-Jordan J, Galea G, Tukuitonga C, Beaglehole R. Preventing chronic diseases: taking stepwise action. *Lancet* 2005; **366**:1667–71.

53. Lopez A. The evolution of the Global Burden of Disease framework for disease, injury and risk factor quantification: developing the evidence base for national, regional and global public health action. *Globalization and Health* 2005; **1**(5).

54. Setel P, Macfarlane SB, Szreter S, et al. A scandal of invisibility: making everyone count by counting everyone. *Lancet* 2007; **370**:1569–77.

55. Ahsan K, Alam N, Kim P. Epidemiological transition in rural Bangladesh, 1986–2006. *Global Health Action* 2009; **19**(2).

56. Walker R, McLarty DG, Kitange HM, et al. Stroke mortality in urban and rural Tanzania. *Lancet* 2000; **355**(9216):1684–7.

57. Joshi R, Cardona M, Iyengar S, et al. Chronic diseases now a leading cause of death in rural India—mortality data from the Andhra Pradesh Rural Health Initiative. *International Journal of Epidemiology* 2006; **35**(6):1522–9.

58. Doak C, Adair LS, Monteiro C, Popkin BM. Overweight and underweight coexist within households in Brazil, China and Russia. *Journal of Nutrition* 2000; **130**:2965–71.

59. Florencio T, Ferreira H, de Franca AP, Cavalcante JC, Sawya AL. Obesity and undernutrition in a very-low-income population in the city of Maceio, northeastern Brazil. *British Journal of Nutrition* 2001; **86**:277–83.

60. Goudge J, Gilson L, Russell S, Gumede T, Mills A. Affordability, availability and acceptability barriers to healthcare for the chronically ill: Longitudinal case studies from South Africa. *BMC Health Services Research* 2009; **9**(1):75.

61. Dror D, van Putten-Rademaker O, Koren R. Cost of illness: evidence from a study in five resource-poor locations in India. *Indian Journal of Medical Research* 2008; **127**(4):347–61.

62. World Health Organization. *Global Health Risks: Mortality and burden of disease attributable to selected major risks.* Geneva: WHO, 2009. (See also reference 8).

62a. Bradford-Hill A. The environment and diseases: association or causation? *Proc R Soc Med* 1965; **58**:295–300.

63. Wedel J. *Collision and Collusion: The strange case of Western aid to Eastern Europe.* New York: St. Martin's, 2001.

64. Doll R, Hill AB. Lung cancer and other causes of death in relation to smoking: A second report on the mortality of British doctors. *British Medical Journal* 1956; **2**(5001):1071–81.

65. Yusuf S, Hawken S, Ounpuu S, et al. Effect of potentially modifiable risk factors associated with myocardial infarction in 52 countries (the INTERHEART study): case-control study. *Lancet* 2004; **364**:937–52.

66. Bruzzi P, Green SB, Byar DP, Brinton LA, Schairer C. Estimating the population attributable risk for multiple risk factors using case-control data. *American Journal of Epidemiology* 1985; **122**(5):904–14.

67. Walter S. Calculation of attributable risks from epidemiologic data. *International Journal of Epidemiology* 1978; **7**:175–82.

68. Lock K, Pomerleau J, Causer L, Altmann DR, McKee M. The global burden of disease attributable to low consumption of fruit and vegetables: implications for the global strategy on diet. *British Medical Journal* 2005; **83**(2):100–8.

69. Jha P, Jacob B, Gajalakshmi V, et al. A nationally representative case-control study of smoking and death in India. *New England Journal of Medicine* 2008; **358**(11):1137–47.

70. Chow C, Lock K, Teo K, Subramanian SV, McKee M, Yusuf S. Environmental and societal influences acting on cardiovascular risk factors and disease at a population level: a review. *International Journal of Epidemiology* 2009; **38**(6):1580–94.

71. Monsivais P, Drewnowski A. The rising cost of low-energy-density foods. *Journal of the American Dietetic Association* 2007; **107**:2071–6.

72. Novotny T, Mamudu HM. Progression of tobaccos control policies: Lessons from the United States and implications for global action. *Health, Nutrition and Population (HNP) Discussion Paper.* Washington, DC: The International Bank for Reconstruction and Development, 2008.

73. Armstrong T. *Food industry.* Geneva: WHO, 2010.

74. Bleich S, Cutler D, Murray C, Adams A. Why is the developed world obese? *Annual Review of Public Health* 2008; **29**:273–95.

75. Cutler D, Glaeser EL, Shapiro J. Why have Americans become more obese? *Journal of Economic Perspectives* 2003; **17**:93–118.

76. Nielsen SJ, Popkin BM. Patterns and trends in food portion sizes, 1977–1998. *Journal of the American Medical Association* 2003; **289**(4):450–3.

77. Diliberti N, Bordi PL, Conklin MT, Roe LS, Rolls BJ. Increased portion size leads to increased energy intake in a restaurant meal. *Obesity Research* 2004; **12**(3):562–8.

78. McKee M, Colagiuri R. What are governments for? *Medical Journal of Australia* 2007; **187**(11/12):654–5.

79. Pucher J, Peng Z-R, Mittal N, Zhu Y, Korattyswaroopan N. Urban transport trends and policies in China and India: Impacts of rapid economic growth. *Transport Reviews.* 2007; **27**(4):379–410.

80. Hawkes C. *Marketing activities of global soft drink and fast food companies in emerging markets: a review.* Geneva: WHO, 2002.

81. Watts D, Peretti J, Frumin M. Viral marketing for the real world. *Harvard Business Review.* 2007; **85**(5), 22–3.

82. Hawkes C. *Marketing of food to children: the global regulatory environment.* Geneva: WHO, 2004.

83. Brownell K, Warner, KE. The perils of ignoring history: Big Tobacco played dirty and millions died. How similar is Big Food? *Milbank Quarterly* 2009; **87**(1):259–94.

84. Borghans L, Golsteyn BH. Time discounting and body mass index: evidence from the Netherlands. *Economics & Human Biology* 2006; **4**(1):39–61.

85. Komlos J, Smith PK, Bogin B. Obesity and the rate of time preference: is there a connection? *Journal of Biosocial Science* 2004; **36**(2):209–19.

86. Witkowski T. Food marketing and obesity in developing countries: Analysis, ethics and public policy. *Journal of Macromarketing* 2007; **27**(2):126–37.

87. The Coca-Cola Company. *Coca-Cola Company Annual Report.* Atlanta, GA: The Coca-Cola Company, 1995.

88. Mac boss is hungry for more. *The Straits Times* (Singapore) 4 July, 1999.

89. Drinking to Coke. *Malaysian Business* 16 October 2001.

90. *Coca-Cola and Pepsi Look to Developing Countries to Maintain Sales.* 2011. Available at: http://www. dumpsoda.org/SodaSalesPattern.pdf

91. Fast food franchisers feed on teenagers. *Budapest Business Journal* 3 March 1995.

92. Coca-Cola. *Coca-Cola India and NFO-MBL explore the teen mindscape.* Coca-Cola Company Press Release, September 2001.

93. Pepsi, Coke duke it out in India, China. *Ad Age Global* October 2000.

94. Chou S, Rashad I, Grossman M. Fast-food restaurant advertising on television and its influence on childhood obesity. *Journal of Law and Economics* 2008; **51**(4):599–618.

95. Patel R. *Stuffed and starved: the hidden battle for the world food system.* Brooklyn, NY: Melville House, 2008.

96. Obstfeld M, Taylor AM. *Global capital markets: integration, crisis and growth.* Cambridge: Cambridge University Press, 2004.

97. Gourinchas P, Jeanne O. The elusive gains from international financial integration. *Review of Economic Studies* 2006; **72**(3).

98. Bordo M, Meissner C, Stuckler D. Foreign currency debt, financial crises and economic growth: A long-run view. *Journal of International Money and Finance* 2010; 1–24.

99. World Health Organization. *Final report of the Globalization and Health Knowledge Network*. Geneva: WHO, 2007.

100. Gourinchas P, Jeanne O. Capital flows to developing countries: the allocation puzzle. NBER Working Paper W13602, 2007.

101. Chang H. *Kicking away the ladder - development strategy in historical perspective*. London: Anthem Press, 2002.

102. Arias M, Kergoat A, Kortlandt J, van Hoof H, Lawson M. *From donorship to ownership? Moving towards PRSP round two*. Oxford: Oxfam, 2004.

103. Hawkes C. Agricultural and food policy for cardiovascular health. *Prevention and Control* 2006; 2:137–47.

104. Wahl P. *Food speculation: the main factor of the price bubble in 2008*. Berlin: Ford Foundation, 2009.

105. Lock K, Stuckler D, Charlesworth K, McKee M. Potential causes and health effects of rising global food prices. *British Medical Journal* 2009; 339:b2403.

106. Food and Agriculture Organization. *Briefing paper: Hunger on the rise*. Rome: FAO, 2008.

107. Food and Agriculture Organization. *World food situation. Food price indices*. Rome: FAO, 2008.

108. Cassels S. Overweight in the Pacific: links between foreign dependence, global food trade, and obesity in the Federated States of Micronesia. *Globalization and Health* 2006; 2(10).

109. Suhrcke M, Nugent R, Stuckler D, et al. *Chronic disease: An economic perspective*. London: Oxford Health Alliance, 2006.

110. Gilmore A, Collin J, McKee M. "Unless health decree 30 is amended satisfactorily it will not be possible for this transaction to proceed": British American Tobacco's erosion of health legislation in Uzbekistan. *British Medical Journal* 2006; 332(7537):355–8.

111. Gilmore A, McKee M. Exploring the impact of foreign direct investment on tobacco consumption in the former Soviet Union. *Tobacco Control* 2005; 14:13–21.

112. Schrecker T, Labonte R, De Vogli R. Globalization and health: the need for a global vision. *Lancet* 2008; 372(9659):1670–6.

113. Davis M. Planet of slums. New York: Verso, 2006.

114. Anderson P, Butcher KF, Levine PB. Maternal employment and overweight children. *Journal of Health Economics* 2003; 22(3):477–504.

115. Hawkes C. Uneven dietary development: linking the policies and processes of globalization with the nutrition transition, obesity and diet-related chronic diseases. *Globalization and Health* 2006; 2(4).

116. Popkin B. What is unique about the experience in lower- and middle-income less-industrialised countries compared with the very-high income countries? The shift in the stages of the nutrition transition differ from past experiences! *Public Health Nutrition* 2002; 5:205–14.

117. Stuckler D, Basu S, Gilmore A, et al. An evaluation of the International Monetary Fund's claims about public health. *International Journal of Health Services* 2010; 40(2):327–32.

118. Williamson J. What washington means by policy reform. In: Williamson J (ed). *Latin American adjustment: How much has happened?* Washington, DC: Institute for International Economics, 1990.

119. Woods N. *The Globalizers: The IMF, the World Bank and their borrowers*. Ithaca, NY: Cornell University Press, 2006.

120. IMF. Articles of agreement of the International Monetary Fund, 27 December 1945.

121. Stuckler D, Basu S. The International Monetary Fund's effects on global health: before and after the 2008 financial crisis. *International Journal of Health Services* 2009; 39(4):771–81.

122. Friedman M. *Capitalism and freedom*. Chicago, IL: University of Chicago Press, 1962.

123. Hayek F. *The road to serfdom*. London: Routledge, 1994.

124. Klein N. *The shock doctrine*. Harmandsworth: Penguin, 2008.

125. Sachs J. *Accelerating privatization in Eastern Europe: The case of Poland. World Bank Annual Conference on Development Economics*, April 25–26, 1991.

126. Lieberman I, Kopf DJ. *Privatization in Transition Economies: the Ongoing Story*. Emerald Group Publishing Limited, 2007.

127. Summers L. "Comment." In: Blanchard O, Froot K, Sachs J (eds). *The Transition in Eastern Europe. Volume 1: Country Studies*, pp. 252–5. Chicago, IL: University of Chicago Press, 1994.

128. Adeyi O, Chellaraj G., Goldstein E., Preker A., Ringold D. Health status during the transition in Central and Eastern Europe: development in reverse? *Health Policy and Planning* 1997; **12(2)**:132–45.

129. Zatonski W, Didkowska J. Closing the gap: Cancer in central and Eastern Europe (CEE). *European Journal of Cancer* 2008; **44**:1425–37.

130. Valkonen T, Martikainen P, Jalovaara M, Koskinen S, Martelin T, Makela, P. Changes in socioeconomic inequalities in mortality during an economic boom and recession among middle-aged men and women in Finland. *European Journal of Public Health* 2000; **10**(4):274–80.

131. Stuckler D, Basu S, Suhrcke M, Coutts A, McKee M. The public health impact of economic crises and alternative policy responses in Europe. *Lancet* 2009; **374**(9686):315–23.

132. Garfield R, Santana S. The impact of the economic crisis and the US embargo on health in Cuba. *American Journal of Public Health* 1997; **87**(1):15–20.

133. Kondo N, Subramanian S, Kawachi I, Takeda Y, Yamagata Z. Economic recession and health inequalities in Japan: an analysis with a national sample, 1986–2001. *Journal of Epidemiology and Community Health* 2008; **62**:869–75.

134. Stuckler D, Basu S, McKee M. How government spending cuts put health at risk. *Nature* 2010; **465**:289.

135. King H, Rewers M. Diabetes in adults is now a Third World problem. *Ethnicity and disease* 1993; 3:S67–74.

136. Secretariat of the Pacific Community. *Obesity in the Pacific now too big to ignore.* New Caledonia: WHO Regional Office, Manila, 2002.

137. World Health Organization. *Western Pacific Region databank on socioeconomic and health indicators.* Manila: WHO Regional Office for the Western Pacific, 1995.

138. Stuckler D, Basu S, Coutts A, McKee M. The health implications of financial crisis: A review of the evidence. *Ulster Medical Journal* 2009; **78**(3):142–5.

139. Marks J, McQueen DV. *Chronic diseases.* In: Koop C, Pearson CE, Schwarz MR (eds). *Critical issues in global health.* San Francisco, CA: Jossey-Bass; 2002.

140. Mathers C, Loncar D. Projections of global mortality and burden of disease from 2002 to 2030. *PLoS Medicine* 2006; **3**(11):e442.

141. Roglic G, Unwin N. Global mortality attributable to diabetes: Time for a realistic estimate. *Diabetes Voice* 2005; **50**(10):33–4.

142. Strong K, Mathers C, Bonita R. Preventing stroke: Saving lives around the world. *Lancet Neurology* 2007; **6**(2):182–7.

143. Centers for Disease Control (CDC). Public health and aging: trends in aging—United States and worldwide. *Morbidity and Mortality Weekly Report* 2003; **52**(6):101–6.

144. Friedman T. *The world is flat: A brief history of the twenty-first century.* New York: Farrar, Straus and Giroux, 2005.

145. Ooms G, Hammond R. Scaling up global social health protection: Prerequisite reforms to the International Monetary Fund. *International Journal of Health Services* 2009; **39**(4):795–801.

146. Rose G. Sick individuals and sick populations. *International Journal of Epidemiology* 1985; **14**(1):32–8.

147. Aral S, Holmes KK, Padian NS, Cates W. Individual and population approaches to the epidemiology and prevention of sexually transmitted diseases and human immunodeficiency virus infection. *Journal of Infectious Diseases* 1996; **174**(S2):S127–33.

148. Durkheim E. *Suicide.* Glencoe: Free Press, 1951.

149. Subramanian S, Jones K, Kaddour A, Krieger N. Revisiting Robinson: The perils of individualistic and ecologic fallacy. *International Journal of Epidemiology* 2009; **38**:342–60.

150. Selvin H. Durkheim's suicide and problems of empirical research. *American Journal of Sociology* 1958; **63**:607–19.

151. Diez-Roux A. Multilevel analysis in public health research. *Annual Review of Public Health* 2000; **21**:171–92.

152. Kafka M. *An appalling waste of life marks the automobile. The New York Times* 28 August 1932.

153. Perrott S, Collins SD. Sickness and the depression. *Milbank Quarterly* 1933; **11**:281–98.

154. World Bank. *Investing in Health*. Washington, DC: World Bank, 1993.

155. World Health Organization. *Macroeconomics and health: investing in health for economic development*. Geneva: World Health Organization Commission on Macroeconomics and Health, 2001.

156. Philip Morris. *Public finance balance of smoking in Czech Republic*. Prague: Arther D. Little International, 2000.

157. Sloan F, Ostermann J, Picone G, Conover C, Taylor D. *The price of smoking*. Cambridge, MA: MIT Press, 2003.

158. Diethelm P, Rielle JC, McKee M. The whole truth and nothing but the truth? The research that Philip Morris did not want you to see. *Lancet* 2005; **366**(9479):86–92.

159. Ong E, Glantz SA. Constructing "sound science" and "good epidemiology": tobacco, lawyers, and public relations firms. *American Journal of Public Health* 2001; **91**(11):1749–57.

160. Neuhann H, Warter-Neuhann C, Lyaruu I, Msuya L. Diabetes care in Kilimanjaro region: clinical presentation and problems of patients of the diabetes clinic at the regional referral hospital—an inventory before structured intervention. *Diabetic Medicine* 2001; **19**:509–13.

161. Chale S, Swai AB, Mujinja PG, McLarty DG. Must diabetes be a fatal disease in Africa? Study of the costs of treatment. *British Medical Journal* 1992; **304**(6836):1215–18.

162. Beran D, Yudkin JS. Diabetes care in sub-Saharan Africa. *Lancet* 2006; **368**(9548):1689–95.

163. Su T, Kouyate B, Flessa S. Catastrophic household expenditure for health care in a low-income society: a study from Nouna District, Burkina Faso. *Bulletin of the World Health Organization* 2006; **84**(1):21–7.

164. Somkotra T, Lagrada LP. Which households are at risk of catastrophic health spending: experience in Thailand after universal coverage. *Health Affairs* 2009; **28**:w467–8.

165. Sabri B. Health, poverty and development. *Eastern Mediterranean Health Journal* 2007; **13**(6).

166. Pelkowski J, Berger MC. The impact of health on employment, wages and hours worked over the life cycle. *Quarterly Review of Economics and Finance* 2004; **44**(1):102–21.

167. Djutaharta T, Surya HV. *Research on tobacco in Indonesia*. Washington, DC: World Bank, 2003.

168. Mete C, Schultz TP. *Health and labour-force participation of the elderly in Taiwan. Allocation public and private resources across generations: riding the age waves*, pp.163–200. Netherlands: Springer, 2006.

169. Narayan D. *Voices of the poor: can anyone hear us?* Washington, DC: World Bank, 2000.

170. Bogale T, Mariam DH, Ali A. Costs of illness and coping strategies in a coffee-growing rural district of Ethiopia. *Journal of Health, Population and Nutrition* 2005; **23**(2):192–9.

171. Kabir M, Rahman A, Salway S, Pryer J. Sickness among the urban poor: a barrier to livelihood security. *Journal of International Development* 2000; **12**(5):707–22.

171a. Schwimmer JB, Burwinkle TM, Varnii JW. Health-related quality of life of severely obese children and adolescents. *JAMA* 2003; **289**(14):1813–9.

172. Furber A, Maheswaran R, Newell JN, Carroll C. Is smoking tobacco an independent risk factor for HIV infection and progression to AIDS? A systematic review. *Sexually Transmitted Infections* 2007; **83**:41–6.

173. World Health Organization. *Commission on Macroeconomics and Health*. Geneva: WHO, 2001.

174. Efroymson D, Ahmed S, Townsend J, et al. Hungry for tobacco: an analysis of the economic impact of tobacco consumption on the poor in Bangladesh. *Tobacco Control* 2001; **10**(2001):212–17.

175. Ali Z, Rahman A, Rahman T. *Appetite for nicotine: An economic analysis of tobacco control in Bangladesh*. Washington, DC: World Bank, 2003.

176. Bonu S, Rani M, Jha P, Peters DH, Nguyen, SN. Household tobacco and alcohol use and child health: an exploratory study from India. *Health Policy and Planning* 2004; **70**:67–83.

177. Bonu S, Rani M, Jha P, Peters DH, Nguyen SN. Does use of tobacco or alcohol contribute to impoverishment from hospital costs in India? *Health Policy and Planning* 2005; **20**(1):41–9.

178. Barcelo A, Aedo C, Rajpathak S, Robles S. The cost of diabetes in Latin America and the Carribean. *Bulletin of the World Health Organization* 2003; **81**:19–27.

179. Becker G. *The economic approach to human behavior.* Chicago, IL: University of Chicago Press, 1978.

180. Levine R, Renelt, D. A sensitivity analysis of cross-country growth regressions. *American Economic Review* 1992; **82**(4):942–63.

181. Pritchett L. The quest continues. *Finance and Development* 2006; **43**(1):18–22.

182. Abegunde D, Mathers CD, Adam T, Ortegon M, Strong K. The burden and costs of chronic diseases in low-income and middle-income countries. *Lancet* 2007; **370**(9603):1929–38.

183. Tan-Torres T, Baltussen R, Adam T, Hutubessy R, Acharya A, Evans DB. *Making choices in health: WHO guide to cost-effectiveness analysis.* Geneva: WHO, 2003.

184. Easterly W. *The elusive quest for growth: economsits' adventures and misadventures in the tropics.* Boston, MA: MIT Press, 2002.

185. Acemoglu D, Johnson S. Disease and development: the effect of life expectancy on economic growth. *Journal of Political Economy* 2007; **115**(6):925–85.

186. Suhrcke M, Sauto-Arce R, McKee M, Rocco L. *The economist costs of ill health in the European Region.* Talinn: WHO and European Observatory on Health Systems and Policies, 2008.

187. Becker G, Philipson, TJ, Soares, RR. The quantity and quality of life and the evolution of world inequality. *American Economic Review* 2005; **95**(1):277–91.

188. Gonzalez-Pier E, Gutierrez-Delgado C, Stevens G, et al. Priority setting for health interventions in Mexico's system of social protection in health. *Lancet* 2006; **368**(9547):1608–18.

189. Husseini A, Abu-Rmeileh, NME, Mikki, N, et al. Cardiovascular diseases, diabetes mellitus, and cancer in the occupied Palestinian territory. *Lancet* 2009; **373**(9668):1041–9.

190. Berry L, Mirabito AM, Berwick DM. A healthcare agenda for business. *MIT Sloan Management Review* 2004; **45**(4):56–64.

191. Business Roundtable. *Economic Outlook Survey, December 2003* Washington, DC: Business Roundtable, 2003.

192. World Economic Forum. *Global Risks 2009: A world economic forum report.* Geneva: World Economic Forum, 2009.

193. Becker G, Murphy KM. A theory of rational addiction. *Journal of Political Economy* 1988; **96**(4):675.

194. Gruber J, Koszegi B. *A modern economic view of tobacco taxation. Paris: International Union Against Tuberculosis and Lung Disease,* 2008. Available at: http://www.emmodesign.com/wlfnew/downloads/report_Gruber.pdf.

195. Offer A. *The challenge of affluence: Self-control and well-being in the United States and Britain since 1950.* New York: Oxford University Press, 2006.

196. Gilmore A, Radu-Loghin C, Zatushevski I, McKee M. Pushing up smoking incidence: plans for a privatised tobacco industry in Moldova. *Lancet* 2005; **365**(9467):1354–9.

197. Lipsey R, Lancaster K. The general theory of second best. *Review of Economic Studies* 1956; **24**(1):11–32.

198. Koplow D. *Smallpox: the fight to eradicate a global scourge.* Berkeley, CA: University of California Press, 2003.

199. Foege W, Millar JD, Henderson DA1. Smallpox eradication in West and Central Africa. *Bulletin of the World Health Organization* 1975; **52**(3341):209–22.

200. Pennington H. Smallpox and bioterrorism. *Bulletin of the World Health Organization* 2003; **81**(10): 762–7.

201. Brauman R. Controversies within health and human rights. New York: Carnegie Council, 2001.

202. Centers for Disease Control and Prevention. *Unrealized prevention opportunities: Reducing the health and economic burden of chronic disease.* Bethesda, MD: CDC, 1997.

203. Yach D, Rowley W, Cha S, et al. *Barriers to chronic disease care in the United States: The case of diabetes and its consequences.* New Haven, CT: Institute of Alternative Futures and Yale School of Public Health, 2005.

204. Starr P. *The social transformation of American Medicine.* New York: Basic Books, 1982.

205. Bara A, van den Heuvel JAW, Maarse JAM. Reforms of healthcare system in Romania. *Croatian Medical Journal* 2002; **43**(2002):446–52.

206. Andreev E, Nolte E, Shkolnikov VM, Varavikova E, McKee M. The evolving pattern of avoidable mortality in Russia. *International Journal of Epidemiology* 2003; **32**(3):437–46.

207. Freire P. *Pedagogy of the oppressed.* New York: Continuum, 1970.

208. Wagner E, Groves T. Care for chronic diseases: the efficacy of coordinated and patient centred care is established, but now is the time to test its effectiveness. *British Medical Journal* 2002; **325**:913–14.

209. Institute of Medicine. *Crossing the quality chasm: a new health system for the 21st century.* Washington, DC: IOM, 2001.

210. Link B, Phelan JC, Bresnahan M, Stueve A, Pescosolido BA. Public conceptions of mental illness: Labels, causes, dangerousness, and social distance. *American Journal of Public Health* 1999; **89**(9):1328–33.

211. McCormick J. Health promotion: the ethical dimension. *Lancet* 1994; **344**:390–1.

212. Berenson R, Horvath J. Confronting the barriers to chronic care management in Medicare. *Health Affairs* 2003; **22**:w37–w53.

213. Cueto M. The origins of primary health care and selective primary health care. *American Journal of Public Health* 2004; **94**(11):1864–74.

214. Gish O. Selective primary health care: old wine in new bottles. *Social Science & Medicine* 1982; **16**:1049–63.

215. Walsh J, Warren KS. Selective Primary Health Care: An interim strategy for disease control in developing countries. *Social Science & Medicine* 1980; **14**:145–63.

216. PAHO. *Salud para todos en el Siglo Veitinuno.* Washington, DC: Pan American Health Organization, 1997.

217. Harries A, Jahn A, Zachariah R, Enarson D. Adapting the DOTS framework for tuberculosis control to the management of non-communicable diseases in sub-Saharan Africa. *PLoS Medicine* 2008; **5**(6):e124.

218. World Health Organization. *Global Tuberculosis Control-Surveillance, Planning, Financing.* Geneva: WHO, 2008.

219. Luntz G. Tuberculous diabetics: the Birmingham Regional Service. *Lancet* 1954; **266**:973–4.

220. Nolte E, McKee M. Measuring the health of nations: Updating an earlier analysis. *Health Affairs* 2008; **27**(1):58–71.

221. McKee M, Nolte E. Responding to the challenge of chronic disease: ideas from Europe. *Clinical Medicine* 2004; **4**:336–42.

222. World Health Organization. *Health systems: improving performance.* Geneva: WHO, 2000.

223. NHANES. *National Health and Nutrition Examination Survey.* Atlanta, GA: Center for Disease Control and Prevention (CDC), 2008.

224. Tarrow S. *Power in movement: Collective action, social movements, and politics.* Cambridge: Cambridge University Press, 1994.

225. Krugman P. Why markets can't cure healthcare. *The New York Times* 25 July, 2009.

226. Reich M. Reshaping the state from above, below and within: implications for public health. *Social Science & Medicine* 2002; **54**:1669–75.

227. Niefeld M, Braunstein JB, Wu AW, et al. Preventable hospitalization among elderly Medicare beneficiaries with type 2 diabetes. *Diabetes Care* 2003; **26**(5):1344–9.

228. Gawande A. The cost conundrum. *The New Yorker* 1 June, 2009.

229. Wennberg J, Fisher ES, Stukel TA, Sharp SM. Use of Medicare claims data to monitor provider-specific performance among patients with severe chronic illness. *Health Affairs* 2004; Suppl Web Exclusives:VAR5-18.

230. Legorreta A, Liu, X, Zaher, CA, Jatulis, DE. Variation in managing asthma: experience at the medical group level in California. *American Journal of Managed Care* 2000; **6**:445–53.

231. Schuster M, McGlynn E, Brook R. How good is the quality of health care in the United States? *Milbank Quarterly* 1998; **76**:517–63.

232. Starfield B. Is US health really the best in the world? *Journal of the American Medical Association* 2000; **284**:483–5.

233. IOM. *To err is human: Building a safer health system.* Washington, DC: National Academy Press, 1999.

234. Lazarou J, Pomeranz B, Corey P. Incidence of adverse drug reactions in hospitalized patients. *Journal of the American Medical Association* 1998; **279**:1200–5.

235. Phillips D, Christenfeld, N, Glynn, L. Increase in US medication-error deaths between 1983 and 1993. *Lancet* 1998; **351**:643–4.

236. Leape L. Unnecessary surgery. *Annual Review of Public Health* 1992; **13**:363–83.

237. Gura T. Obesity drug pipeline not so far. *Science* 2003; **299**:849–52.

238. Santry H, Gillen DL, Lauderdale DS. Trends in bariatric surgical procedures. *Journal of the American Medical Association* 2005; **294**:1909–17.

239. Lee W, Wang W. Bariatric surgery: Asia-Pacific perspective. *Obesity Surgery* 2005; **15**:751–7.

240. Families USA. Profiting from pain: where prescription drug dollars go. Washington, DC: Families USA Foundation, 2002.

241. McKeown T. *The role of medicine: dream, mirage or nemesis.* In: Soothill K, Melia K (eds). *Classic Texts in Health Care*, pp. 31–4. Oxford: Butterworth-Heineman, 1998.

242. Cochrane A, St Leger A, Moore SF. Health service 'input' and mortality 'output' in developed countries. *Journal of Epidemiology and Community Health* 1978; **32**:200–5.

242a. World Diabetes Foundation 2010.

243. Martinez-Gonzalez MA, Bes-Rastrollo M, Serra-Majem L, Lairon D, Estruch R, Trichopoulou A. Mediterranean food pattern and the primary prevention of chronic disease: recent developments. *Nutr Rev.* 2009 May; **67**(Suppl 1):S111–6.

244. USDHHS. *Physical Activity Guidelines Advisory Committee Report.* Washington, DC: US Department of Health and Human Services, 2008.

245. Critchley J, Capewell S. Smoking cessation for the secondary prevention of coronary heart disease. *Cochrane Database of Systematic Reviews* 2003; **4**:CD003041.

246. Appel L, Anderson C. Compelling evidence for public helath action to reduce salt intake. *New England Journal of Medicine* 2010; **362**(7):650–2.

247. Alderman M. Reducing dietary sodium: the case for caution. *Journal of the American Medical Association* 2010; **303**(5):448–9.

248. Narayan KM. A case of well-intentioned public health reductionism. *BMJ Blog Group*; 2010.

249. Ebrahim S, Beswick, A, Burke, M, Davey Smith, G. Multiple risk factor interventions for primary prevention of coronary heart disease (review). *Cochrane Database of Systematic Reviews* 2006; **4**:CD001561.

250. Wald NJ, Law MR. A strategy to reduce cardiovascular disease by more than 80%. *British Medical Journal* 2003; **326**(7404):1419.

251. Franco OH, Bonneux L, de Laet C, Peeters A, Steyerberg EW, Mackenbach JP. The Polymeal: a more natural, safer, and probably tastier (than the Polypill) strategy to reduce cardiovascular disease by more than 75%. *British Medical Journal* 2004; **329**(7480):1447–50.

252. Drope J, Chapman S. Tobacco industry efforts at discrediting scientific knoweldge of environmental tobacco smoke: A review of internal industry documents. *Journal of Epidemiology and Community Health* 2001; **55**:588–94.

253. Crandall JP, Knowler WC, Kahn SE, et al. The prevention of type 2 diabetes. *Nature Clinical Practice Endocrinology & Metabolism* 2008; **4**(7):382–93.

254. Paulweber B, Valensi P, Lindstrom J, et al. A European evidence-based guideline for the prevention of type-2 diabetes. *Hormone and Metabolic Research* 2010; **42**(S1):S3–36.

255. Monteiro CA, Conde WL, Popkin BM. Income-specific trends in obesity in Brazil: 1975–2003. *American Journal of Public Health* 2007; **97**(10):1808–12.

256. Dolan P, Hallsworth W, Halpern D, King D, Vlaev I. *Mindspace: influencing behaviour through public policy.* London: Institute for Government and the UK Cabinet Office, 2010.

257. Bolton J, Cox B, Clara I, Sareen J. Use of alcohol and drugs to self-medicate anxiety disorders in a nationally representative sample. *Journal of Nervous and Mental Disease* 2006; **194**(11):818–25.

258. Gine X, Karlan D, Zinman J. *Put your money where your butt is: A commitment contract for smoking cessation.* Washington, DC: World Bank, 2008.

259. Williams B, Bezner, J, Chesbro, SB, Leavitt, R. The effect of a behavioiural contract on adherence to a walking program in postmenopausal African American women. *Topics in Geriatric Rehabilitation* 2005; **21**(4):332–42.

260. Jha P, Chaloupka FJ. *Tobacco control in developing countries.* Washington, DC: World Bank, 2000.

261. Jha P, Chaloupka F, Moore J, et al. Tobacco addiction. In: Jamison DT, Breman JG, Measham AR, et al. (eds). *Disease Control Priorities in Developing Countries*, 2nd edn, pp. 869–85. Oxford: Oxford University Press, 2006.

262. Sunley et al. The design, administration, and potential revenue of tobacco excises. In: Jha P, Chaloupka FJ (eds). *Tobacco control in developing countries*, pp. 409–26. Oxford: Oxford University Press, 2000.

263. French SA, Jeffery RW, Story M, et al. Pricing and promotion effects on low-fat vending snack purchases: the CHIPS Study. *American Journal of Public Health* 2001; **91**(1):112–17.

264. Sargent R, Shepard R, Glantz S. Reduced incidence of admissions for myocardial infarction associated with public smoking ban: before and after study. *British Medical Journal* 2004; **328**(7446):977–80.

265. Cesaroni G, Forastiere F, Agabiti N, Valente P, Zuccaro P, Perucci C. Effect of the Italian smoking ban on population rates of acute coronary events. *Circulation* 2008; **117**(9):1183–8.

266. White S. *Russia goes dry.* Cambridge: Cambridge University Press, 1996.

267. Roberto C, Agnew H, Brownell KD. An observational study of consumers' accessing of nutrition information in chain restaurants. *American Journal of Public Health* 2009; **99**:820–1.

268. Elbel B, Kersh R, Brescoll VL, Dixon LB. Calorie labeling and food choices: a first look at the effects on low-income people in New York City. *Health Affairs.* 2009; **28**(6):w1110–21.

269. Bollinger B, Leslie P, Sorensen A. Calorie Posting in Chain Restaurants. Stanford University and NBER, 2010.

270. Tandon PS, Wright J, Zhou C, Rogers CB, Christakis DA. Nutrition menu labeling may lead to lower-calorie restaurant meal choices for children. *Pediatrics* 2010; **125**(2):244–8.

271. Wiecha J, Peterson KE, Ludwig DS, Kim J, Sohol A, Gortmaker SL. When children eat what they watch: the impact of television viewing on dietary intake in youth. *Archives of Pediatrics & Adolescent Medicine* 2006; **160**:436–42.

272. Stahl T, Wismar M, Ollila E, Lahtinen E, Leppo K. Health in all policies: prospects and potentials. Brussels: European Observatory on Health Systems and Policies, 2006.

273. World Health Organization. *Promoting physical activity and active living in urban environments: the role of local governments.* Copenhagen: WHO Europe, 2006.

274. World Health Organization. *Interventions on Diet and Physical Activity: What Works.* Geneva: WHO; 2009.

275. Rabinovitch J. Innovative land use and public transport policy: The case of Curitiba, Brazil. *Land Use Policy* 1996; **13**(1):51–67.

276. Willett WC, Koplan JP, Nugent R, Dusenbury C, Puska P, Gaziano TA. *Prevention of Chronic Disease by Means of Diet and Lifestyle Changes. Disease Control Priorities for Developing Countries*, pp. 833–50. Washington, DC: The World Bank, 2006.

277. Davis B, Carpenter C. Proximity of fast-food restaurants to schools and adolescent obesity. *American Journal of Public Health* 2009; **99**:505–10.

278. Austin S, Meliy SJ, Sanchez BN, Patel A, Buka S, Gortmaker SL. Clustering of fast-food restaurants around schools: a novel application of spatial statistics to the the study of food environments. *American Journal of Public Health* 2005; **95**:1575–81.

279. Marmot M. Social determinants of health inequalities. *Lancet* 2005; **365**:1099–104.

280. Stuckler D, Basu S, McKee M. Budget crises, health, and social welfare programmes. *British Medical Journal* 2010; **340**:77–9.

281. Gray B. Conditions facilitating interorganizational collaboration. *Human Relations* 1985; **38**(10):911–36.

282. Reich M. The politics of agenda setting in international health: child health versus adult health in developing countries. *Journal of International Development* 1995; **7**(3):489–502.

283. Halstead S, Walsh JA, Warren KS. *Good health at low cost.* New York: Rockefeller Foundation, 1985.

284. Murray C, Frenk J. World Health Report 2000: a step towards evidence-based health policy. *Lancet* 2001; **357**(9269):1698–700.

285. Navarro V. Assessment of the World Health Report. *Lancet* 2000; **356**(9241):1598–601.

286. Jamison D, Breman JG, Measham AR, et al. *Disease control priorities in developing countries.* Washington, DC: World Bank, 2006.

287. Asaria P, Chisholm D, Mathers C, Ezzati M, Beaglehole R. Chronic disease prevention: health effects and financial costs of strategies to reduce salt intake and control tobacco use. *Lancet* 2007; **370**(9604):2044–53.

288. Israel B, Eng E, Schulz AJ, Parker EA. *Methods in community-based participatory research for health.* San Francisco, CA: Jossey-Bass, 2005.

289. Economos D, Irish-Hauser S. Community interventions: a brief overview and their application to the obesity epidemic. *Journal of Law, Medicine & Ethics* 2007; **35**(1):131–7.

290. McLaren L, Ghali LM, Lorenzetti D, et al. Out of context? Translating evidence from the North Karelia project over place and time. *Health Education Research* 2007; **22**(3):414.

291. Sarrafzadegan N, Kelishadi R, Esmaillzadeh A, et al. Do lifestyle interventions work in developing countries? Findings from the Isfahan Healthy Heart Program in the Islamic Republic of Iran. *Bulletin of the World Health Organization* 2009; **87**(1):39–50.

292. Sallis JF, Bowles HR, Bauman A, et al. Neighborhood environments and physical activity among adults in 11 Countries. *American Journal of Preventive Medicine* 2009; **36**(6):484–90.

293. Van Baal PHM, Polder JJ, de Wit GA, et al. Lifetime medical costs of obesity: prevention no cure for increasing health expenditure. *PLoS Medicine* 2008; **5**(2):e29.

294. Pan XR, Li GW, Hu YH, et al. Effects of diet and exercise in preventing NIDDM in people with impaired glucose tolerance. The Da Qing IGT and Diabetes Study. *Diabetes Care* 1997; **20**(4):537–44.

295. Tuomilehto J, Lindstrom J, Eriksson JG, et al. Prevention of type 2 diabetes mellitus by changes in lifestyle among subjects with impaired glucose tolerance. *New England Journal of Medicine* 2001; **344**(18):1343–50.

296. Diabetes Prevention Program Research G. 10-year follow-up of diabetes incidence and weight loss in the Diabetes Prevention Program Outcomes Study. *Lancet* 2009; **374**(9702):1677–86.

297. Kosaka K, Noda M, Kuzuya T. Prevention of type 2 diabetes by lifestyle intervention: a Japanese trial in IGT males. *Diabetes Research and Clinical Practice* 2005; **67**(2):152–62.

298. Ramachandran A, Ramachandran S, Snehaltha C, et al. Increasing expenditure on health care incurred by diabetic subjects in a developing country: a study from India. *Diabetes Care* 2007; **30**(2):252–6.

298a. Ebrahim S. Chronic diseases and calls to action. *Int J Epidemiology* 2008; **37**(2): 225–230.

298b. McCoy D, Chand S, Sridhar D. Global health funding: how much, where it comes from and where it goes. *Health Policy Plan* 2009; **24**(7):407–417. (See also reference 301).

299. McCoy D, Kembhavi G, Patel J, Luintel A. The Bill & Melinda Gates Foudnation's grant-making programme for global health. *Lancet* 2009; **373**:1645–53.

299a. Nye J. Soft power. *Foreign Policy* 2004; **80**: 153–71.

299b. Lukes S. *Power: A radical view.* London: Macmillan Press, 1974.

299c. Stuckler D, Basu S, McKee M. Global health philanthropy and institutional relationships: How should conflicts of interest be addressed? *PLoS Medicine* 2011; **8**(4):e1001020.

300. Easterly W, Pfutze T. Where does the money go? Best and worst practices in foreign aid. *Journal of Economic Perspectives* 2008; **22**(2):1–24.

301. McCoy D, Chand S, Sridhar D. Global health funding: how much, where it comes from and where it goes. *Health Policy and Planning* 2009; **24**(7):407–17. (See also reference 298b).

302. Ravishankar N, Gubbins P, Cooley RJ, et al. Financing of global health: Tracking development assistance for health from 1990 to 2007. *Lancet* 2009; **373**(9681):2113–24.

303. Yach D, Hawkes C. *Towards a WHO long-term strategy for prevention and control of leading chronic diseases.* Geneva: WHO, 2004.

304. Farag M, Nandakumar AK, Wallack SS, Gaumer G, Hodgkin D. Does funding from donors displace government spending for health in developing countries? *Health Affairs* 2009; **28**(4): 1045–55.

305. Stuckler D, Basu S, McKee M. International Monetary Fund and aid displacement. *International Journal of Health Services* 2011; **41**(1):67–76.

306. Easterly W. The white man's burden. *Lancet* 2006; **367**(9528):2060.

307. Stuckler D, King L, Robinson H, McKee M. WHO's budgetary allocations and burden of disease: a comparative analysis. *Lancet* 2008; **372**(9649):1563–9.

308. Sridhar D, Batniji R. Misfinancing global health: a case for transparency in disbursements and decision making. *Lancet* 2009; **372**:1185–91.

308a. World Health Organization. Roll Back Malaria Partnership: Conflict of interest policy and procedure. Available at http://www.rbm.who.int/docs/constituencies/RBMcoiPolicy.pdf. Accessed 10 March 2011.

309. Renz L, Atienza J. *International grantmaking update: a snapshot of US Foundation trends.* New York: Foundation Centre, 2006.

310. McNeil D. Gates Foundation's influence criticized. *The New York Times* 16 February 2008.

311. MarketWatch. *PepsiCo tries to appeal to our better angels* [commentary]. 22 April 2010.

312. Piller C. Gates Foundation causing harm with same money it used to do good. *Democracy Now* 9 January 2007.

313. Reuters. Merck gives malaria drug to non-profit group. *Reuters* 18 March 2009.

313a. World Health Organization. *Parties to the WHO Framework Convention on Tobacco Control.* Geneva: WHO, 2010. (See also reference 672).

314. Merck. *African comprehensive HIV/AIDS Partnerships.* Merck, 2010.

315. The Lancet. What has the Gates Foundation done for global health? *Lancet* 2009; **373**(9675):1577.

316. World Economic Forum. *Global Risks 2010: A Global Risk Network Report.* Geneva: World Economic Forum, 2010.

317. Delamothe T. Aid agencies neglect non-communicable diseases, international health organisations warn. *British Medical Journal* 2009; **338**:b2102.

318. Institute of Medicine. *The U.S. commitment to global health: recommendations for the new administration.* Washington, DC: IOM, 2009.

319. Campbell E, Weissman JS, Ehringhaus S, et al. Institutional academic-industry relationships. *Journal of the American Medical Association* 2007; **298**:1779–86.

320. Nabel E, Stevens S, Smith R. Combating chronic disease in developing countries. *Lancet* 2009; **373**:2004–6.

320a. Nugent R, Feigl A. *Scarce donor funding for non-communicable diseases: Will it contribute to a health crisis?* Washington, DC: Center for Global Development, 2010.

321. Daar A, Singer PA, Persad DL, et al. Grand challenges in chronic non-communicable diseases. *Nature* 2007; **450**:494–6.

322. Hotez P, Molyneux DH, Fenwick A. Control of neglected tropical diseases. *New England Journal of Medicine* 2007; **357**:1018–27.

323. Feachem R, Kjellstrom T, Murray CL, Over M, Phillips MA. *The health of adults in the developing world*. New York: Oxford University Press for the World Bank, 1992.

324. Gwatkin D, Guillot, M. *The burden of disease among the global poor: current situation, future trends, and implications for strategy*. Washington, DC: World Bank, 2000.

325. Camdessus M. Statement before the United Nations Economic and Social Council in Geneva. 11 July 1990.

326. Sachs S, Sachs JD. Mental health in the Millennium Development Goals: Not ignored. *PLoS Medicine* 2007; **4**:e56.

327. SciDev. Gates Foundation increases spending for 2009. *SciDev* 28 January 2009.

328. Stuckler D, Robinson HR, McKee M, King L. World Health Organization budget and burden of disease: a comparative anlaysis. *Lancet* 2008; **372**(9649):1563–9.

329. Magnusson R. Non-communicable diseases and global health governance: enhancing global processes to improve health development. *Globalization and Health* 2007; **3**(2):1–16.

330. Rehm J, Mathers C, Popova S, Thavorncharoensap M, Teerawattananon Y, Patra J. Global burden of disease and injury and economic cost attributable to alcohol use and alcohol-use disorders. *Lancet* 2009; **373**:2223–33.

331. Bonita R, Beaglehole R. Stroke prevention in poor countries: Time for action. *Stroke* 2007; **38**(11):2871–2.

332. Beaglehole R, Ebrahim S, Reddy S, Voute J, Leeder S. Prevention of chronic diseases: a call to action. *Lancet* 2007; **370**(9605):2152–7.

333. Beaglehole R, Yach D. Globalisation and the prevention and control of non-communicable disease: the neglected chronic diseases of adults. *Lancet* 2003; **362**:903–8.

334. Stuckler D. Population causes and consequences of leading chronic diseases: a comparative analysis of prevailing explanations. *Milbank Quarterly* 2008; **86**(2):273–326.

335. Aikins A. Ghana's neglected chronic disease epidemic: a developmental challenge. *Ghana Medical Journal* 2007; **41**(4):154–9.

336. TheyRule. TheyRule Database. 2004.

337. NNDB. *NNDB Mapper: Tracking the entire world*. 2010.

338. Smelser N. *Theory of collective behaviour*. New York: Free Press, 1962.

339. Shiffman J. Has donor prioritization of HIV/AIDS displaced aid for other health issues? *Health Policy and Planning* 2008; **23**(2):95–100.

340. Tilly C. *Social movements, 1768–2004*. Boulder, CO: Paradigm Publishers, 2004.

341. McAdam D. *Political process and the development of black insurgency, 1930–1970*. Chicago, IL: University of Chicago Press, 1982.

342. Tilly C. *From mobilization to revolution*. Reading, MA: Addison-Wesley, 1978.

342a. Ryan C, Gamson WW. The Art of Reframing Political Debates *Contexts* 2006; **5**(1):13–18.

343. Schmidt H. Transport policy, food policy, obese people, and victim blaming. *Lancet* 2008; **372**(9639):627.

344. Marx K. *The grundrisse: foundations of the critique of political economy*. New York: Harper & ow, 1971.

345. Koch R. Über den augenblicklichen Stand der bakteriologischen Choleradiagnose [in German]. *Zeitschrift für Hygiene und Infectionskrankheiten* 1893; **14**:319–33.

346. Grant J. Children's needs climb toward top of world agenda. *Forum for Applied Research and Public Policy* 1992; **7**:66–72.

347. Scheper-Hughes N. *The cultural politics of child survival*. In: Scheper-Hughes N (ed). *Child survival: Anthropological perspectives on the treatment and maltreatment of children*, pp. 1–29. Boston, MA: D. Reidel Publishing Co; 1987.

348. Philips M, Feachem RGA, Koplan JP. *The emerging agenda for adult health.* New York: Oxford University Press, 1992.

349. Nicoll A, Laukamm-Josten, U, Mwizarubi, B, et al. Lay health beliefs concerning HIV and AIDS—a barrier for control programmes. *AIDS Care* 1993; 5(2):223–33.

350. Nicoll A. Contraindications to whooping-cough immunisation—myths or realities? *Lancet* 1985:679–81.

351. Diethelm P, McKee M. Denialism: what is it and how should scientists respond? *European Journal of Public Health* 2009; 19(1):2–4.

352. World Health Organization. *A WHO/The Union Monograph on TB and Tobacco Control.* Geneva: WHO, 2007.

353. Barry C, Brescoll VL, Brownell KD, Schlesinger M. Obesity metaphors: how beliefs about the causes of obesity affect support for public policy. *Milbank Quarterly* 2009; 87(1):7–47.

353a. Farmer P. *Pathologies of Power: Health, Human Rights and the New War on the Poor.* Berkeley, CA: University of California Press, 2004.

353b. Stuckler D, Basu S, McKee M. Public health in Europe: Power, politics, and where next? *Public Health Reviews* 2010; 31: 213–42.

354. Gollust S, Lantz PM, Ubel PA. The polarizing effect of news media messages about the social determinants of health. *American Journal of Public Health* 2009; 99:2160–7.

355. Attaran A, Freedberg KA, Hirsch M. Dead wrong on AIDS. *Washington Post* 15 June 2001; Sect. A33.

356. Lamb W. Keep America Beautiful: grassroots non-profit or tobacco front group? *PR Watch Archives* 2001; 8:3.

357. Novotny T, Lum K, Smith E, Wang V, Barnes R. Cigarettes butts and the case for an environmental policy on hazardous cigarette waste. *International Journal of Environmental Research and Public Health* 2009; 6(5):1691–705.

358. Epstein S. *Impure science: AIDS, activism and the politics of knowledge.* San Diego, CA: University of California Press, 1996.

359. Mahler H. *The political struggle for health:* Address of the Director General at the 29th session of the regional committee for the Western Pacific, August 21 1978. World Health Organization, 1978.

360. Goodfield J. *A chance to live.* New York: McMillan International, 1991.

361. World Health Organization. *World Health Statistics 2008.* Geneva: WHO, 2008.

362. FAO/UNPF. Food Needs and Population. World Food Summit, Food for All; 13–17 November 1996; Rome.

363. Black RE, Allen LH, Bhutta ZA, et al. Maternal and child undernutrition: global and regional exposures and health consequences. *Lancet* 2008; 371(9608):243–60.

364. Wilkinson R, Pickett K. *The spirit level: Why greater equality makes societies stronger.* New York: Bloomsbury Press, 2009.

365. McKee M. Alcohol in Russia. *Alcohol and Alcoholism* 1999; 34(6):824–9.

366. World Health Organization. *Global Burden of Disease Study (2004).* Geneva: WHO, 2009.

367. WHO. *Preventing Chronic Diseases: A Vital Investment.* Geneva: WHO, 2005.

368. Mirmiran P, Noori N, Zavareh M, Azizi F. Fruit and vegetable consumption and risk factors for cardiovascular disease. *Metabolism* 2009; 58(4):460–8.

369. Lichtenstein A, Appel L, Brands M. Diet and lifestyle recommendations revision 2006: a scientific statement from the American Heart Association Nutrition Committee. *Circulation* 2006; 114(1):82–96.

370. Stampfer MJ, Hu FB, Manson J, Rimm E, Willett W. Primary prevention of coronary heart disease in women through diet and lifestyle. *New England Journal of Medicine* 2000; 343(1):16–22.

371. Vorster H, Kruger A, Venter C, Margetts B, Macintyre U. Cardiovascular disease risk factors and socio-economic position of Africans in transition: the THUSA study. *Cardiovasc Journal of Africa* 2007; 18(5):282–9.

372. Thow AM, Hawkes C. The implications of trade liberalization for diet and health: a case study from Central America. *Global Health* 2009; 5:5.

373. Popkin BM. The nutrition transition: an overview of world patterns of change. *Nutrition Reviews* 2004; **62**(7 Pt 2):S140–3.

374. Ramakrishnan U. Prevalence of micronutrient malnutrition worldwide. *Nutrition Reviews* 2002; **60**(5 Pt 2):S46–52.

375. Food and Agricultural Organization. *The State of Food Insecurity in the World.* Geneva: FAO, 2008.

376. Delisle H. Poverty: the double burden of malnutrition in mothers and the intergenerational impact. *Annals of the New York Academy of Sciences* 2008; **1136**:172–84.

377. Shafique S, Akhter N, Stallkamp G, de Pee S, Panagides D, Bloem M. Trends of under- and overweight among rural and urban poor women indicate the double burden of malnutrition in Bangladesh. *International Journal of Epidemiology* 2007; **36**(2):449–57.

378. Sawaya A, Sesso R, Florencio T, Fernandes M, Martins P. Association between chronic undernutrition and hypertension. *Maternal & Child Nutrition* 2005; **1**(3):155–63.

379. van Rooyen J, Kruger H, Huisman H, Schutte A, Malan N, Schutte R. Early cardiovascular changes in 10- to 15-year-old stunted children: the Transition and Health during Urbanization in South Africa in Children study. *Nutrition* 2005; **21**(7–8):808–14.

380. Mackay J. The fight against tobacco in developing countries. *Tubercle and Lung Disease* 1994; **75**:8–24.

381. Shetty P, Schmidhuber J. Introductory lecture the epidemiology and determinants of obesity in developed and developing countries. *Internatinal Journal for Vitamin and Nutrition Research* 2006; **76**(4):157–62.

382. Yusuf S, Hawken S, Ounpuu S, et al. Effect of potentially modifiable risk factors associated with myocardial infarction in 52 countries (the INTERHEART study): case-control study. *Lancet* 2004; **364**(9438):937–52.

383. University of Liverpool. Anti-obesity drugs unlikely to provide lasting benefit, according to scientists. *ScienceDaily.* March 1 2010.

384. Stuckler D, Hawkes C, Yach D. Governance of chronic diseases. In: Buse K, Drager N (eds). *Making sense of global health governance—a policy primer.* Houndsmills: Palgrave MacMillan Press and WHO, 2009.

385. Shamah T, Villalpando S. The role of enriched foods in infant and child nutrition. *British Journal of Nutrition* 2006; **96**(Suppl 1):S73–7.

386. Hertrampf E, Cortes F. Folic acid fortification on wheat flour: Chile. *Nutrition Reviews* 2004; **62**(6 Pt 2):S44–S8.

387. Xu J, Kochanek K, Tejada-Vera B. *Deaths: Preliminary Data for 2007.* National Vital Statistics Reports. Hyattsville, MD: National Center for Health Statistics, 2009.

388. Winslow R. *Some Success Fighting Heart Disease. The Wall Street Journal* 6 April 2010.

389. World Health Organization. *Health systems: improving performance.* Geneva: WHO, 2000.

390. Young I. Is healthy eating all about nutrition. *British Journal of Nutrition: Nutrition Bulletin.* 2002; **27**:7–12.

391. Study FH. *Framingham Heart Study.* 1948 [cited 2010 April 14]; Available at: http://www.framinghamheartstudy.org.

392. Tuomilehto J, Jousilahti P, Rastenyte D, et al. Urinary sodium excretion and cardiovascular mortality in Finland: a prospective study. *Lancet* 2001; **357**(9259):848–51.

393. Sharkey J, Horel S, Han D, Huber JJ. Association between neighborhood need and spatial access to food stores and fast food restaurants in neighborhoods of colonias. *International Journal of Health Geographics* 2009; **16**(8):9.

394. Centre Y. Yunus Centre: Grameen Danone. 2009. Available from: http://www.muhammadyunus.org/Social-Business/grameen-danone/ (Accessed 2010 April 8).

395. IOM, Committee on Prevention of Obesity in Children and Youth. *Preventing Childhood Obesity: Health in the Balance.* Washington, DC: National Academies Press, 2005.

396. IOM. *Food Marketing to Children and Youth: Threat or Opportunity?* Washington, DC: National Academies Press, 2005.

397. New York Times. The Bittersweet History of Sugar Substitutes. *The New York Times* 29 March 1987.

398. Kerner J, Cazap E, Yach D, et al. Comprehensive cancer control-research & development: knowing what we do and doing what we know. *Tumori* 2009; **95**(5):610–22.

399. World Health Organization/World Economic Forum. *Preventing Noncommunicable Diseases in the Workplace through Diet and Physical Activity: WHO/World Ecoomic Forum Report of a Joint Event.* Geneva: WHO/WEF, 2008.

400. Dresler C, Leon M, Straif K, Baan R, Secretan B. Reversal of risk upon quitting smoking. *Lancet* 2006; **368**:348–9.

401. Ozminkowski R, Dunn R, Goetzel R, Cantor R, Murnane J, Harrison M. A return on investment evaluation of the Citibank, N.A. Health Management Program. *American Journal of Health Promotion* 1999; **14**(1):31–43.

402. Naydeck B, Pearson J, Ozminkowski R, Day B, Goetzel R. The impact of the highmark employee wellness programs on 4-year healthcare costs. *Journal of Occupational and Environmental Medicine* 2008; **50(2)**:146–56.

403. Alliance IFaB. *Progress Report on the Food and Beverage Alliance's Five Commitments to Action under the 2004 Global Strategy on Diet, Physical Activity, and Health,* IFBA, 2009.

404. Association AB. *Alliance School Beverage Guidelines Final Progress Report.* Washington, DC: American Beverage Association, 2010.

405. PepsiCo. *PepsiCo Annual Report 2007.* Purchase, NY: PepsiCo, 2007.

406. Xu J, Eilat-Adar S, Loria C. Dietary fat intake and risk of coronary heart disease: the Strong Heart Study. *American Journal of Clinical Nutrition* 2006; **84**(4):894–902.

407. Agency UFS. *Industry Activity.* 2010. Available from: http://www.salt.gov.uk/industry_activity.html (Accessed April 12 2010).

408. Federation UFaD. *Recipe for Change.* 2009. Available from: http://www.fdf.org.uk/publicgeneral/ Recipe_for_change_Jul09.pdf (Accessed April 12 2010).

409. He FJ, MacGregor GA. *A comprehensive review on salt and health and current experience of worldwide salt reduction programmes. Journal of Human Hypertension* 2009; **23**(6):363–84.

410. He F, MacGregor GA. Salt, blood pressure and cardiovascular disease. *Current Opinion in Cardiology* 2007; **22**(4):298–305.

411. Kraft Foods Press release. *Kraft Foods Plans to Reduce Sodium in North American Products an Average of 10 Percent by 2012.* 2010. Available from: http://phx.corporate-ir.net/phoenix.zhtml?c=129070&p= irol-newsArticle&ID=1403344 (Accessed March 19 2010).

412. Unilever. *Unilever salt reduction commitment.* 2010. Available from: http://www.unilever.com/brands/ nutrition/unileversaltreduction/commitment/ (Accessed March 19 2010).

413. Food labeling: health claims, soluble fiber from certain foods and risk of coronary heart disease. Final rule. *Federal Register* 2008; **73**(85):23947–53.

414. Braaten J, Wood P, Scott F. Oat beta-glucan reduces blood cholesterol concentration in hypercholesterolemic subjects. *European Journal of Clinical Nutrition* 1994; **48**(7):465–74.

415. Wolever T, Jenkins D, Mueller S. Method of administration influences the serum cholesterol-lowering effect of psyllium. *American Journal of Clinical Nutrition* 1994; **59**(5):1055–9.

416. Sprecher D, Harris B, Goldberg A. Efficacy of psyllium in reducing serum cholesterol levels in hypercholesterolemic patients on high- or low-fat diets. *Annals of Internal Medicine* 1993; **119**(7 Pt 1):545–54.

417. Delaney B, Nicolosi R, Wilson T. Beta-glucan fractions from barley and oats are similarly antiatherogenic in hypercholesterolemic Syrian golden hamsters. *Journal of Nutrition* 2003; **133**(2):468–75.

418. Shimizu C, Kihara M, Aoe S. Effect of high beta-glucan barley on serum cholesterol concentrations and visceral fat area in Japanese men—a randomized, double-blinded, placebo-controlled trial. *Plant Foods for Human Nutrition* 2008; **63**(1):21–5.

419. Keenan J, Goulson M, Shamliyan T, Knutson N, Kolberg L, Curry L. The effects of concentrated barley beta-glucan on blood lipids in a population of hypercholesterolaemic men and women. *British Journal of Nutrition* 2007; **97**(6):1162–8.

420. St-Onge M, Aban I, Bosarge A, Gower B, Hecker K, Allison D. Snack chips fried in corn oil alleviate cardiovascular disease risk factors when substituted for low-fat of high-fat snacks. *American Journal of Clinical Nutrition* 2007; **85**(6):1503–10.

421. Rudkowska I, Roynette C, Nakhasi D, Jones P. Phytosterols mixed with medium-chain triglycerides and high-oleic canola oil decrease plasma lipids in overweight men. *Metabolism* 2006; **55**(3):391–5.

422. Lukaczer D, Liska D, Lerman R. Effect of a low glycemic index diet with soy protein and phytosterols on CVD risk factors in postmenopausal women. *Nutrition* 2006; **22**(2):104–13.

423. Binkowski A, Kris-Etherton P, Wilson T, Mountain M, Nicolosi R. Balance of unsaturated fatty acids is important to a cholesterol-lowering diet: comparison of mid-oleic sunflower oil and olive oil on cardiovascular disease risk factors. *Journal of the American Dietetic Association* 2005; **105**(7):1080–6.

424. Judd J, Baer D, Clevidence B. Effects of margarine compared with those of butter on blood lipid profiles related to cardiovascular disease risk factors in normolipemic adults fed controlled diets. *American Journal of Clinical Nutrition* 1998; **68**(4):768–77.

425. St-Onge M, Lamarche B, Mauger J, Jones P. Consumption of a functional oil rich in phytosterols and medium-chain triglyceride oil improves plasma lipid profiles in men. *Journal of Nutrition* 2003; **133**(6):1815–20.

426. Bourque C, St-Onge M, Papamandjaris A, Cohn J, Jones P. Consumption of an oil composed of medium chain triacyglycerols, phytosterols, and N-3 fatty acids improves cardiovascular risk profile in overweight women. *Metabolism* 2003; **52**(6):771–7.

427. Dyerberg J, Eskesen D, Andersen P. Effects of trans- and n-3 unsaturated fatty acids on cardiovascular risk markers in healthy males. An 8 weeks dietary intervention study. *European Journal of Clinical Nutrition* 2004; **58**(7):1062–70.

428. Davison K, Coates A, Buckley J, Howe P. Effect of cocoa flavanols and exercise on cardiometabolic risk factors in overweight and obese subjects. *International Journal of Obesity* 2008; **32**(8):1289–96.

429. Snoek H, Huntjens L, Van Gemert L, De G, Weenen H. Sensory-specific satiety in obese and normal-weight women. *American Journal of Clinical Nutrition* 2004; **80**(4):823–31.

430. Gerstein D, Woodward-Lopez G, Evans A, Kelsey K, Drewnowski A. Clarifying concepts about macronutrients' effects on satiation and satiety. *Journal of the American Dietetic Association* 2004; **104**(7):1151–3.

431. Havermans R, Janssen T, Giesen J, Roefs A, Jansen A. Food liking, food wanting, and sensory-specific satiety. *Appetite* 2009; **52**(1):222–5.

432. Yach D, Feldman ZA, Bradley DG, Khan M. Can the food industry help tackle the growing global burden of under nutrition? *American Journal of Public Health* doi/10.2105/AJPH.2009.174359.

433. Cincera M, Ortega-Argiles R, Moncada-Paterno-Castello P. *The performance of top R&D investing companies in the stock market.* IPTS Working Paper on Corporate R&D and Innovation. Luxembourg: European Commission, 2009.

434. Tuebke A. *Monitoring industrial research: The 2008 EU Survey on R&D Investment Business Trends.* Luxembourg: European Commission, 2009.

435. NIH. *Estimates of Funding for Various Research, Condition, and Disease Categories (RCDC).* Washington, DC: National Institutes of Health, 2010.

436. Anand G. Green Revolution in India Wilts as Subsidies Backfire. *The Wall Street Journal* February 22, 2010.

437. Qaderi M, Reid D. In: Singh S (ed). *Climate Change and Crops*, pp. 1–9. Berlin: Springer-Verlag, 2009.

438. Zahm S, Ward M. Pesticides and childhood cancer. *Environmental Health Perspectives* 1998; **106**:893–908.

439. Andreotti G, Freeman L, Hou L, et al. Agricultural pesticide use and pancreatic cancer risk in the Agricultural Health Study Cohort. *International Journal of Cancer* 2009; **124**(10):2495–500.

440. Kamel F, Tanner C, Umbach D, et al. Pesticide exposure and self-reported Parkinson's disease in the agricultural health study. *American Journal of Epidemiology* 2007; **165**(4):364–74.

441. Alayanja M, Sandler D, Lynch C, et al. Cancer Incidence in the Agricultural Health Study. *Scandinavian Journal of Work, Envirionment and Health* 2005; **31**(S1):39–45.

442. Andon M, Anderson J. State of the Art Reviews: The Oatmeal-Cholesterol Connection: 10 Years Later. *American Journal of Lifestyle Medicine* 2008; **2**:51–7.

443. Hickman M. *Unilever drops major palm-oil producer. The Independent* 22 February 2010.

444. Khan M, Mensah GA. *Changing Practices to Improve Dietary Outcomes and Reduce Cardiovascular Risk: A Food Company's Perspective.* Washington, DC: Institute of Medicine; 2009.

445. Sharma L, Teret SP, Brownell KD. The food industry and self-regulation: standards to promote success and to avoid public health failures. *American Journal of Public Health* 2010; **100**:240–6.

446. Lewin A, Lindstrom L, Nestle M. Food industry promises to address childhood obesity: preliminary evaluation. *Journal of Public Health Policy* 2006; **27**(4):327–48.

447. Ludwig D, Nestle M. Can the food industry play a constructive role in the obesity epidemic? *Journal of the American Medical Association* 2008; **300**(15):1808–11

448. Yach D. Invited editorial: A personal view. Food companies and nutrition for better health. *Public Health Nutrition* 2008; **11**(2):109–11.

449. Verduin P, Agarwal S, Waltman S. Solutions to obesity: perspectives from the food industry. *American Journal of Clinical Nutrition* 2005; **82**(1 Suppl):259S–61S.

450. Science-Based Solutions to Obesity: What are the Roes of Academia, Government, Industry, and Health Care? Proceedings of a symposium, Boston, MA, USA, March 10–11, 2004 and Anaheim, California, USA, October 2, 2004. *American Journal of Clinical Nutrition* 2004; **82**(1 Suppl):207S–73S.

451. Moss R. Transforming giants: what kind of company makes it its business to make the world a better place? *Harvard Business Review* 2008.

452. Brownell KD, Warner KE. The perils of ignoring history: big tobacco played dirty and millions died. *How Similar Is Big Food? Milbank Quarterly* 2009; **87**(1):259–94.

453. Hamburger T, Geiger K. Beverage industry douses tax on soft drinks. *Los Angeles Times* 7 February 2010.

454. Retailers, NGOs and Food and Beverage Industry Launch National Initiative to Help Reduce Obesity. *PR Newswire* 5 October 2009.

455. Zerhouni E, Sanders C, von Eschenbach A. The Biomarkets Consortium: public and private sectors working in partnership to improve the public health. *Oncologist* 2007; **12**(3):250–2.

456. Bradley DG. Beyond product: the private sector drive to perform with the purpose of alleviating global under-nutrition. *Global Forum for Health Research* 2008; **5**:171–173.

457. Vartanian LR, Schwartz MB, Brownell KD. Effects of soft drink consumption on nutrition and health: a systematic review and meta-analysis. *American Journal of Public Health* 2007; **97**(4):667–75.

458. Nestle M. *Food politics: how the food industry influences nutrition and health.* Berkeley, CA: University of California Press, 2002.

459. Simon M. *Appetite for profit: How the food industry undermines our health and how to fight back.* New York: Nation Books, 2006.

460. Monteiro A, Gomes FS, Cannon G. The snack attack. *American Journal of Public Health* 2010; doi/10.2105/AJPH.2009.187666.

461. Kassirer J. *On the take: How medicine's complicity with big business can endanger your health.* New York: Oxford University Press, 2005.

462. Brody H. *Hooked: ethics, the medical profession, and the pharmaceutical industry.* Lanham, MD: Rowman & Littlefield Publishers, 2007.

463. Chopra M, Darnton-Hill, I. Tobacco and obesity epidemics: not so different after all? *British Medical Journal* 2004; **328**:1558–60.

464. Wiist W. The corporation: An overview of what it is, its tactics, and what public health can do. In: Wiist W (ed). *The bottom line or public health.* New York: Oxford University Press, 2010.

465. Monardi F, Glantz SA. Are tobacco industry campaign contributions influencing state legislative behavior? *American Journal of Public Health* 1998; **88**:918–23.

466. Warner K. Tobacco industry scientific advisors: Serving society or selling cigarettes? *American Journal of Public Health* 1991; **81**(7):839–42.

467. Chapman S. Research from tobacco industry affiliated authors: need for particular vigilance. *Tobacco Control* 2005; **14**:217–9.

468. Apollonio D, Bero LA. The creation of industry front groups: The tobacco industry and 'Get government off our back'. *American Journal of Public Health* 2007; **97**:419–27.

469. Lesser L, Ebbeling CB, Goozner M, et al. Relationship between funding source and conclusion among nutrition-related scientific articles. *PLoS Medicine* 2007; **4**(1):e5.

470. Nestle M. Soft drink pouring rights: Marketing empty calories. *Public Health Reports* 2000; **115**(4):308–19.

471. Warner K. US: Is Fast Food Just What the Doctor Ordered? New York Times, 2010. Retrieved April 16, 2005 from http://www.corpwatch.org/article.php?id=12193.

472. Byrnes N. Pepsi brings in the health police. *Bloomberg Business Week* 14 January 2010. Retrieved April 22, 2010 from http://www.businessweek.com/magazine/content/10_04/b4164050511214.htm

473. Norum K. Invited commentary to Yach editorial: PepsiCo recruitment strategy challenged. *Public Health Nutrition* 2008; **11**(2):112–3.

474. Yach D, Bialous SA. Junking science to promote tobacco. *American Journal of Public Health* 2001; **91**(11):1745–8.

475. Center for Media and Democracy. Daniel J. Edelman, Inc. Retrieved Apr 20, 2010 from http://www.sourcewatch.org/index.php?title=Edelman

476. Malone R. The tobacco industry. In: Wiist W (ed). *The bottom line or public health.* New York: Oxford University Press, 2010.

477. Tesler L, Malone RE. Corporate philanthropy, lobbying, and public health policy. *American Journal of Public Health* 2008; **98**(12):2123–33.

478. Center for Responsive Politics. *PepsiCo annual lobbying.* 2010. Retrieved April 27, 2010 from http://www.opensecrets.org/lobby/clientsum.php?lname=PepsiCo+Inc&year=2009

479. Center for Responsive Politics. *Food and beverage industry profile.* 2010. Retrieved April 27, 2010 from http://www.opensecrets.org/lobby/indusclient.php?lname=N01&year=2009

480. Center for Responsive Politics. *PepsiCo Inc Fundraising/Spending by Cycle.* 2010. Retrieved April 27, 2010 from http://www.opensecrets.org/pacs/lookup2.php?strID=C00039321&cycle=2008

481. PepsiCo. PepsiCo human rights workplace policy. Retrieved from http://www.pepsico.com/codeofconduct/2009_human_rights_english_.pdf. Retrieved April 16, 2010 from http://www.pepsico.com/investors/corporate-governance/policies.html

482. Securities and Exchange Commission. PepsiCo Inc (Filer) CIK: 0000077476. PepsiCo Inc Income Taxes. 2010. Retrieved April 15, 2010 from http://www.sec.gov/cgi-bin/viewer?action=view&cik=77476&accession_number=0001193125-10-036385

483. Citizens for Tax Justice. *Why we have a corporate minimum tax.* CTJ Publications, 2001. Retrieved April 27, 2010 from http://www.ctj.org/html/whyamt.htm

484. The Guardian. How to save a packet. *The Guardian* 5 February 2009. Retrieved April 16, 2010 from http://www.guardian.co.uk/business/2009/feb/05/tax-gap-walkers

485. PepsiCo. *Performance with purpose: The promise of PepsiCo 2009 Annual report.* Purchase, NY: PepsiCo, 2009. Retrieved April 19, 2010 from http://www.pepsico.com/download/pepsico_ar.pdf

486. Crow M. The human rights responsibilities of multinational tobacco companies. *Tobacco Control* 2005; **14**(S2):ii14–8.

486a. Enlazando Alternativas Bi-regional Europe, Latin America and Caribbean Network. Profit before people and human rights: European transnational corporations in Latin America and the Caribbean. Report to the Consultation on Business and Human Rights organized by the Office of the High Commission of the United Nation for Human Rights. Geneva, Switzerland, 2009. Retrieved October 7, 2009 from http://www2.ohchr.org/english/issues/globalization/business/docs/BiRegional.pdf.

487. Multinational Monitor. The corporate hall of shame: PEPSI: boycott. *The Multinational Monitor* December 1994. Retrieved April 16, 2010 from http://www.multinationalmonitor.org/hyper/mm1294.html

488. Burma Campaign UK. *Pepsi ends Burma business British Burma campaign gathers momentum*, 27 January 1997. Retrieved April 29, 2010 from http://www.burmacampaign.org.uk/index.php/news-and-reports/news-stories/Pepsi-ends-Burma-Business-British-Burma-campaign-gathers-momentum

489. Interfaith Center on Corporate Responsibility. *Split in beverage industry: PepsiCo faces resolution on global HIV/AIDS policies; CocaCola decides to work with shareholders.* ICCR, 2004. Retrieved April 16, 2010 from http://www.iccr.org/news/press_releases/2004/pr_pepsi050304.htm

490. Luce E. India: Pepsi and Coca-Cola deny pesticide claims. *Financial Times* 6 August 2003. Retrieved April 16, 2010 from http://www.corpwatch.org/article.php?id=7909

491. Gardner S. *Lori Perlow, individually and on behalf of all similarly situated individuals v. PepsiCo Inc, Frito-Lay North America, Inc. and Frito-Lay, Inc.:* Center for Science in the Public Interest, 2006. Retrieved April 16, 2010 from http://www.cspinet.org/new/pdf/olestra_demand.pdf

491a. PR Watch (2002). $4.6 million to fight biotech food labels. Retrieved April 20, 2010 from http://www.prwwatch.org/node/1451.

492. Nestle M. Can PepsiCo help alleviate world hunger? www.foodpolitics.com, 16 April 2010. Retrieved April 16, 2010 from http://www.foodpolitics.com/2010/04/can-pepsico-help-alleviate-world-hunger/

493. Khan M. *We recognize our responsibility to provide balanced nutrition.* Purchase, NY: PepsiCo; 2010. Retrieved April 12, 2010 from http://www.pepsico.com/purpose/sustainability/sustainability-report/human-sustainabilty.html#block_introduction

493a. Association of Schools of Public Health. PepsiCo announcemes global nutrition, environment and workplace goals. Friday Letter, 2010. Retrieved April 12, 2010 from http://fridayletter.asph.org/article)view.cfm?FLE_index=12301%FL_index=1614.

494. Nooyi I. *Worldwide code of conduct: PepsiCo.* Purchase, NY: PepsiCo, 2008. Retrieved May 2, 2010 from http://www.pepsico.com/codeofconduct/english_09.pdf

495. Harms J, Knapp T. The new economy: what's new, what's not. *Review of Radical Political Economics* 2003; **35**:413–36.

496. Giroux H. Beyond the biopolitics of disposability: rethinking neoliberalism in the New Gilded Age. *Social Identities* 2008; **14**(5):587–620.

497. Citizens for Tax Justice. United States remains one of the least taxed industrial countries. CTJ Publications, 2007. Retrieved March 2, 2009 from http://www.ctj.org/pdf/oecd07.pdf

498. General Accountability Office. *Comparison of the reported tax liabilities of Foreign- and U.S.-Controlled corporations, 1998–2005.* Washington, DC: GAO-08-957; 2008. Retrieved April 29, 2010 from http://www.gao.gov/new.items/d08957.pdf

499. Institute on Taxation and Economic Policy. State corporate tax disclosure: Why it is needed. Policy Brief # 16. Washington, DC: Institute on Taxation and Economic Policy, 2005. Retrieved April 29, 2010 from http://docs.google.com/viewer?a=v&q=cache:uQi2qovRxvYJ:www.itepnet.org/pb16corp.pdf+corporate+taxes&hl=en&gl=us&pid=bl&srcid=ADGEESgzM3dgq-3mQ7U9ebimVE8FmOqhwWnyWao2_7TciWSTbAF737cgmiFiXFelbxWuPpPK69N4dTSGNDJIL-nM8ocY2mf9-Rs8m2zjVIA0q6qi12o5gKHR2oTU7NSbZltJWp2AdPC8&sig=AHIEtbQn8cqH_0-J7x_DONXRjKpuWp2uzQ

500. Jacobson M. Lifting the veil of secrecy from industry funding of nonprofit health organizations. *International Journal of Occupational and Environmental Health* 2005; **11**:349–55.

501. Komisar L. Corporate tax evasion via offshore subsidiaries: A primer. *Pacific News Service* 2004. Retrieved April 27, 2010 from http://www.reclaimdemocracy.org/articles_2004/corporate_tax_evasion_offshore.html

502. *Center for Responsive Politics. Food & Beverage: Long-term contribution trends.* Center for Responsive Politics, 2009. Retrieved April 29, 2010 from http://www.opensecrets.org/industries/indus.php?ind=N01

503. *Citizens United v Federal Elections Commission. No. 130 US 876.* Supreme Court of the United States, 2010.

504. Rutkow L, Vernick, JS, Teret, SP. The potential health effects of Citizens United. *New England Journal of Medicine* 2010; **362**(15):1356–8.

504a. Wiist, W.H. Citizens United, public health, and democracy: the Supreme Court ruling, its implications, and proposed actions. *Am J Public Health* 2011; **101**:1172–9.

505. Hartmann T. *Unequal protection: The rise of corporation dominance and the theft of human rights.* San Francisco, CA: Berrett-Koehler, 2002.

506. Nace T. *Gangs of America: The rise of corporate power and the disabling of democracy.* San Francisco, CA: Berrett-Koehler, 2003.

507. Mayer C. Personalizing the impersonal: corporations and the bill of rights. *Hastings Law Journal* 1990; **557**:1–82.

507a. Revolving Door Working Group. (2005). A Matter of Trust: How the revolving door undermines public confidence in government—and what to do about it. Available from http://www.cleanupwashington.org/documents/RevovDoor.pdf.

508. Wettstein F. *Multinational corporations and global justice: Human rights obligations of a quasi-governmental institution.* Palo Alto, CA: Stanford University Press, 2009.

509. Udayagiri M, Walton J. Global transformation and local counter movements: The prospects for democracy under neoliberalism. *International Journal of Comparative Sociology* 2003; **44**:309–43.

510. Clapp J, Fuchs D. Agrifood corporations, global governance, and sustainability: a framework for analysis. In: Clapp J & Fuchs D (eds). *Corporate power in global agrifood governance.* Cambridge, MA: MIT Press, 2009.

511. Shue H. Global accountability: Transnational duties towards economic rights. In: Coicaud J, Doyle MW, Gardner AM (eds). *The globalization of human rights.* New York: United Nations Press, 2003.

512. Blouin C, Chopra M, van der Hoeven R. Trade and social determinants of health. *Lancet* 2009; **373**:502–7.

513. Peet R. *Unholy trinity: The IMF, World Bank and WTO.* London: Zed Books, 2003.

514. United States Trade Representative. Advisory committees. 2010. Retrieved April 29, 2010 from http://www.ustr.gov/about-us/intergovernmental-affairs/advisory-committees

515. Shaffer E, Waitzkin W, Brenner J, Jasso-Aguilar R. Global trade and public health. *American Journal of Public Health* 2005; **95**(1):23–34.

516. Broad R. The Washington Consensus meets the global backlash: Shifting debates and policies. *Globalizations* 2004; **1**(2):129–54.

517. Dembele D. The International Monetary Fund and World Bank in Africa: A disastrous record. *International J of Health Services* 2005; **35**(2):389–98.

518. Michalowski R, Kramer RC. *State-corporate crime: Wrongdoing at the intersection of business and government.* New Brunswick, NJ: Rutgers University Press, 2006.

519. Reich R. *Supercapitalism: The transformation of business, democracy, and everyday life.* New York: Knopf, 2007.

520. Levine B. Are Americans a broken people? Why we've stopped fighting back against the forces of oppression. *Alternet* 11 December 2009. Retrieved December 15, 2009 from http://www.alternet.org/news/144529/are_americans_a_broken_people_why_we've_stopped_fighting_back_against_the_forces_of_oppression/

521. Yach D, Bettcher D. The Globalization of public health I: Threats and opportunities. *American Journal of Public Health* 1998; **88**(5):735–8.

522. Yach D, Bettcher D. The globalization of public health, II: The convergence of self-interest and altruism. *American Journal of Public Health* 1998; **88**(5):738–41.

522a. Yach D, Brinchmann S, Bellet S. Healthy Investments and Investing in Health. *Journal of Business Ethics,* 2001; **33**(3):191–8.

523. Organization for Economic Cooperation and Development. *Transparency and integrity in lobbying.* Paris: OECD, 2010. Retrieved March 22, 2010 from http://www.oecd.org/dataoecd/14/57/44641288.pdf

523a. Ludwig DS, Peterson KE, Gortmaker SL. Relation between consumption of sugar-sweetened drinks and childhood obesity: a prospective, observational analysis. *Lancet* 2001; **357**:23–262.

524. Hill S. Europe's answer to Wall Street. *The Nation* 2010; **290**(18):669–89.

525. Marx M, Margil M, Cavanagh J, et al. *Strategic corporate initiative: Toward a global citizens movement to bring corporations back under control.* Portland: Corporate Ethics International, 2007. http://corpethics.org/downloads/SCI_Report_September_2007.pdf

526. Korten F. Ten ways to stop corporate dominance of politics. *Yes!magazine* 25 January 2010. Retrieved February 1, 2010 from http://www.alternet.org/rights/145441/10_ways_to_stop_corporate_dominance_of_politics

526a. Shamir R. The De-Radicalization of corporate social responsibility. *Critical Sociology* 2010; **290**(18):23–262.

527. U.S. Department of Labor. *U.S. Department of Labor's OSHA issues record-breaking fines to BP.* US Department of Labor news release, 30 October 2009. Retrieved April 29, 2010 from http://www.osha.gov/pls/oshaweb/owadisp.show_document?p_table=NEWS_RELEASES&p_id=16674

527a. Eif J. *World trends in social welfare and human rights.* Seoul, Korea: Human Right Conference, 2001.

528. Ratner S. Corporations and human rights. *The Yale Law Journal* 2001; **111**(443–545).

529. Wiist W. *The bottom line or public health: tactics corporations use to influence health and health policy, and what we can do to counter them.* New York: Oxford University Press, 2010.

530. Wiist W. Public health and the anticorporate movement: Rationale and recommendations. *American Journal of Public Health* 2006; **96**:1370–5.

530a. Public Health Leadership Society. Principles of the Ethical Practice of Public Health. 2002. Available at: http://www.apha.org/codeofethics/ethicsbrochure.pdf. Accessed December 30, 2004.

531. Gostin L. *Public health law: Power, duty, restraint.* Berkeley, CA: University of California Press, 2000.

531a. International Council on Human Rights Policy (2003). Human rights and global social justice. Retrieved February 3, 2010 from http://www.ichrp.org/files/reports/43/108_report_en.pdf

532. Wilson D, Purushothaman R. *Dreaming With BRICs: The Path to 2050.* Goldman Sachs Global Economics Paper No: 99, 2003.

533. Chang H-J. *Kicking Away the Ladder: Policies and Institutions for Economic Development in Historical Perspective First edition ed.* London: Anthem Press, 2003.

534. World Bank. *World Development Indicators.* Washington, DC: World Bank, 2009.

535. UN-Human Settlements Programme. *Millenium Development Goals Indicators.* Geneva: UN-HABITAT, 2008.

536. United Nations University, Institute for Water, Environment and Health. *Sanitation as a Key to Global Health: Voices from the Field.* Hamilton, ON: UNU-INWEH, 2010.

537. Sridhar D, Gomez EJ. Health Financing in Brazil, *Russia and India: What Role Does the International Community Play? Health Policy and Planning* 2010; 1–16.

538. FAOSTAT. *Food Balance Sheets 2004.* 20 July 2005 Available at: http://www.fao.org/faostat (Accessed March 25 2010).

539. Murray C, Yang G, Qiao X. Adult mortality: levels, patterns, and causes. In: Feachem R, Kjellstrom T, Murray CL, Over M, Phillips MA (eds). *The health of adults in the developing world*, pp. 23–111. Oxford: Oxford University Press, 1992.

540. Stevens D, Siegel K, Smith R. Global interest in addressing non-communicable disease. *Lancet* 2007; **370**(9603):1901–2.

541. SustainAbility. *Brazil—Country of Diversities and Inequalities.* London: SustainAbility, 2007.

542. *The Pan American Health Organization Promoting Health in the Americas.* 2005. Available at: www.paho.org/English/DD/AIS/cp_076.htm (Accessed April 8 2010).

543. Chackiel J. *El envejecimiento de la población latinoamericana: hacia una relacion de dependencia favorable?* Santiago de Chile: CEPAL/CELADE, 2000.

544. World Health Organization and IDF. *Screening for type-2 diabetes.* Geneva: WHO, 2003.

545. da Costa Ribeiro I, Taddei JAA, Colugnatti F. Obesity among children attending elementary public schools in São Paulo, Brazil: a case–control study. *Public Health Nutrition* 2003; **6**(07):659–63.

546. Granville-Garcia AF, de Menezes VA, de Lira PI, Ferreira JM, Leite-Cavalcanti A. Obesity and dental caries among preschool children in Brazil. *Rev Salud Publica (Bogota)* 2008; **10**(5):788–95.

547. Ministério da Saúde. *Saúde Brasil 2008: 20 anos de Sistema Único de Saùde (SUS) no Brasil.* Brasilia DF, 2009.

548. INCA. *Atlas de Mortalidade por Cancer 1970–2007.* Brasilia: Ministèrio da Saùde, Instituto Nacional de Cancer (INCA), 2010.

549. Iglesias R, Jha P, Pinto M, da Costa e Silva VL, Godinho J. *Tobacco Control in Brazil.* Washington, DC: The World Bank, 2007.

550. Knuth AG, Bacchieri G, Victora CG, Hallal PC. Changes in physical activity among Brazilian adults over a five-year period. *Journal of Epidemiology & Community Health* 2010; **64**:591–5.

551. Food and Agricultural Organization. *The State of Food Insecurity in the World.* Rome: FAO, 2004.

552. Levy-Costa RB, Sichieri R, Pontes Ndos S, Monteiro CA. [Household food availability in Brazil: distribution and trends (1974–2003)]. *Rev Saude Publica* 2005; **39**(4):530–40.

553. Jaime PC, Monteiro CA. Fruit and vegetable intake by Brazilian adults, 2003. *Cadernos de Saúde Pública* 2005; **21**(Suppl):19–24.

554. Jaime PC, Figueiredo IC, de Moura EC, Malta DC. Factors associated with fruit and vegetable consumption in Brazil, 2006. *Revista de Saúde Pública* 2009; **43**(Suppl 2):57–64.

555. Monteiro AC, Conde W, Matsudo S, Matsudo V, Bensenor I, Lotufo PA. A descriptive epidemiology of leisure-time physical activity in Brazil (1996/97). *Revista Panamericana de Salud Pública* 2003; **14**:246–54.

556. Jacoby E, Hawkes C. Agriculture and food policies can promote better health and mitigate the burden of chronic non-communicable diseases in the Americas. 5th Meeting Pan American Commission on Food Safety (COPAIA), June 10, 2008; Rio de Janeiro, Brazil, 2008.

557. Luxner L. *Golden arches over Brazil. Latin CEO: Executive Strategies for the Americas.* FindArticlescom, 2002.

558. Reardon T, Berdeguè JA. The Rapid Rise of supermarkets in Latin America: Challenges and opportunities for development. *Development Policy Review* 2002; **20**(4):371–88.

559. Brazil Go. *Brazil—Atlas sócio econômico do Rio Grande do Sul 2010.* Available at: http://www.scp.rs.gov.br/atlas/atlas.asp?menu=266

560. Nascimento S. *A Bancada do Tabaco.* Brasilia: Correio Brasiliense, 2007.

561. Monteiro CA, Conde WL, Popkin BM. Independent effects of income and education on the risk of obesity in the Brazilian adult population. *Journal of Nutrition* 2001; **131**(3):881S–6S.

562. Sichieri R, Nascimento S, Coutinho W. The burden of hospitalization due to overweight and obesity in Brazil. *Cadernos de Saùde Pùblica* 2007; **23**(7):1721–7.

563. Leeder S, Raymond S, Greenberg H, Liu H. *A Race Against Time: The Challenge of Cardiovascular Disease in Developing Economies.* New York: The Center for Global Health and Economic Development, Columbia University, 2004.

564. Nucci L, Toscano C, Maia A, et al. A nationwide population screening program for diabetes in Brazil. *Pan American Journal of Public Health* 2004; **16**(5):320–7.

565. Jurberg C. Brazil and tobacco use: a hard nut to crack. *Bulletin of the World Health Organization* 2009; **87**(11):812–13.

566. Menezes MFB. *Personal Communication with Marcelo Fisch B Menezes, Representative of the Ministry of Finance in the National Commission for FCTC implementation.* In: Cavalcante T (ed). 2010.

567. FCA. *Technology and the Fight against Tobacco Trade: Media Briefing.* Framework Convention Alliance, 2008.

568. Coitinho D, Monteiro CA, Popkin BM. What Brazil is doing to promote healthy diets and active lifestyles. *Public Health Nutrition* 2002; **5**(1a):263–7.

569. Simoes EJ, Hallal P, Pratt M, et al. Effects of a community-based, professionally supervised intervention on physical activity levels among residents of Recife, Brazil. *American Journal of Public Health* 2009; **99**(1):68–75.

570. SustainAbility. *China—New Landscapes*. London: SustainAbility, 2007.

571. China Office of the World health Organization Representative in China and Social Development Department of China State Council Development research Center. *China: health, poverty and economic development*. Beijing, 2005.

572. Liu Y. *Shrinking arable lands jeopardizing China's food security*. Beijing: China Watch, World Watch Institute, 2006.

573. Whyte MK, Zhongxin S. The Impact of China's Market Reforms on the Health of Chinese Citizens: Examining Two Puzzles. *China: An International Journal* **8**(1):1–32.

574. Health Mo. *Chinese Health Statistical Digest*. Beijing: Ministry of Health, 2009.

575. Yang G, Kong L, Zhao W, et al. Emergence of chronic non-communicable diseases in China. *Lancet* 2008; **372**(9650):1697–705.

576. Health Mo. *China Health Statistics Yearbook 2009*. Beijing: Chinese Academy Science & Peking Union Medical College Press, 2009.

577. ADA. *National Diabetes Fact Sheet*. 2007. Available at: http://www.diabetes.org/diabetes-basics/diabetes-statistics/ (Accessed 22 April 2010).

578. Bibbins-Domingo K, Chertow GM, Coxson PG, et al. Projected effect of dietary salt reductions on future cardiovascular disease. *New England Journal of Medicine* 2010; **362**(7):590–9.

579. Gu D, Kelly TN, Wu X, et al. Mortality attributable to smoking in China. *New England Journal of Medicine* 2009; **360**:150–9.

580. Liu B-Q, Peto R, Chen Z-M, et al. Emerging tobacco hazards in China: 1. Retrospective proportional mortality study of one million deaths. *British Medical Journal* 1998; **317**(7170):1411–22.

581. Office of the Leading Small Group for Implementation of the Framework Convention on Tobacco Control, Ministry of Health, PRC. *2007 China Tobacco Control Report—Create a Smoke-Free Environment, Enjoy a Healthy Life*. Beijing: Chinese Centers for Disease Prevention and Control, 2007.

582. Wu Y. Overweight and obesity in China. *British Medical Journal* 2006; **333**:362–3.

583. Kong L, Hu S. *2005 Report on Cardiovascular Diseases in China*. Beijing: National Center for Cardiovascular Diseases, CHINA(NCCD), 2006.

584. China National Bureau of Statistics. *China Statistics Yearbook 2009*. Beijing: China Statistics Press, 2009.

585. Leeder S, Raymond S, Greenberg H, Liu H, Esson K. *A race against time: the challenge of cardiovascular disease in developing economies*. New York: Colombia University, 2005.

586. Yani L. Social analysis on reasons of childhood obesity in China cities. *Studies in Preschool Education* 2008; **3**:37–40.

587. Popkin B. Will China's nutrition transition overwhelm its health care system and slow economic growth? *Health Affairs* 2008; **27**(4):1064–76.

588. Etchells P, Jackson D. *Coca-Cola China 2007 Sustainability Report*. Coca-Cola Beverages Ltd, 2007.

589. Decree of the State Council of the People's Republic of China. Interim Regulation of the People's Republic of China on Consumption Tax (2008) 2008. Available at: http://www.gov.cn/zwgk/2008-11/14/content_1149528.htm (Accesses 29 August 2009).

590. World Bank. *Dying too Young: Addressing premature mortality and ill health due to non-communicable diseases and injuries in the Russian Federation*. Washington, DC: World Bank, 2005.

591. Du YX, Cha Q, Chen XW, et al. An epidemiological study of risk factors for lung cancer in Guangzhou, China. *Lung Cancer* 1996; **Suppl**(1):S9–37.

592. Galeone C, Pelucchi C, La Vecchia C, Negri E, Bosetti C, Hu J. Indoor air pollution from solid fuel use, chronic lung diseases and lung cancer in Harbin, Northeast China. *European Journal of Cancer Prevention* 2008; **17**(5):473–8.

593. Eggleston K, Ling L, Qingyue M, Lindelow M, Wagstaff A. Health service delivery in China: a literature review. *Health Econ.* 2008; **17**(2):149–65.

594. Zhu C. "Health China 2020" strategic program. 2008. Available at: http://epaper.rmzxb.com.cn/2008/20080304/t20080304_182130.htm.

595. World Health Organization. *WHO report on the global tobacco epidemic, 2008: MPOWEER.* Geneva: WHO, 2008.

596. Gai C, Hao L, Yi Y. Effect of "Take 10!" Intervention on the related indexes of obese pupils. *Chinese Journal of Chronic Diseases Prevention* 2009; **17**(5):505–7.

597. Shi-Chang X, Xin-Wei Z, Shui-Yang X, et al. Creating health-promoting schools in China with a focus on nutrition. *Health Promotion International* 2004; **19**(4):409–18.

598. Shi-Chang X, Xin-Wei Z, Shui-Yang X, et al. Effectiveness evaluation of the Program—School Health Promotion Focusing on Nutrition Education of China/WHO. *Chinese Journal of Health Education* 2006; **22**(9):703–6.

599. Wen C. China's plans to curb cervical cancer. *Lancet* 2005; **6**(3):139–41.

600. Limited AN. Philip Morris gets China approval for full production of Marlboro brand. *Forbescom* 21 December 2005.

601. Coca-Cola. *Move: Enjoy a Healthy Lifestyle through Physical Activity and Nutrition.* 2009. Available from: http://www.thecoca-colacompany.com/citizenship/move.html (Accessed 29 August 2009).

602. PepsiCo. *Health Care Reform: Our Health Care Commitment.* 2009. Available from: http://www.pepsico.com/Purpose/Health-and-Wellness/Health-Care-Reform.html (Accessed 29 August 2009).

603. Backman G, Hunt, P, Khosla, R, et al. Health systems and the right to health: an assessment of 194 countries. *Lancet* 2008; **372**(9655):2047–85.

604. UN-Habitat. *State of the World's Cities 2008/2009: Harmonious Cities.* London: UN Habitat, 2008.

605. Nutrition Foundation of India. *Double burden of malnutrition: Case study from India.* New Delhi: Food and Agricultural Organization, 2005.

606. Das G. *India Unbound: The Social and Economic Revolution from Independence to the Global Information Age.* New York: Anchor Books, 2002.

607. World Health Organization. *Global Infobase.* 2009. Available from: http://www.who.int

608. Sicree R, Shaw J, Zimmet P. *The Global Burden: Diabetes and impaired glucose tolerance.* 2010. Available at: http://www.diabetesatlas.org/sites/default/files/Diabetes%20and%20Impaired%20Glucose%20Tolerance_1201.pdf (Accessed 17 March 2010).

609. Jindal SK. Emergence of chronic obstructive pulmonary disease as an epidemic in India. *Indian Journal of Medical Research* 2006; **124**:619–30.

610. Reddy KS, Prabhakaran D, Shah P, Shah B. Differences in body mass index and waist: hip ratios in North Indian rural and urban populations. *Obesity Reviews* 2002; **3**(3):197–202.

611. International Institute for Population Sciences, Macro International. *National Family Health Survey (NFHS-3) 2005–06: India.* Mumbai: IIPS; 2007.

612. Wang Y, Chen H-J, Shaikh S, Mathur P. Is obesity becoming a public health problem in India? Examine the shift from under- to overnutrition problems over time. *Obesity Reviews* 2009; **10**(4):456–74.

613. Thankappan KR, Mini GK. Case-control study of smoking and death in India. *New England Journal of Medicine* 2008; **358**(26):2842–3.

614. International Institute for Population Sciences, World Health Organization, World Health Organization-India WRO. *World Health Survey, 2003 INDIA.* Mumbai: IIPS; 2006.

615. Food and Agriculture Organization. *Food Security Statistics.* Rome: FAO, 2009.

616. Pingali P, Khwaja Y. *Globalisation of Indian Diets and the Transformation of Food Supply Systems. ESA Working Paper no 04–05.* Hyderabad: Agricultural Development Economics Division, 2004.

617. Mohan V, Radhika G, Vijayalakshmi P, Sudha V. Can the diabetes/cardiovascular disease epidemic in India be explained, at least in part, by excess refined grain (rice) intake? *Indian Journal of Medical Research* 2010; **131**:369–72.

618. Dohlman E, Persaud S, Landes R. *India's Edible Oil Sector: Imports Fill Rising Demand*. Washington DC: United States Department of Agriculture, 2003.

619. Mohan V, Sandeep S, Deepa R, Shah B, Varghese C. Epidemiology of type 2 diabetes: Indian scenario. *Indian Journal of Medical Research* 2007; **125**(3):217–30.

620. Thankappan KR, Shah B, Mathur P, et al. Risk factor profile for chronic non-communicable diseases: results of a community-based study in Kerala, India. *Indian Journal of Medical Research* **131**:53–63.

621. Park D, Desai P, Aiyengar J, Balladur A. Geographic differences in the characteristics of coronary artery disease in India. *International Journal of Cardiology* 1998; **67**:187–9.

622. Ajay VS, Prabhakaran D, Jeemon P, Thankappan KR, Mohan V, Ramakrishnan L, et al. Prevalence and determinants of diabetes mellitus in the Indian industrial population. *Diabetic Medicine* 2008; **25**(10):1187–94.

623. Subramanian SV, Nandy S, Kelly M, Gordon D, Davey Smith G. Patterns and distribution of tobacco consumption in India: cross sectional multilevel evidence from the 1998–9 national family health survey. *British Medical Journal* 2004; **328**(7443):801–6.

624. Shetty P. Nutrition transition in India. *Public Health Nutrition* 2002; **5**(1A):175–82.

625. Prime Minister's Council on Trade & Industry. *Report on Food & Agro Industries Management Policy*. 2010. Available at: http://indiaimage.nic.in/pmcouncils/reports/food/mreport.htm (Accessed 11 April 2010).

626. Planning Commission of India, Government of India. *State Development Report of Punjab*, 2002.

627. Ministry of Housing and Urban Poverty Alleviation and UNDP. *India: Urban Poverty report*. India: Oxford University Press, 2009.

628. Ebrahim S, Kinra S, Bowen L, et al. The effect of rural-to-urban migration on obesity and diabetes in India: a cross-sectional study. *PLoS Medicine* 2010; **7**(4):e1000268.

629. Chabra A. Smooth traffic flow, safer roads: cycle tracks to be laid across the city. *Hindustan Times* 9 December 2002.

630. Errol Y, Morrison S. Diabetic foot amputations as the most frequent diabetes complication in developing countries. *IDF Bulletin* 1997; **42**:14–7.

631. Srinath Reddy K, Shah B, Varghese C, Ramadoss A. Responding to the threat of chronic diseases in India. *Lancet* 2005; **366**(9498):1744–9.

632. Shobhana R, Rama, RP, Lavanya, A, Williams, R, Vijay, V, Ramachandra, A. Expenditure on health care incurred by diabetic subjects in a developing country - a study from Southern India. *Diabetes Research & Clinical Practice* 2000; **48**(1):37–42.

633. Mohan V, Madan Z, Jha R, Deepa R, Pradeepa R. Diabetes: Social and Economic Perspectives in the New Millenium. *International Journal of Diabetes in Developing Countries* 2004; **24**:29–35.

634. Xavier D, Pais P, Devereaux PJ, et al. Treatment and outcomes of acute coronary syndromes in India (CREATE): a prospective analysis of registry data. *Lancet* 2008; **371**(9622):1435–42.

635. Raab R, Fezeu L, Mbanya J. Cost and availability of insulin and other diabetes supplies: IDF survey 2002-03. *Diabetes Voice* 2004; **49**(3):24–9.

636. Correspondent S. BP, diabetes check for 70 million. *The Telegraph* 8 July 2010. Available at: http://www.telegraphindia.com/1100709/jsp/nation/story_12663504.jsp.

637. India Government. *Report of the Working Group in Communicable and Non-communicable diseases for the eleventh five year plan*. 2006.

638. FSSAI. Welcome To Food Safety and Standards Authority of India. Available at: http://www.fssai.gov.in/, accessed May 20, 2010.

639. Prasad R. Alcohol use on the rise in India. *Lancet* 2009; **373**(9657):17–8.

640. Ministry of Urban Development. *National Urban Transport Policy*. Government of India, 2005.

641. Siegel K, Narayan KM, Kinra S. Finding a Policy Solution to India's Diabetes Epidemic. *Health Affairs* 2008; **27**(4):1077–90.

642. Mohan V, Shanthirani C, Deepa M, Datta M, Williams O, Deepa R. Community Empowerment—A Successful Model for Prevention of Non-communicable Diseases in India—the Chennai Urban Population Study (CUPS–17). *Journal of Association of Physicians of India* 2006; **54**.

643. Ministry of Health and Family Welfare, Government of India. *Report of the National Commission on Macroeconomics and Health.* New Delhi: Ministry of Health and Family Welfare, 2005.

644. Hazarika S, Yadav A, Reddy K. Public health law in India: A framework for its application as a tool for social change. *National Medical Journal of India* 2009; **22**(44):199–200.

645. World Health Organization. *World health report 2006—working together for health.* Geneva: WHO, 2006.

646. Patel R. *Stuffed and Starved: Markets, Power, and the Hidden Battle for the World's Food System.* London: Portobello Books Ltd, 2007.

647. Secretaría de Salud. *Programa Nacional de Salud 2007–2012. Por un Mexico sano: construyendo alianzas para una mejor salud* [Spanish]. Report No.: Primera edicion. Mexico: Secretaría de Salud, 2007.

648. Rivera J, Barquera, S, Campirano, F, Campos, I, Safdie, M, Tovar, V. Epidemiological and nutritional transition in Mexico: rapid increase of non-communicable chronic diseases and obesity. *Public Health Nutrition* 2006; **5**(1A):113–22.

649. Sepulveda J, Bustreo F, Tapia R, et al. Improvement of child survival in Mexico: the diagonal approach. *Lancet* 2006; **368**(9551):2017–27.

650. Acosta-Cazares B, Arando-Alvarez JG, Reyes-Morales H. ENCOPREVENIMISS 2004: Patrones de actividad fisica de la mujer y del hombre. *Revista medica del Instituto Mexicano del Seguro Social* 2006; **44**(Suppl 1):S79–86.

651. del Carmen Morales-Ruán M, Hernández-Prado B, Gómez-Acosta LM, et al. Obesity, overweight, screen time and physical activity in Mexican adolescents. *Salud Publica de Mexico* 2009; **51**(suppl 4): S613–S20.

652. Shamah-Levy T, Villalpando-Hernandez S, Rivera-Dommarco JA. *Resultados de Nutricion de la ENSANUT 2006.* Cuernavaca, Mexico: Instituto Nacional de Salud Publica, 2007.

653. Fernald LC, Neufeld LM. Overweight with concurrent stunting in very young children from rural Mexico: prevalence and associated factors. *European Journal of Clinical Nutrition* 2007; **61**:623–32.

654. Hawkes C. Uneven dietary development: linking the policies and processes of gloablization with the nutrition transition, obesity and diet-related chronic diseases. *Globalization and Health* 2006; **2**(4).

655. Secretaría de Salud, Subsecretaría de Prevención y Promoción de la Salud. *PROGRAMA DE ACCION ESPECIFICO 2007–2012. Diabetes Mellitus.* Report No.: Primera edicion. Mexico: Secretaría de Salud, 2008.

656. Reardon T, Timmer P, Berdegue J. The rapid rise of supermarkets in developing countries: induced organizational, institutional, and technological change in agrifood systems. *Electronic Journal of Agricultural and Development Economics* 2004; **1**(2):168–83.

657. Andino J, Taylor RD, Koo WW. The Mexican sweeteners market and sugar exports to the United States. Agribusiness & Applied Economics Report No. 579. North Dakota State University, Fargo: Center for Agricultural Policy and Trade Studies, 2006.

658. Schmitz A, Seale JL, Schmitz TG. Sweetener-Ethanol Complex in Brazil, the United States, and Mexico: Do Corn and Sugar Prices Matter? Report No.: PBTC 03-9. Gainesville, FL: IATPC, University of Florida, 2003.

659. Zahniser S, Young E, Wainio J. *Recent Agricultural Policy Reforms in North America* United States: Department of Agriculture (USDA), p. 35. 2005.

660. Sawaya AL, Martins P, Hoffman D, Roberts SB. The link between childhood undernutrition and risk of chronic diseases in adulthood: A case study of Brazil. *Nutrition Reviews* 2003; **61**(5):168–75.

661. Central Intelligence Agency. *The World Factbook 2009.* Washington, DC: CIA, 2009.

662. Hippert C. Multinational corporations, the politics of the world economy, and their effects on women's health in the developing world: A review. *Health Care for Women International* 2002; **23**(8):861–9.

663. Ridaura RL, Barquera S, Prado BH, Rivera J. *Preventing Obesity in Mexican Children and Adolescents. Joint US-Mexico Workshop on Preventing Obesity in Children and Youth of Mexican Origin*, pp. 81–127. Washington, DC: The National Academies Press, 2007.

664. Jennings-Aburto N, Nava F, Bonvecchio A, et al. Physical activity during the school day in public primary schools in Mexico City. *Salud Pública de México* 2009; **51**:141–7.

665. Fernald LCH. Socio-economic status and body mass index in low-income Mexican adults. *Social Science & Medicine* 2007; **64**:2030–42.

666. Secretaría de Salud, Subsecretaría de Prevención y Promoción de la Salud. *PROGRAMA DE ACCION ESPECIFICO 2007–2012. Escuela y salud* [Spanish]. Report No.: Primera edicion. Mexico: Secretaría de Salud, 2007.

667. Arredondo A, de Icaza E. Financial requirements for the treatment of diabetes in Latin America: implications for the health system and for patients in Mexico. *Diabetologia* 2009; **52**(8):1693–5.

668. Arredondo A, Zuniga A. Economic consequences of epidemiological changes in diabetes in middle-income countries: The Mexican case. *Diabetes Care* 2004; **27**:104–9.

669. Arredondo A, Barcelo A. The economic burden of out-of-pocket medical expenditures for patients seeking diabetes care in Mexico. *Diabetologia* 2007; **50**:2408–9.

670. Arochi R, Tessmann KH, Galindo O. Advertising to children in Mexico. *Young Consumers* 2005; **6**(4):82–5.

671. Secretaría de Salud. NORMA Oficial Mexicana Nom-043-SSA2-2005, Servicios Básicos de salud. Promoción y educación para la salud en materia alimentaria. Criterios para brindar Orientación. Mexico: Secretaría de Salud, 2006.

672. World Health Organization. *Parties to the WHO Framework Convention on Tobacco Control*. Geneva: WHO, 2010. (See also reference 313a).

673. World Health Organization. *WHO Report On The Global Tobacco Epidemic, 2009: Implementing smoke-free environments*. Geneva: WHO, 2009.

673a. Amosun S, Reddy P, Kambaran N, Omardien R. Are students in public high schools in South Africa physically active? Outcome of the 1st South African National Youth Risk Behaviour Survey. *Canadian Journal of Public Health* 2007; **98**(4):254–8. (See also reference 685).

673b. Department of Health. *South African Demographic and Health Survey 1998: Full Report*. Pretoria, Department of Health, 2002

673c. Department of Health. *South African Demographic and Health Survey 2003: Full Report*. Pretoria: Department of Health, 2007. (See also reference 683).

673d. Norman R, Bradshaw D, Steyn K, Gaziano T. Estimating the burden of disease attributable to high cholesterol in South Africa in 2000. *South African Medical Journal* 2007; **97**(8 Pt 2):708–15. (See also reference 679).

673e. Reddy S, Panday S, Swart D, Jinabhai C, Amosun S, James S. *Umthenthe Uhlaba Usamila—The South African Youth Risk Behaviour Survey 2002*. Cape Town: South African Medical Research Council, 2003. (See also reference 693).

673f. Reddy S, James S, Sewpaul R, et al. *Umthente Uhlaba Usamila—The South African Youth Risk Behaviour Survey 2008*. Cape Town: South African Medical Research Council; 2010. (See also reference 686).

673g. Schneider M, Norman R, Steyn N, Bradshaw D. Estimating the burden of disease attributable to low fruit and vegetable intake in South Africa in 2000. *South African Medical Journal* 2007; **97**(8 Pt 2):717–23.

673h. World Health Organization. *The Diabetes Declaration and Strategy for Africa: A Call to Action and Plan of Action to Prevent and Control Diabetes and Related Chronic Diseases*. Geneva: WHO AFRO Region, 2006. (See also reference 705).

674. Sanders D, Chopra M. Key challenges to achieving health for all in an inequitable society: the case of South Africa. *American Journal of Public Health* 2006; **96**(1):73–8.

675. Statistics South Africa. *Mid-year Population Estimates: Statistical Release P0302.* Pretoria: Statistics South Africa; 2008.

676. World Health Organization. *Global tuberculosis control—surveillance, planning, financing*. Geneva: WHO, 2008.

677. Bradshaw D, Groenwald P, Laubscher R, Nannan N, Nojilana B, Norman R. Initial burden of disease estimates for South Africa, 2000. *South African Medical Journal* 2003; **93**:682–8.

678. Bradshaw D, Nannan N, Groenwald P, et al. Provincial mortality in South Africa, 2000: priority-setting for now and a benchmark for the future. *South African Medical Journal* 2005; **95**(7):496–503.

679. Norman R, Bradshaw D, Steyn K, Gaziano T. Estimating the burden of disease attributable to high cholesterol in South Africa in 2000. *South African Medical Journal* 2007; **97**(8 Pt 2):708–15. (See also reference 673d).

680. Puoane T, Steyn K, Bradshaw D, et al. Obesity in South Africa: the South African demographic and health survey. *Obesity Research* 2002; **10**(10):1038–48.

681. Steyn K, Bradshaw D, Norman R, Laubscher R, Saloojee Y. Tobacco use in South Africans during 1998: the first demographic and health survey. *Journal of Cardiovascular Risk* 2002; **9**(3):161–70.

682. Peer N, Bradshaw D, Laubscher R, Steyn K. Trends in adult tobacco use from two South African Demographic and Health Surveys conducted in 1998 and 2003. *South African Medical Journal* 2009; **99**(10):744–9.

683. Department of Health. *South African Demographic and Health Survey 2003: Full Report*. Pretoria: Department of Health, 2007. (See also reference 673c).

684. Joubert J, Norman R, Lambert EV, et al. Estimating the burden of disease attributable to physical inactivity in South Africa in 2000. *South African Medical Journal* 2007; **97**(8 Pt 2):725–31.

685. Amosun S, Reddy P, Kambaran N, Omardien R. Are students in public high schools in South Africa physically active? Outcome of the 1st South African National Youth Risk Behaviour Survey. *Canadian Journal of Public Health* 2007; **98**(4):254–8. (See also reference 673a).

686. Reddy S, James S, Sewpaul R, et al. *Umthente Uhlaba Usamila—The South African Youth Risk Behaviour Survey 2008*. Cape Town: South African Medical Research Council; 2010. (See also reference 673f).

687. Lu C, Schneider MT, Gubbins P, Leach-Kemon K, Jamison D, Murray CJL. Public financing of health in developing countries: a cross-national systematic analysis. *Lancet* 2010; **6736**(10):60233–4.

688. Charlton K, Steyn K, Levitt N, et al. Diet and blood pressure in South Africa: intake of foods containing sodium, potassium, calcium and magnesium in three ethnic groups. *Nutrition* 2005; **21**:39–50.

689. Norman R, Barnes B, Mathee A, Bradshaw D. Estimating the burden of disease attributable to indoor air pollution from household use of solid fuels in South Africa in 2000. *South African Medical Journal* 2007; **97**(8 Pt 2):764–71.

690. Joubert J, Bradshaw D, Dorrington R. Population ageing and older persons' health in South Africa. International Union of the Scientific Studies of Populations Conference; September 2009, Marrakech.

691. Cook I, Alberts M, Lambert E. Relationship between adiposity and pedometer-assessed ambulatory activity in adult, rural women. *International Journal of Obesity* 2008; **32**(8):1327–30.

692. SBFF. *Standard Bank Franchise Factor*. 2008. Available at: http://www.franchize.co.za/statistics.

693. Reddy S, Panday S, Swart D, Jinabhai C, Amosun S, James S. *Umthenthe Uhlaba Usamila—The South African Youth Risk Behaviour Survey 2002*. Cape Town: South African Medical Research Council, 2003. (See also reference 673e).

694. BFAP. *Bureau of Food and Agricultural Policy Baseline Report: Consumer Trends 2009*. Pretoria: Agricultural Annex Building, Department of Agricultural Economics, Extension & Rural Development, 2009.

695. Associated Press. Africa Faces Growing Obesity Problem. *The New York Times* November 29 2006.

696. Mvo Z, Dick J, Steyn K. Perceptions of overweight African women about acceptable body size of women and children. *Curationis* 1999; **22**(2):27–31.

697. Puoane T, Tsolekile L, Steyn N. Perceptions about body image and sizes among Black African girls living in Cape Town. *Ethnicity & Disease* 2010; **20**(1):29–34.

698. Norman R, Cairncross E, Witi J, Bradshaw D. Estimating the burden of disease attributable to urban outdoor air pollution in South Africa in 2000. *South African Medical Journal* 2007; **97**(8 Pt 2):782–90.

699. Pestana JA, Steyn K, Leiman A, Hartzenberg GM. The direct and indirect costs of cardiovascular disease in South Africa in 1991. *South African Medical Journal* 1996; **86**(6):679–84.

700. Steyn K, Gaziano T, Bradshaw D, Laubscher R, Fourie J. Hypertension in South African adults: results from the Demographic and Health Survey, 1998. *Journal of Hypertension* 2001; **19**(9):1717–25.

701. Anand SS, Islam S, Rosengren A, Franzosi MG, Steyn K, Yusufali AH, et al. Risk factors for myocardial infarction in women and men: insights from the INTERHEART study. *European Heart Journal* 2008; **29**(7):932–40.

702. Motala AA, Esterhuizen T, Gouws E, Pirie FJ, Omar MAK. Diabetes and other disorders of glycemia in a rural South African community. *Diabetes Care* 2008; **31**(9):1783–8.

703. Levitt NS, Katzenellenbogen J, Bradshaw D, Hoffman M, Bonnici F. The prevalence and identification of risk factors for NIDDM in urban Africans in Cape Town, South Africa. *Diabetes Care* 1993; **16**(4):601–7.

704. Department of Health. *National Department of Health: Strategic Plan.* 2009 Available at: http://www.doh.gov.za/docs/misc/stratplan.

705. World Health Organization. *The Diabetes Declaration and Strategy for Africa: A Call to Action and Plan of Action to Prevent and Control Diabetes and Related Chronic Diseases.* Geneva: WHO AFRO Region, 2006. (See also reference 673h).

706. RSA. Tobacco Products Control Amendment. B7-2008; 2004.

707. Charlton K, Steyn K, Levitt N, et al. A food-based randomised controlled trial to assess the impact of dietary manipulation of medications on blood pressure in hypertensive South Africans. *Public Health Nutrition* 2008; **11**(12):1397–406.

708. Mayosi BM, Flisher AJ, Lalloo UG, Sitas F, Tollman SM, Bradshaw D. The burden of non-communicable diseases in South Africa. *Lancet* 2009; **374**(9693):934–47.

709. Labadarios D, Steyn N, Maunder E, et al. (eds). *The National Food Consumption Survey (NFCS): Children aged 1-9 years, South Africa, 1999.* Pretoria; Directorate: Nutrition, Department of Health, 2000.

710. Navarro V. Politics and health: a neglected area of research. *European Journal of Public Health* 2008; **18**(4):354–6.

711. Ling P, Haber LA, Wedl S. Branding the rodeo: a case study of tobacco sports sponsorship. *American Journal of Public Health* 2010; **100**(1):32–41.

712. McKee M. Competing interests: the importance of transparency. *European Journal of Public Health* 2003; **13**:193–4.

713. Ling P, Glantz SA. Why and how the tobacco industry sells cigarettes to young adults: Evidence from industry documents. *American Journal of Public Health* 2002; **92**(6):908–16.

714. RJ Reynolds. *The importance of younger adults.* Legacy Tobacco Documents Library, 1988.

715. Muggli M, Forster JL, Hurt RD, Repace JL. The smoke you don't see: uncovering tobacco industry scientific strategies aimed at environmental tobacco smoke policies. *American Journal of Public Health* 2001; **91**(9):1419–23.

716. Ciresi M, Walburn RB, Sutton TD. Decades of deceit: document discovery in the Minnesota tobacco litigation. *Mitchell Legal Review* 1999; **25**:477–566.

717. Parsigian K, Williams UG. *Obesity litigation—the next "Tobacco"?* Goodwin Procter LLP, 2010.

718. McKee M, Suhrcke, M, Nolte, E, et al. Health systems, health, and wealth: a European perspective. *Lancet* 2009; **373**:349–51.

719. Nussbaum M. Human rights and human capabilities. *Harvard Human Rights Journal* 2007; **20**:21–4.

720. Sen A. Why and how is health a human right? *Lancet* 2008; **372**(9655):2010.

721. Glantz SA, Barnes DE, Bero L, et al. Looking through a keyhole at the tobacco industry: The Brown and Williamson Documents. *Journal of the American Medical Association* 1995; **274**(3): 219–24.

Index